T0291781

Immune Checkpoint Inhibitors in Cancer

Immune Checkpoint Inhibitors in Cancer

FUMITO ITO, MD, PHD
Associate Professor of Oncology
Department of Surgical Oncology, Center for Immunotherapy
Roswell Park Comprehensive Cancer Center
Buffalo, New York
United States
Associate Professor of Surgery
Department of Surgery
Jacobs School of Medicine and Biomedical Sciences
State University of New York at Buffalo
Buffalo, New York
United States

MARC S. ERNSTOFF, MD
Professor and Katherine Anne Gioia Chair of Medicine
Senior Vice President for Clinical Investigation
Roswell Park Comprehensive Cancer Center
Buffalo, New York
United States
Professor and Section Chief
Hematology Oncology
Department of Medicine
Jacobs School of Medicine and Biomedical Sciences
State University of New York at Buffalo
Buffalo, New York
United States

ELSEVIER

ELSEVIER

3251 Riverport Lane
St. Louis, Missouri 63043

IMMUNE CHECKPOINT INHIBITORS IN CANCER

ISBN: 978-0-323-54948-6

Copyright © 2019 Elsevier, Inc. All rights reserved.

No part of this publication may be reproduced or transmitted in any form or by any means, electronic or mechanical, including photocopying, recording, or any information storage and retrieval system, without permission in writing from the publisher. Details on how to seek permission, further information about the Publisher's permissions policies and our arrangements with organizations such as the Copyright Clearance Center and the Copyright Licensing Agency, can be found at our website: www.elsevier.com/permissions.

This book and the individual contributions contained in it are protected under copyright by the Publisher (other than as may be noted herein).

Notices

Practitioners and researchers must always rely on their own experience and knowledge in evaluating and using any information, methods, compounds or experiments described herein. Because of rapid advances in the medical sciences, in particular, independent verification of diagnoses and drug dosages should be made. To the fullest extent of the law, no responsibility is assumed by Elsevier, authors, editors or contributors for any injury and/or damage to persons or property as a matter of products liability, negligence or otherwise, or from any use or operation of any methods, products, instructions, or ideas contained in the material herein.

Content Strategist: Robin Carter
Content Development Manager: Christine McElvenny
Content Development Specialist: Jennifer Horigan
Publishing Services Manager: Jameel Shereen
Project Manager: Nadhiya Sekar
Designer: Gopalakrishnan Venkatraman

Working together
to grow libraries in
developing countries

www.elsevier.com • www.bookaid.org

Printed in United States of America
Last digit is the print number: 9 8 7 6 5 4 3 2 1

This book is dedicated to scientists who were involved with the discovery of immune checkpoint proteins and inhibitors, funding resources for their support in cancer research, healthcare professionals who were committed to cancer treatment, and many patients who kindly participated in clinical trials that provided significant progress in the field of cancer immunotherapy.

List of Contributors

Jame Abraham, MD, FACP
Director, Breast Medical Oncology
Professor of Medicine
Hematology and Medical Oncology
Cleveland Clinic
Cleveland, OH, United States

Anjali Advani, MD
Staff Physician
Director of the Inpatient Leukemia Program
Hematology and Medical Oncology
Cleveland Clinic
Cleveland, OH, United States

Per Basse, MD, PhD, DM.Sci
Assistant Member
Department of Medicine
Roswell Park Comprehensive Cancer Center
Buffalo, NY, United States

Shailender Bhatia, MD
Associate Professor
Medical Oncology
Department of Medicine
University of Washington
Fred Hutchinson Cancer Research Center
Seattle, WA, United States

Patrick M. Boland, MD
Assistant Professor of Oncology
Department of Medicine
Roswell Park Comprehensive Cancer Center
Buffalo, NY, United States

Assistant Professor of Medicine
Department of Medicine
Jacobs School of Medicine and Biomedical Sciences
State University of New York at Buffalo
Buffalo, NY, United States

Hongbin Chen, MD, PhD
Associate Professor of Oncology
Department of Medicine
Roswell Park Comprehensive Cancer Center
Buffalo, NY, United States

Clinical Assistant Professor (HS) of Medicine
Department of Medicine
Jacobs School of Medicine and Biomedical Sciences
State University of New York at Buffalo
Buffalo, NY, United States

Grace K. Dy, MD
Associate Professor of Oncology
Department of Medicine
Roswell Park Comprehensive Cancer Center
Buffalo, NY, United States

Marc S. Ernstoff, MD
Professor and Katherine Anne Gioia Chair of Medicine
Senior Vice President for Clinical Investigation
Roswell Park Comprehensive Cancer Center
Buffalo, NY, United States

Professor and Section Chief
Hematology Oncology
Department of Medicine
Jacobs School of Medicine and Biomedical Sciences
State University of New York at Buffalo
Buffalo, NY, United States

Christos Fountzilas, MD
Assistant Professor of Oncology
Department of Medicine
Roswell Park Comprehensive Cancer Center
Buffalo, NY, United States

Gregory K. Friedman, MD
Associate Professor
Pediatric Hematology and Oncology
University of Alabama at Birmingham
Birmingham, AL, United States

G. Yancey Gillespie, PhD
Professor
Department of Neurosurgery
University of Alabama at Birmingham
Birmingham, AL, United States

Ahmad Hanif, MD
Hematology and Oncology Fellow
Department of Medicine
Roswell Park Comprehensive Cancer Center
Buffalo, NY, United States

Michael R. Harrison, MD
Assistant Professor of Medicine
Division of Medical Oncology
Duke Cancer Institute
Durham, NC, United States

Brant A. Inman, MD, MS
Associate Professor of Surgery
Division of Urology
Duke Cancer Institute
Durham, NC, United States

Fumito Ito, MD, PhD
Associate Professor of Oncology
Department of Surgical Oncology
Center for Immunotherapy
Roswell Park Comprehensive Cancer Center
Buffalo, NY, United States

Associate Professor of Surgery
Department of Surgery
Jacobs School of Medicine and Biomedical Sciences
State University of New York at Buffalo
Buffalo, NY, United States

Renuka V. Iyer, MD
Professor of Oncology
Co-Director, Liver and Pancreas Tumor Center
Section Chief for Gastrointestinal Oncology
Department of Medicine
Roswell Park Comprehensive Cancer Center
Buffalo, NY, United States

Professor of Medicine
Department of Medicine
Jacobs School of Medicine and Biomedical Sciences
State University of New York at Buffalo
Buffalo, NY, United States

Pawel Kalinski, MD, PhD
Rustum Family Professor for Molecular Therapeutics
  and Translational Research
Vice Chair for Translational Research and Professor of
  Oncology
Department of Medicine
Director of Cancer Vaccine and Dendritic Cell
  Therapies
Center for Immunotherapy
Co-Leader, Tumor Immunology & Immunotherapy
  Program
Roswell Park Comprehensive Cancer Center
Buffalo, NY, United States

Sumera Khan, MD
Department of Educational Affairs
Roswell Park Comprehensive Cancer Center
Buffalo, NY, United States

Megan Kruse, MD
Associate Staff
Hematology and Medical Oncology
Cleveland Clinic
Cleveland, OH, United States

Sunyoung S. Lee, MD, PhD
Hematology and Oncology Fellow
Department of Medicine
Roswell Park Comprehensive Cancer Center
Buffalo, NY, United States

Sylvia Lee, MD
Assistant Professor
Medical Oncology
Department of Medicine
University of Washington
Fred Hutchinson Cancer Research Center
Seattle, WA, United States

Matthew Loecher, MD
Jacobs School of Medicine and Biomedical Sciences
State University of New York at Buffalo
Buffalo, NY, United States

Ali A. Maawy, MD
Surgical Oncology Fellow
Department of Surgical Oncology
Roswell Park Comprehensive Cancer Center
Buffalo, NY, United States

Paul Mayor, MD, MS
Gynecologic Oncology Fellow
Department of Gynecologic Oncology
Roswell Park Comprehensive Cancer Center
Buffalo, NY, United States

Megan A. McNamara, MD
Medical Instructor
Division of Medical Oncology
Duke Cancer Institute
Durham, NC, United States

Igor Puzanov, MD, MSCI, FACP
Professor of Oncology
Director, Early Phase Clinical Trials Program
Chief of Melanoma
Department of Medicine
Roswell Park Comprehensive Cancer Center
Buffalo, NY, United States

Professor of Medicine
Department of Medicine
Jacobs School of Medicine and Biomedical Sciences
State University of New York at Buffalo
Buffalo, NY, United States

Eric K. Ring, MD
Hematology and Oncology Fellow
Pediatric Hematology and Oncology
University of Alabama at Birmingham
Birmingham, AL, United States

Yazeed Sawalha, MD
Hematology Oncology Fellow
Hematology and Medical Oncology
Cleveland Clinic
Cleveland, OH, United States

Kristen Starbuck, MD
Gynecologic Oncology Fellow
Department of Gynecologic Oncology
Roswell Park Comprehensive Cancer Center
Buffalo, NY, United States

Tian Zhang, MD
Assistant Professor of Medicine
Division of Medical Oncology
Duke Cancer Institute
Durham, NC, United States

Emese Zsiros, MD, PhD
Assistant Professor of Oncology
Department of Gynecologic Oncology
Roswell Park Comprehensive Cancer Center
Buffalo, NY, United States

Clinical Assistant Professor
Department of Obstetrics and Gynecology
Jacobs School of Medicine and Biomedical Sciences
State University of New York at Buffalo
Buffalo, NY, United States

Preface

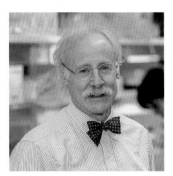 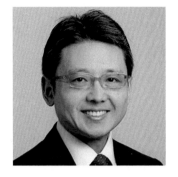

Harnessing the immune system in treating cancer has long been pursued. The concept that the immune system plays an important role in cancer can be traced back to the 1890s when William H. Coley, an American surgeon, used bacterial products as an immune stimulant to treat cancer. While occasional remarkable successes including durable complete responses were observed, his works were overlooked due to the lack of consistency in response and soon overwhelmed by the development of more effective treatments such as chemotherapy and radiotherapy. After years of germination phase, a better understanding of the mechanisms governing the relationship or cross talk between neoplastic and immune cells has led to the novel strategy of targeting the immune system, not the tumor itself. These mechanisms are the immune cell—intrinsic checkpoints that are induced on T-cell activation.

The discovery of these checkpoints, cytotoxic T-lymphocyte—associated antigen 4 (CTLA-4) and programmed death 1 (PD-1), has led to the development of new promising drugs, immune checkpoint inhibitors (ICIs). The increasing occurrence of significant clinical responses with these ICIs has transformed conventional treatment paradigms. Furthermore, clinical trials combining blockade of CTLA-4 and PD-1 have provided the framework for future approaches to immuno-oncology combination therapy. Emergent technologies that have enhanced our understanding of genomic,

transcriptional, proteomic, and epigenetic mechanisms in immune systems and tumor microenvironment have further motivated scientists to develop new immuno-modulatory agents that may open promising therapeutic options. These advances, however, come with unforeseen challenges for healthcare professionals who did not have formal training of tumor immunology when they evaluate treatment response and toxicity, which are distinct from conventional treatment such as chemotherapy and radiotherapy.

We anticipate that *Immune Checkpoint Inhibitors in Cancer* will be a strong reference for medical professionals and trainees (students, residents, and fellows) and scientists in academic institutions and industries who seek current evidence, indications, and clinical trials for the treatment of hematologic and solid malignancies with ICIs. This book includes contributions from experts internationally acclaimed for their outstanding research and oncology care in their fields and provides an up-to-date and comprehensive summary of tumor immunology and ICI therapies.

Mechanisms of T-cell activation and inhibition and immune homeostasis are discussed in depth. Several reviews also provide insight into why patients do not respond to ICIs or develop therapeutic resistance after initial response to ICIs (primary and acquired resistance). There is tremendous potential for synergistic combinations of immunotherapy agents and for combining immunotherapy agents with conventional cancer treatments. The importance of the combinatory use of ICIs for inducing synergistic antitumor reactivity is described in detail by several leading authorities. Particularly interesting is the continuing discovery of other immune modulators that will afford opportunities for future combination therapy with ICIs. Therefore, although the title of this book says "immune checkpoint inhibitors," some chapters briefly describe emerging immune costimulatory molecules and agents, adoptive T-cell therapy, and vaccines.

We hope that the readers will enjoy reading this book and find useful information that will inspire future immunotherapeutic strategies and provide guidance for the treatment of cancer.

Contents

CHAPTER 1

Immune Checkpoint Inhibitors: Mechanisms and Emerging Therapeutic Opportunities

PAWEL KALINSKI, MD, PHD • PER BASSE, MD, PHD, DMSCI

INTRODUCTION

Modern efforts to fight cancer by activating the immune system date back to the work of William Coley[4,5] in the 19th century. After decades of inconsistent clinical results of different immune approaches[6] and multiple studies showing dissociation between the levels of systemic immunization against tumor-associated antigens and cancer progression,[7,8] recent studies have focused on immune events in the tumor microenvironment (TME), as the determinant of the effectiveness of cancer immunity during cancer progression and response to treatment. The change of the focus from immunization to modulation of effector phase of immunity in TME allowed the design of consistently effective immune therapies, such as immune checkpoint (IC) inhibitor (ICI) therapies [alternatively referred to as IC blockade (ICB)]. Compared with the therapeutic activity of Bacille Calmette−Guérin (BCG) (in bladder cancer)[9] and IL-2 and IFNα for melanoma and renal cell carcinoma,[10] ICI therapies show higher response rates and often result in long-lasting responses, even in patients with advanced cancer. Ipilimumab [Yervoy; cytotoxic T-lymphocyte-associated antigen-4 (CTLA-4) blocker], the first ICI approved by the Food and Drug Administration in 2010, provided a new treatment option for patients with metastatic melanoma, which allowed for durable clinical responses in up to 20% of patients with metastatic melanoma,[11−16] who previously lacked any effective treatment options.[17]

So far, the most effective ICIs are PD-1-blocking agents that have been shown effective (and subsequently approved) for the treatment of melanoma,[18−24] non-small-cell lung cancer (NSCLC),[25−31] microsatellite-instability-high (MSI^{high}) colorectal cancer (CRC) and other MSI^{high} cancers,[32−35] renal cell carcinoma (RCC),[36] Hodgkin's lymphoma,[37,38] urothelial (bladder) cancer,[39−45] head and neck squamous cell carcinoma (HNSCC),[46,47] Merkel-cell carcinoma,[48] hepatocellular carcinoma,[49] and gastric cancer[50] (reviewed in Ref. 51).

However, the effectiveness of ICIs in different tumor types and individual patients is strongly affected by the tumor's mutation load and two elements of local TME[1,2,52−61]: the presence of cytotoxic T cells [cytotoxic T lymphocytes (CTLs)] and the associated expression of checkpoint molecules, which are typically induced by CTL-produced immune mediators.[1−3,34,56,57,62−65] As a result, even in melanoma, the majority of patients show limited or only transient benefit of checkpoint blockade,[64,65] while large groups of patients with such common cancers as breast, prostate, and MSI^{low} CRC benefit from ICIs only sporadically,[3,59,61−68] despite strong evidence that immune surveillance is an important element controlling the rate of recurrence and progression of these cancers.[69−72]

IMMUNE CHECKPOINT INHIBITION: MOLECULES AND MECHANISMS

The presence of IC molecules on activated immune cells, and their inducible ligands on most of the healthy cells of human body (Fig. 1.1), represents a basic homeostatic mechanism, providing a negative feedback to activated T cells, preventing uncontrolled activation of the immune system and damage to healthy tissues. PD-1-deficient mice or the animals treated with PD-1-blocking antibodies develop multiple autoimmune phenomena[73−76] and fertility problems,[77] showing critical importance of ICI molecules in multiple aspects of healthy organism.

IC molecules are typically absent on resting T cells and induced upon activation. The kinetics of their expression depends on the cell history (naïve or memory) and

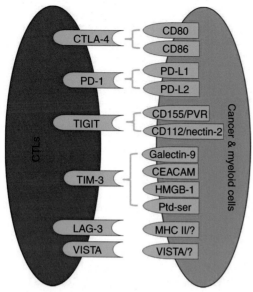

FIG. 1.1 Key immune checkpoints and their ligands in tumor and lymphoid tissues: **CTLs**: cytotoxic T lymphocytes. **CTLA-4**: cytotoxic T-lymphocyte-associated antigen-4 is known to interact with two members of the B.7 family, CD80 (B7.1) and CD86 (B.7.2), expressed mainly on antigen-presenting cells in lymphoid and tumor tissues. **PD-1** (program cell death-1; CD279) has two known ligands, PD-L1 (CD274) and PD-L2 (CD273), which are expressed on both nonimmune and immune cells. **TIGIT** [T-cell immunoglobulin and immunoreceptor tyrosine inhibitory motif (ITIM) domain] is another member of the CD28 family-like receptors expressed by T cells. Its suppressive activity is triggered by at least two known ligands: CD155 [poliovirus receptor (PVR)] and CD112 (PVRL2/nectin-2). **TIM-3** [T-cell immunoglobulin-3; hepatitis A virus cellular receptor-2 (HAVRC2)] is known to interact with cancer cell-expressed galectin-9, **HMGB-1** (high mobility group box-1), phosphatidylserine, and **CEACAM**-1 (carcinoembryonic antigen-related cell adhesion molecule-1). **LAG-3** (lymphocyte activation gene-3; CD223) is known to interact with **MHC** [major histocompatibility complex] class II molecules. **VISTA** (V-domain Ig suppressor of T-cell activation; programmed death-1 homolog; PD-1H/B7-H5), another member of the CD28/B7 family is activated by homotypic interactions, although alternative ligands may exists.

the conditions of activation. Upon the initial T-cell receptor (TCR) priming, T cells rapidly acquire surface PD-1,[78] with the PD-1 expression affecting the magnitude of primary T-cell responses.[79]

Depending on the type of IC, their interaction with the respective ligands and the delivery of the inhibitory signal may occur automatically (hardwired inhibition), for example, in case of CLTA-4 which reacts to the same CD80 and CD86 molecules which provide the initial

costimulation at early phases of activation of the same cells, or in more specific condition, such as entry into TMEs expressing high levels of PD-1 ligands.

Similarly, the consequences of the inhibition differ from the termination of T-cell proliferation and abrogation of effector functions (in case of CTLA-4) to eliminate the activated cells (in case of PD-1 signaling).

CTLA-4 is absent from naïve and memory T cells and acquired only after their activation. It has at least two ligands, B7.1 (CD80) and B7.2 (CD86), expressed on dendritic cells (DCs) and other activated antigen-presenting cells, although typically lacking from cancer cells. In result, naïve and memory T cells initially benefit from the interaction between CD80/CD86 molecules and CD28, which represents an alternative receptor for these molecules, which is expressed constitutively and cooperates with TCR, providing the costimulatory signal (signal 2) which synergizes with antigen-TCR interaction (signal 1) in inducing expansion and functional development of antigen-specific T cells. This interaction is critical, since in the absence of CD28-mediated costimulation, TCR-activated T cells are anergized and deleted.

At later stages, the appearance of CTLA-4 on the cell surface reverses the role of CD80/CD86 from costimulatory to inhibitory. Since CTLA4 has a significantly higher affinity for both these molecules, it effectively competes with CD28 for both of them.[17]

CTLA-4 belongs to the immunoglobulin superfamily. The CTLA-4 molecule has an extracellular region (V domain), a transmembrane domain, and a cytoplasmic tail. Membrane-bound CTLA-4 is a homodimer, while soluble CTLA-4 is monomeric. CTLA-4 is not expressed on naïve and resting T cells, but it can be detected as early as 4 h after T-cell activation.[80] Peak expression is reached after 1–3 days. The stronger the TCR signal during T-cell activation, the higher the levels of CTLA-4 induction.[81] CTLA-4 binds CD80 and CD86, the same antigen-presenting cell (APC)-expressed ligands as CD28, the T-cell co-stimulatory receptor, but the affinity of CTLA-4 for both these ligands is roughly 100-fold higher than that of CD28.[82] Although CTLA-4 resembles a classic membrane-expressed ligand-binding receptor,[83] it is mainly found on intracellular membranes close to the nucleus.[84] However, upon T-cell activation, it traffics to the cell membrane near the site of TCR engagement.[85] Its focal presence on the surface of the T cell is far from static as it continuously cycles between the cell surface and the intracellular compartment.[85]

CD28 ligation by its B7 family ligands results in a positive co-stimulatory signal needed by the T cells for optimal IL-2 production, proliferation, and development of effector functions. In contrast, CD80/CD86 binding to CTLA-4 results in an inhibitory signal. The induction of high levels of CTLA4 at later stages of T-cell activation, together with a higher affinity of CTLA-4 compared with CD28 for CD80/CD86 results in effective competition and eventual termination of CTL activity. Surprisingly, experiments in chimeric mice where CTLA-4 expression is only present on half of CTLs[86] showed no differences between CTLA-4-expressing and CTLA-4-nonexpressing T cells with respect to numbers or function, indicating that direct CTLA-4-dependent inhibition can occur even in the absence of direct signaling in CTLs. Apart from the direct negative signaling through CTLA-4 in T cells, CTLA-4 inhibition may also involve regulatory CD4+ T cell (Treg) activation which then suppress CTL functions independently of the CTLA-4 expression on CTLs, by "stripping" CD80/CD86 from APCs.[87,88] This process requires physical contact between Tregs, APC, and CTL and is most likely to occur in lymph nodes, rather than TME, consistent with the lymph nodes being the primary targets of CTLA-4 inhibition. This "central" mode of action may also explain the more severe autoimmune reactions to CTLA-4 blockade, compared with anti-PD-1 treatment, which is believed to affect CTLs in the TME.

The mechanism of action of CTLA-4 blockade still remains only partially understood, with a recent report by Du et al. indicating an important role of Treg depletion in anti-CTLA-4-driven tumor rejection.[89]

PD-1 molecule is also expressed on T cells upon their activation[90]; however, its two known ligands, PD-L1 (CD274) and PD-L2 (CD273), have no costimulatory roles, selectively driving the suppression of T-cell responses and the elimination of PD-1-expressing T cells. PD-L1 and PD-L2 are expressed on both nonimmune and immune cells. They are present on the surface of myeloid cells, including macrophages, DCs, myeloid-derived suppressor cells (MDSCs) and mast cells, as well as on lymphoid cells, such as T cells, B cells, and natural killer (NK) cells (reviewed in Ref. 51). Importantly, it is also inducible on nonhematopoietic cells present in healthy tissues, such as epithelia (including keratinocytes), pancreatic islet cells, astrocytes, placental cells, as well as stromal fibroblast. Importantly, PD-L1 and PD-L2 are also often expressed on cancer cells and multiple noncancer cells in tumor stroma.

Interestingly, although the interaction between PD-1 and PD-L2 in tumor tissues can contribute to PD-1-mediated inhibition of CTL responses,[91] there is no evidence that antibodies against PD-1 show higher clinical activity than antibodies against PD-L1, suggesting

that PD-L1 is the dominant inhibitory ligand of PD-1 on T cells in the human TME.

PD-1 and PD-L1 are type I transmembrane proteins of the immunoglobulin (Ig) superfamily. PD-1 contains one Ig-V-like extracellular domain, a transmembrane domain, and a cytoplasmic domain with two tyrosine signaling motifs.[90,92] PD-L1 contains two extracellular domains (Ig-V- and Ig-C-like), a transmembrane domain, and a cytoplasmic tail which lacks known signaling motifs.[93–95] Interactions between the PD-1's immunoreceptor tyrosine inhibitory motif (ITIM) and its immune receptor tyrosine-based switch motif result in the recruitment of the SHP-2 and SHP-1 protein tyrosine phosphatases, which blocks T-cell-activating signals.[96–98]

PD-1/PD-L1 binding was shown to block both the TCR signal delivery[99–101] and the delivery of the co-stimulatory signals mediated by CD28 ligation,[102,103] resulting in the inhibition of T-cell proliferation, cytokine production, and CTL killer functions, and eventual death of activated T cells.[93,104–109]

The key suppressive actions of PD-1 and its ligands are related to their direct inhibition of T-cell activation. However, ICIs also affect the activity of other immune cells. PD-1 expression and its suppressive function have been observed in activated NK cells and NK cells from cancer patients.[110,111] PD-1/PD-L1 blockade counteracts the suppressive function of PD-1-expressing B cells[112] and enhances the antitumor function of PD-1+ macrophages.[113]

Although the cytoplasmic tail of PD-L1 lacks known signaling motifs, there is evidence of "reverse signaling" through PD-L1. Binding of PD-L1 by PD-1 has been proposed to deliver survival signals to cancer cells, enhancing their resistance to proapoptotic effects of Fas, interferons, and CTLs.[114,115] It also reduces mTOR activity and their glycolytic pathway of metabolism in cancer cells.[116] The cytoplasmic domain of PD-L1 has been shown to be critical for these effects, although the relevant signaling pathway remains unknown.[114]

TIGIT (T-cell immunoglobulin and ITIM domain) is another member of the CD28 family-like receptors expressed by T cells. Its ligation directly suppresses T-cell activation and promotes the release of suppressive cytokine, IL-10.[117,118] The known agonists for TIGIT include CD155 [poliovirus receptor (PVR)] and CD112 (PVRL2/nectin-2), which are expressed by both cancer cells and stromal and inflammatory components of the TME.[119] TIGIT is typically coexpressed with PD-1, T-cell immunoglobulin (TIM)-3, and

LAG-3, suggesting their coordinate induction on exhausted T cells at late stages of their activation.[120]

TIM-3 known to interact with cancer cell-expressed galectin-9, HMGB-1, phosphatydyl serine, and CEA-CAM-1[121] provides direct negative regulator of T cells enhancing their apoptosis.[122–127] In addition, TIM-3 has also been implicated in the expansion of MDSCs, acting as indirect suppressor of T-cell immunity.[128] Its levels are particularly high on exhausted T cells which lack effector functions.[124–127]

LAG-3 is present on T cells and NK cells and delivers inhibitory signal after binding to the after major histocompatibility complex (MHC) class II molecules.[121,129] Although its mechanism remains unclear, its modulation causes a negative regulatory effect over T-cell function, preventing tissue damage and autoimmunity.[130–132] LAG-3 and PD-1 are frequently coexpressed on tumor-infiltrating lymphocytes (TILs) indicative of their immune exhaustion and associated with tumor progression.[121]

VISTA (V-domain Ig suppressor of T-cell activation; programmed death-1 homolog; PD-1H/B7-H5) is also a member of the CD28/B7 family (with significant similarities with PD-1, CD28, and, particularly, CTLA-4), expressed on immune effector cells (CD4+ and CD8+ T cells and NK cells), as well as on myeloid cells (monocytes, macrophages, DCs, and granulocytes), and acting as both inhibitory receptor and its ligand.[128,133–135] Its ligation has been shown to suppress T activation, proliferation, and cytokine production.[136] VISTA blockade has been shown to result in improved T-cell activation and enhanced tumor-specific T-cell responses in TME and peripheral blood,[137] showing synergy with PD-1 blockade.[138] In addition to its homotypic interaction, VISTA is likely to have additional ligands, although their identity remains unknown.[128,133–135]

REGULATION OF THE IMMUNE CHECKPOINT MOLECULES ON ACTIVATED T CELLS

The regulation of two prototypal checkpoint molecules, CTLA-4 and PD-1, has been extensively evaluated, helping in the rational design of the clinical trials of their respective blockers and the eventual approval of their blockers for clinical use.

Naïve and resting memory T cells lack CTLA-4 and acquire its expression only at later stages of activation.[11,139–141] The CTLA-4 expression is reduced during the conversion of effector cells into memory cells, allowing their reactivation. However, chronically activated T cells keep high levels of CTLA-4 and often loose CD28, becoming nonresponsive to their

targets.[11,139–141] Ag priming also results in T-cell acquisition of PD-1.[17] PD-1-positive T cells in TME and peripheral blood mononuclear cells (PBMCs) have been shown to be enriched in tumor-specific cells, consistent with the need for expression.[142,143] However, PD-1 expression is also enhanced by tumor-associated suppressive factors, such as IL-10[144] and TGF-β.[145] Similar to PD-1, the expression of LAG-3 and TIM-3 is induced upon activation, while the expression of VISTA has been also noted on naïve T cells.[121,128]

REGULATION OF THE EXPRESSION OF IMMUNE CHECKPOINT LIGANDS

The presence of IC molecule ligands for CTLA-4 (and CD28), B7.1 (CD80), and B7.2 (CD86) are selectively expressed at low levels on "professional" APCs, such as immature DCs, but are overexpressed on DCs (and other APC types) upon their activation by endogenous or exogenous danger signals. These include pathogen-associated molecular pattern (PAMP) sensors, such as (cell surface and endosomal) toll-like receptors (TLRs) and other pattern recognition receptors (PRRs, such as cytosolic helicases), which all recognize elements of bacteria and viruses, which constitute TLR ligands (TLR-Ls) and helicase ligands.

The second type of "danger" receptors, leading to the activation of DCs is the recognition of endogenous sensors of "danger" or tissue damage, so called damage-associated molecular patterns (DAMPs). These include sensors of extracellular DNA or high-mobility group protein-1 (HMGB-1), which reflect cell death, uric acid, or caspase activation resulting in the cleavage of IL-1 and its release.

Activation of APCs following the detection of pathogen-associated PAMP tissue damage-reflecting DAMPs typically (with the exception of TLR3, which acts in a MyD88-independent manner) involves MyD88 adaptor molecule and activation of NFkB and resulting production of proinflammatory cytokines (such as TNFα, which activates additional APC in the tissue) and the onset of transcription of a number of surface molecules, including B7.1 and B7.2, as well as enhanced antigen uptake, enhanced transcription of MHC class I and class II genes, and activation of multiple antigen presentation molecules, resulting in effective presentation of the pathogen-derived antigen on the cell surface. It also results in a shift of surface expression of chemokine receptors, which result in the migration of DCs from tissues to draining lymph nodes, and production of endogenous chemokines, which promote interaction with T cells.

Primary (nonimmune-driven) overexpression of PD-1 ligands on cancer cells. PD-L1 and PD-L2 are both located in close proximity to each other on chromosome 9p24.1. Their amplifications and translocations can result in their "primary" overexpression in several types of tumors.[51] Genetic amplification of the PD-L1/PD-L2 locus have been shown in nearly all cases of Hodgkin's lymphoma,[146] consistent with the well-documented responsiveness of Hodgkin's lymphomas to PD-1 blockade.[37,38,147,148] Amplification of the PD-L1/PD-L2 locus has been also described in non-small cell lung cancer (NSCLC),[149] small-cell lung cancer (SCLC),[150] and oral squamous cell carcinoma.[151]

Activation of multiple oncogenic pathways is another cause of the primary PD-L1 overexpression in cancer cells. It can reflect the activation of phosphatidylinositol 3-kinase (PI3K) signaling pathway involving downstream activation of AKT-mTOR cascade, which is known to promote cancer cell survival, proliferation, and formation of metastases. Loss of phosphatase and tensin homolog (PTEN - a negative regulator of PI3K-AKT signaling) has been shown to promote PD-L1 expression in CRC and NSCLC cells,[152,153] with additional reports showing the contribution of the PI3K-AKT pathway in PD-L1 induction in NSCLC, CRC, glioma, breast cancer, and melanoma cells.[152,154-157] Hyperactivation of MEK-ERK pathway, reflecting activation of RAS GTPase and BRAF[22] can directly promote PD-L1 gene expression.[158-162] MEK-dependent increase in PD-L1 expression has been reported in multiple myeloma, bladder cancer, and lymphomas.[158,163-165] PD-L1 over-expression can also reflect activation of KRAS, epidermal growth factor receptor, and anaplastic lymphoma kinase,[161,166,167] as observed in NSCLC, head and neck cancer, breast cancer, lymphomas, and other malignancies.[165,168-171]

In addition, "primary" elevation of PD-L1/PD-L2 levels in cancer tissues can reflect unique biology of the TME, such as tumor-associated hypoxia. Hypoxic TME induces HIF-1α activation, aimed to promote angiogenesis,[172] but also leading to local PD-L1 expression. HIF-1α and HIF-2a are known to interact with the hypoxia responsive element in the PD-L1 promoter.[173,174] HIF-1α-dependent PD-L1 elevation has been demonstrated in different types of murine cancers, as well as in MDSCs.[173,175-177] Activation of STAT3 in TME[178] represents another PD-L1-enhancing pathway. Activated STAT3 directly binds to PD-L1 promoter, increasing PD-L1 expression.[171,179,180] Tumor-associated elevation of PD-L1 expression in human cancer and myeloid cells can also result from the activation of NF-kB, another proliferation-enhancing and antiapoptotic factor

frequently activated in the TME of different cancers.[181-183] Rel-A (p65subunit of NF-kB) binds to the PD-L1 promoter, indicating its direct ability to enhance PD-L1 transcription.[183-185]

These observations explain frequent observations of the elevated levels of PD-L1 and PD-L2, even in the absence of active immune infiltrate and indicate the common role of these molecules in the primary evasion of cancer cells from immune attack.

Induction of PD-L1 and PD-L2 by immune cells: ICIs as a secondary mechanism of cancer-related immune suppression. PD-L1 expression is strongly enhanced in cancer tissues undergoing immune attack, representing one of the "secondary" mechanisms of tumor-related immune suppression.[186] Several mediators secreted by activated immune cells are known to participate in PD-L1 induction. IFNγ, produced by activated CTLs, Th1, and NK cells in the TME is the most potent inflammatory inducer of PD-L1,[187-193] acting through IRF1 activation.[194] Since IFNγ is the most prominent soluble inducer of PD-L1, the expression of PD-L1 typically reflects the levels of CTL infiltration in different tumors.

Elevated expression of PD-L1 in cancer cells, as well as in tumor-associated stroma endothelial cells, monocytes, and inflammatory cells can also reflect local production of type I interferons (IFNα and IFNβ).[195-197]

Other inflammatory stimuli that have been shown to induce PD-L1 are TNFα,[190,198-203] a factor known to cooperate with IFNγ in the induction of other (not checkpoint-dependent) forms of secondary suppression in the TME,[204] inflammatory factors associated with tumor progression, such as IL-17,[200,203] IL-10,[106,200] IL-4,[201] IL-1β,[163] or IL-6,[163,205] and members of IL-12 family, such as IL-27.[206-208] Similar to TNFα, other NFkB activators, such as TLR ligands induce PD-L1 in cancer cells, myeloid cells, and tumor stroma,[164,182,209-213] although it remains to be determined if their PD-L1-inducing effects are direct or mediated by the induction of interferons or TNFα.

FACTORS AFFECTING THE ANTITUMOR EFFECTIVENESS OF IMMUNE CHECKPOINT INHIBITORS

The character, location, and density of TILs are strong predictors of survival of cancer patients, independent of tumor histology, metastatic status, and the stage of disease.[60,69-72,214-220] The prognostic value of CD8+ T cells may also reflect their function (effector, memory, exhausted), which may differ in different tumors. For example, a recent study in gastric cancer showed that infiltration of Tbet-positive T cells (effector CTLs and

Th1 cells) has a stronger predictive value than total levels of infiltrating CD8+ T cells.[221]

Clinical efficacy of ICIs requires tumor-infiltrating CTLs and local PD-L-1 expression. ICB therapies (such as PD-1/PDL-1 or CTLA-4 blockade), which are highly effective in multiple forms of advanced cancer, show only marginal effectiveness in most forms of CRC and ovarian cancer.[61,67,68,222–224] The responsiveness to PD-1/PD-L1 blockers has been shown to critically depend on the presence of intratumoral accumulation of CTLs (and associated local PD-L1 expression in the TME, which is induced by CTL-produced IFNγ).[1–3,34,59,61,62,225] Notably, despite its overall aggressive character, the subset of CRC with mismatch repair deficiency and high microsatellite instability (MSI^{high} tumors) shows surprisingly high responsiveness to PD-1/PD-L1 blockade, compared with MSI^{low} CRC,[3,59,61–63,66] which is associated with its very high CTL infiltration of MSI^{high} tumors at baseline.[223,226]

Although the association between the clinical effectiveness of the PD-1 blockade and the MSI status of CRC is most commonly attributed to the differences in numbers of cancer cell mutations (and resulting numbers of new antigenic targets, *see next paragraph*) MSI^{low} and MSI^{high} CRC also show differences in the intratumoral activation of the WNT/β-catenin pathway,[227–235] which has been recently shown critical to the suppression of chemokine production in subpopulations of melanoma patients (resulting in their resistance to immune attack[236]). Since the β-catenin pathway can be affected by PGE2 levels,[237–240] which are modulated by hypoxia, it remains to be tested if the cross-regulation of the β-catenin pathway may be the common denominator of multiple mechanisms of the regulation of CTL influx in the TME and resulting local expression of different checkpoint molecules and responsiveness to ICIs.

Role of the mutational load and antigenic neoepitopes in cancer cells. The close association between the clinical effectiveness of PD-1/PD-L1 blockade and intratumoral densities of CTLs, raises the questions of the relevant antigens recognized by such TILs. In accord with a possibility that the correlation between variable local CTL infiltrations and clinical outcomes reflects not only the molecular character of the TME[236,241] but also the presence of "actionable" immunogenic epitopes on cancer cells (seen as non-self, due to their mutated character or elevated levels, compared to healthy cells), multiple studies have demonstrated that heavily mutated tumors are generally more responsive to ICI than tumors harboring fewer mutations.[242] The highest rates of clinical responses to anti-PD-1/anti-PD-L1 or anti-CTLA-4 therapies are seen in patients with melanoma[66] and lung cancer,[243] tumors with very high mutational burden. In contrast, most CRCs have very low mutational load and are in general unresponsive to checkpoint blockade. Interestingly, MSI^{high} CRC, characterized by DNA mismatch-repair deficiency and very high mutational burden (at least 20-fold higher than that of DNA mismatch-repair proficient CRCs) show up to 50% objective response-rate to PD-1 blockade,[34] compared with 0% in the patients with mismatch-repair proficient CRCs.[34] Progression-free survival (PFS) and overall survival (OS) were also significantly prolonged in patients with MSI^{high} tumors. An association between mutational and neoantigen burden and PD-1/PD-L1 treatment was also observed in NSCLC, melanoma and urothelial (bladder) cancer.[44]

Recently, Panda et al. analyzed data from more than 30 cancer types to identify a threshold level of mutational burden, intratumoral CTL infiltration, and ICs predicting clinical responses to ICB therapy.[244] In addition to confirming such correlations in melanoma, lung cancer, CRC, and urothelial cancer, the authors found IC-activating mutation (iCAM) threshold in four other tumor types (endometrial cancer, stomach adenocarcinoma, cervical cancer, and estrogen receptor (ER)-positive/HER2-negative breast cancer). Although the iCAM threshold does not always separate responders from nonresponders, it demonstrates that tumors with high mutational burden are generally more infiltrated and show upregulation of IC molecules.

TARGETING THE TUMOR MICROENVIRONMENT TO ENHANCE THE THERAPEUTIC EFFECTIVENESS OF IMMUNE CHECKPOINT INHIBITORS

Although the therapeutic modulation of the frequencies of tumor-associated mutations is not currently feasible (although it may occur incidentally as a side effect of radio- and chemotherapy), emerging evidence indicates that the efficacy of PD1/PD-L1 blockade and additional ICIs may be enhanced by the modulation of the intratumoral signaling to attract CTLs and associated intratumoral expression of IC molecules.

The relevant treatments may target not only cancer cells, which typically constitute only a minor part of the overall tumor mass (and themselves may be poorly response to modulation) but also the stromal (fibroblastoid) and inflammatory components of the TME (Fig. 1.2), which often constitute the main component of overall tumor mass.[57,245]

Tumor-associated inflammatory cells represent myeloid or lymphoid lineages. Myeloid cells include tumor-associated macrophages (TAMs), monocytic

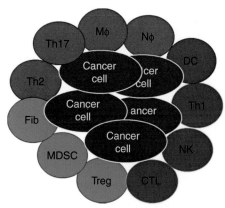

FIG. 1.2 Tumor microenvironment: Key components. **CTL:** cytotoxic T lymphocytes; **DCs** dendritic cells; **Fib:** fibroblasts; **MDSC:** myeloid-derived suppressor cells; **Mɸ:** macrophages; **Nɸ:** neutrophils **NK:** natural killer cells; **Th1:** Type-1T helper cells; **Th2:** Type-2T helper cells; **Th17:** Type-17T helper cells; **Treg:** regulatory T cells. *Blue:* tumor-promoting suppressive cells; *Red:* immune cells with predominant antitumor functions; *Purple:* predominantly tumor promoting, but with antitumor potential.

and granulocytic MDSCs, granulocytes, and DCs. TAMs include type-1 (M1) macrophages which express TNFα and other TNF/TNF-R family members, which have antitumor functions, and type-2 (M2) macrophages, which, similar to MDSCs express multiple suppressive (tumor-promoting) factors, which include adenosine, prostaglandin E2 (PGE2), IL-10, indoleamine 2,3-dioxygenase (IDO), arginase, inducible nitric oxide synthase (iNOS), TGFβ, and vascular endothelial growth factors.[52–55,57,246,247]

Lymphoid cells in the TME, typically referred to as TILs, include T and B lymphocytes and NK cells. Intratumoral T cells include CD8+ T cells (which involve CTLs, the key antitumor effector cells) and CD4+ T cells, whose role is more complex. Type-1 CD4+ T (Th1) cells secrete effector cell-activating cytokines, such as IL-2, TNFα, and IFNγ, and promote effective antitumor immunity by supporting CTL activity and antitumor functions of M1 macrophages. Tregs produce such factors as TGFβ and IL-10 which suppress CTL functions and activate suppressive functions of M2 macrophages and MDSCs. Th2 and Th17 subsets have been shown to have mostly tumor-promoting functions, similar to B cells,[248,249] although their presence in tumor-associated lymphoid structures has also been reported to have a positive prognostic value.[250] NK cells represent another population of tumor-associated lymphoid cells. Although NK cells are a mixed population with different functions, in general, NK cells show a unique

ability to kill cancer cells upon the first encounter, without the need for prior education or "priming," although their antitumor activity can be further enhanced by Th cells and DCs.[251–253a] Lymphoid cells are present in TME as either disseminated cells or as elements of lymph-node-like structures.[215,254–258] Their relative prevalence and localization within TME is regulated by their distinct patterns of chemokine-guided migration (see Fig. 1.3).

Different chemokine receptor usage between type-1 effector cells (CTL, Th1, and NK cells), which typically home to sites of acute inflammation (such as viral infections), versus Tregs and MDSCs, which accumulate at late and chronic stages of inflammation to promote tissue healing and regeneration, make the chemokine system an interesting target for TME reprograming for enhanced therapy outcomes (Fig. 1.3).

Multiple groups, including ours, demonstrated that different types of immune cells show different expression of chemokine receptors and respond to different chemokines. The key chemokines attracting the CCR5- and CXCR3-expressing CTLs, Th1, and NK cells are CCL5 (ligand for CCR5) and CXCL9, CXCL10, and CXCL11 (ligands for CXCR3). In contrast, local production of CCL2, CCL22, and CXCL12 within TME promotes intratumoral attraction of CXCR4+ (and, in some cases, CCR2+) MDSCs and M2 macrophages, as well as CCR4+/CXCR4+ Tregs.

High tumor production of CCL5 (RANTES; ligand for CCR5) and CXCL9 (MIG), CXCL10 (IP10), and CXCL11 interferon-inducible T-cell α chemoattractant, ITAC, the three known ligands for CXCR3, is associated with high CTL infiltration in CRC[259] and other cancers.[260,261] Our own studies showed tight correlation between intratumoral production of CCL5, CXCL9, and CXCL10, and local infiltration with CD8+GrB+ CTLs, with expressing at least one of these chemokine receptors in over 95% of cases.[262]

Both the spontaneously occurring and vaccination-induced tumor-specific CTLs express high levels of CCR5 and CXCR3,[263] and migrate in response to their relevant chemokine ligands produced by inflamed tissues and "hot" tumors.[262–264] For this reason, the therapeutic benefit of ICIs is likely to be enhanced by therapies that selectively enhance CXCL10 (and other CXCR3 ligands) and CCR5 (such as CCL5/RANTES) ligands, thus promoting migration of CTLs and other effector cells to tumor tissues. Mouse studies confirmed the antitumor role of CXCL10 and CTL accumulation in the effectiveness of therapeutic cancer vaccines, combined with ligands for TLR3.[265,266] However, poly-I:C alone is a relatively ineffective inducer of CTL-attracting chemokines and can enhance local production of COX2- and COX2-dependent Treg/MDSC-attracting

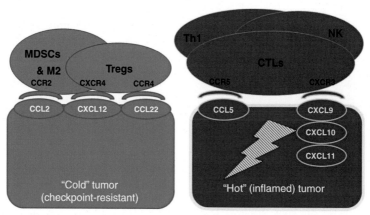

FIG. 1.3 Differential expression of chemokine receptors on antitumor effector cells and tumor-promoting suppressor cells allow for their therapeutic targeting to enhance the effects of cancer immunotherapy and other forms of cancer treatment.

chemokines and suppressive factors.[262,264,267,268] Two options to enhance its potency and selectivity of action are either to combine them with COX2 blockers (and/or with IFNα, which we found to uniformly reprogram the pattern of poly-I:C-induced chemokines in the TMEs of several types of cancer)[187,189,194,195] or, potentially, to use modified TLR ligands which avoid activation of suppressive events (Theodoraki, Kalinski et al., manuscript submitted).

Clinically relevant factors with documented TME-reprogramming activities include ligands for multiple TLRs, such as TLR4-binding monophosphoryl lipid A; the TLR7 agonist imiquimod, or TLR9 agonists CpGs, interferons, and cytokines (e.g., interferon-α, interleukin-2, or granulocyte macrophage colony-stimulating factor), as well as complete microorganisms (e.g., BCG), although their undesirable induction of suppressive factors remains a concern which still needs to be addressed.[267] Enhanced infiltration of CD8+ T cells resulting from intratumoral injection of a STING activator (cGAMP) has been shown to improve the antitumor effectiveness of PD-1 and CTLA-4 blockade in mouse models of CRC and other cancers.[269] Similar to their importance during checkpoint blockade, the levels of intratumoral CTL infiltration can predict patients' clinical response to cancer vaccines,[270] which can trigger different levels of intratumoral CTL accumulation.[270,271]

CONCLUSIONS

Despite the increasing effectiveness of immunotherapy and other forms of comprehensive cancer care which often have high cure rates of multiple patient groups, cancer remains a leading cause of death.[272] Recent developments in the area of cancer immunotherapy, especially the introduction of ICIs as a standard element of comprehensive cancer, and the demonstration of the predictive value of intratumoral accumulation of CTLs and other type 1 immune cells (Th1 and NK cells), in the clinical activity of ICIs, provide multiple actionable targets and different classes of new tools to further enhance the overall success rate of cancer immunotherapy.

Clinical and laboratory evidence showing the importance of the immune composition of the TME in regulating cancer progression and its response to ICIs and other forms of immunotherapy, suggest that modulating TME to selectively enhance CTL infiltration and reduce Treg and MDSC migration, together with limiting secondary suppressive mechanisms induced in the TME by activated CTLs,[204] is likely to enhance the current response rate of ICIs and improve overall outcomes of comprehensive cancer care.

ACKNOWLEDGMENTS AND DISCLOSURES

This work was supported by the National Institutes of Health grant CA159981 and by the Rustum Family Foundation. We thank Ms. Janet Martin for editorial and administrative assistance.

REFERENCES

1. Tumeh PC, Harview CL, Yearley JH, et al. PD-1 blockade induces responses by inhibiting adaptive immune resistance. *Nature.* 2014;515(7528):568–571.
2. Herbst RS, Soria JC, Kowanetz M, et al. Predictive correlates of response to the anti-PD-L1 antibody MPDL3280A in cancer patients. *Nature.* 2014;515(7528):563–567.

3. Taube JM, Klein A, Brahmer JR, et al. Association of PD-1, PD-1 ligands, and other features of the tumor immune microenvironment with response to anti-PD-1 therapy. *Clin Cancer Res*. 2014;20(19):5064–5074.

4. Coley WB. The treatment of inoperable sarcoma by bacterial toxins (the mixed toxins of the streptococcus erysipelas and the *Bacillus prodigiosus*). *Proc R Soc Med*. 1910; 3(Surg Sect):1–48.

5. Nauts HC, Swift WE, Coley BL. The treatment of malignant tumors by bacterial toxins as developed by the late William B. Coley, M.D., reviewed in the light of modern research. *Cancer Res*. 1946;6(4):205–216.

6. Rosenberg SA, Yang JC, Restifo NP. Cancer immunotherapy: moving beyond current vaccines. *Nat Med*. 2004;10(9):909–915.

7. Astsaturov I, Petrella T, Bagriacik EU, et al. Amplification of virus-induced antimelanoma T-cell reactivity by high-dose interferon-alpha2b: implications for cancer vaccines. *Clin Cancer Res*. 2003;9(12):4347–4355.

8. Rosenberg SA, Sherry RM, Morton KE, et al. Tumor progression can occur despite the induction of very high levels of self/tumor antigen-specific CD8+ T cells in patients with melanoma. *J Immunol*. 2005;175(9):6169–6176.

9. Bassi P. BCG (Bacillus of Calmette Guerin) therapy of high-risk superficial bladder cancer. *Surg Oncol*. 2002; 11(1–2):77–83.

10. Kirkwood JM, Butterfield LH, Tarhini AA, Zarour H, Kalinski P, Ferrone S. Immunotherapy of cancer in 2012. *CA Cancer J Clin*. 2012;62(5):309–335.

11. Chambers CA, Kuhns MS, Egen JG, Allison JP. CTLA-4-mediated inhibition in regulation of T cell responses: mechanisms and manipulation in tumor immunotherapy. *Annu Rev Immunol*. 2001;19:565–594.

12. Egen JG, Kuhns MS, Allison JP. CTLA-4: new insights into its biological function and use in tumor immunotherapy. *Nat Immunol*. 2002;3(7):611–618.

13. Eggermont AM, Testori A, Maio M, Robert C. Anti-CTLA-4 antibody adjuvant therapy in melanoma. *Semin Oncol*. 2010;37(5):455–459.

14. Fife BT, Bluestone JA. Control of peripheral T-cell tolerance and autoimmunity via the CTLA-4 and PD-1 pathways. *Immunol Rev*. 2008;224:166–182.

15. Weber J. Immune checkpoint proteins: a new therapeutic paradigm for cancer—preclinical background: CTLA-4 and PD-1 blockade. *Semin Oncol*. 2010;37(5):430–439.

16. Wolchok JD, Saenger Y. The mechanism of anti-CTLA-4 activity and the negative regulation of T-cell activation. *Oncologist*. 2008;13(suppl 4):2–9.

17. Pardoll DM. The blockade of immune checkpoints in cancer immunotherapy. *Nat Rev Cancer*. 2012;12(4): 252–264.

18. Brahmer JR, Drake CG, Wollner I, et al. Phase I study of single-agent anti-programmed death-1 (MDX-1106) in refractory solid tumors: safety, clinical activity, pharmacodynamics, and immunologic correlates. *J Clin Oncol*. 2010;28(19):3167–3175.

19. Larkin J, Chiarion-Sileni V, Gonzalez R, et al. Combined nivolumab and ipilimumab or monotherapy in untreated melanoma. *N Engl J Med*. 2015;373(1):23–34.

20. Ribas A, Puzanov I, Dummer R, et al. Pembrolizumab versus investigator-choice chemotherapy for ipilimumab-refractory melanoma (KEYNOTE-002): a randomised, controlled, phase 2 trial. *Lancet Oncol*. 2015;16(8): 908–918.

21. Robert C, Schachter J, Long GV, et al. Pembrolizumab versus ipilimumab in advanced melanoma. *N Engl J Med*. 2015;372(26):2521–2532.

22. Roberts PJ, Der CJ. Targeting the Raf-MEK-ERK mitogen-activated protein kinase cascade for the treatment of cancer. *Oncogene*. 2007;26(22):3291–3310.

23. Weber JS, D'Angelo SP, Minor D, et al. Nivolumab versus chemotherapy in patients with advanced melanoma who progressed after anti-CTLA-4 treatment (CheckMate 037): a randomised, controlled, open-label, phase 3 trial. *Lancet Oncol*. 2015;16(4):375–384.

24. Weber J, Mandala M, Del Vecchio M, et al. Adjuvant nivolumab versus ipilimumab in resected stage III or IV melanoma. *N Engl J Med*. 2017;377(19):1824–1835.

25. Antonia SJ, Villegas A, Daniel D, et al. Durvalumab after chemoradiotherapy in stage III non-small-cell lung cancer. *N Engl J Med*. 2017;377(20):1919–1929.

26. Borghaei H, Paz-Ares L, Horn L, et al. Nivolumab versus docetaxel in advanced nonsquamous non-small-cell lung cancer. *N Engl J Med*. 2015;373(17):1627–1639.

27. Brahmer J, Reckamp KL, Baas P, et al. Nivolumab versus docetaxel in advanced squamous-cell non-small-cell lung cancer. *N Engl J Med*. 2015;373(2):123–135.

28. Fehrenbacher L, Spira A, Ballinger M, et al. Atezolizumab versus docetaxel for patients with previously treated non-small-cell lung cancer (POPLAR): a multicentre, open-label, phase 2 randomised controlled trial. *Lancet*. 2016;387(10030):1837–1846.

29. Herbst RS, Baas P, Kim DW, et al. Pembrolizumab versus docetaxel for previously treated, PD-L1-positive, advanced non-small-cell lung cancer (KEYNOTE-010): a randomised controlled trial. *Lancet*. 2016;387(10027): 1540–1550.

30. Langer CJ, Gadgeel SM, Borghaei H, et al. Carboplatin and pemetrexed with or without pembrolizumab for advanced, non-squamous non-small-cell lung cancer: a randomised, phase 2 cohort of the open-label KEYNOTE-021 study. *Lancet Oncol*. 2016;17(11):1497–1508.

31. Reck M, Rodriguez-Abreu D, Robinson AG, et al. Pembrolizumab versus chemotherapy for PD-L1-positive non-small-cell lung cancer. *N Engl J Med*. 2016;375(19): 1823–1833.

32. Kok M, Horlings HM, Snaebjornsson P, et al. Profound immunotherapy response in mismatch repair-deficient breast cancer. *JCO Precis Oncol*. 2017;1:1–3.

33. Le DT, Durham JN, Smith KN, et al. Mismatch repair deficiency predicts response of solid tumors to PD-1 blockade. *Science*. 2017;357(6349):409–413.

34. Le DT, Uram JN, Wang H, et al. PD-1 blockade in tumors with mismatch-repair deficiency. *N Engl J Med.* 2015; 372(26):2509−2520.

35. Overman MJ, McDermott R, Leach JL, et al. Nivolumab in patients with metastatic DNA mismatch repair-deficient or microsatellite instability-high colorectal cancer (CheckMate 142): an open-label, multicentre, phase 2 study. *Lancet Oncol.* 2017;18(9):1182−1191.

36. Motzer RJ, Escudier B, McDermott DF, et al. Nivolumab versus everolimus in advanced renal-cell carcinoma. *N Engl J Med.* 2015;373(19):1803−1813.

37. Ansell SM, Lesokhin AM, Borrello I, et al. PD-1 blockade with nivolumab in relapsed or refractory Hodgkin's lymphoma. *N Engl J Med.* 2015;372(4):311−319.

38. Chen R, Zinzani PL, Fanale MA, et al. Phase II study of the efficacy and safety of pembrolizumab for relapsed/refractory classic hodgkin lymphoma. *J Clin Oncol.* 2017; 35(19):2125−2132.

39. Balar AV, Castellano D, O'Donnell PH, et al. First-line pembrolizumab in cisplatin-ineligible patients with locally advanced and unresectable or metastatic urothelial cancer (KEYNOTE-052): a multicentre, single-arm, phase 2 study. *Lancet Oncol.* 2017;18(11):1483−1492.

40. Balar AV, Galsky MD, Rosenberg JE, et al. Atezolizumab as first-line treatment in cisplatin-ineligible patients with locally advanced and metastatic urothelial carcinoma: a single-arm, multicentre, phase 2 trial. *Lancet.* 2017;389(10064):67−76.

41. Bellmunt J, de Wit R, Vaughn DJ, et al. Pembrolizumab as second-line therapy for advanced urothelial carcinoma. *N Engl J Med.* 2017;376(11):1015−1026.

42. Patel MR, Ellerton J, Infante JR, et al. Avelumab in metastatic urothelial carcinoma after platinum failure (JAVELIN Solid Tumor): pooled results from two expansion cohorts of an open-label, phase 1 trial. *Lancet Oncol.* 2018;19(1):51−64.

43. Powles T, O'Donnell PH, Massard C, et al. Efficacy and safety of durvalumab in locally advanced or metastatic urothelial carcinoma: updated results from a phase 1/2 open-label study. *JAMA Oncol.* 2017;3(9):e172411.

44. Rosenberg JE, Hoffman-Censits J, Powles T, et al. Atezolizumab in patients with locally advanced and metastatic urothelial carcinoma who have progressed following treatment with platinum-based chemotherapy: a single-arm, multicentre, phase 2 trial. *Lancet.* 2016;387(10031): 1909−1920.

45. Sharma P, Retz M, Siefker-Radtke A, et al. Nivolumab in metastatic urothelial carcinoma after platinum therapy (CheckMate 275): a multicentre, single-arm, phase 2 trial. *Lancet Oncol.* 2017;18(3):312−322.

46. Ferris RL, Blumenschein Jr G, Fayette J, et al. Nivolumab for recurrent squamous-cell carcinoma of the head and neck. *N Engl J Med.* 2016;375(19):1856−1867.

47. Seiwert TY, Burtness B, Mehra R, et al. Safety and clinical activity of pembrolizumab for treatment of recurrent or metastatic squamous cell carcinoma of the head and neck (KEYNOTE-012): an open-label, multicentre, phase 1b trial. *Lancet Oncol.* 2016;17(7):956−965.

48. Kaufman HL, Russell J, Hamid O, et al. Avelumab in patients with chemotherapy-refractory metastatic Merkel cell carcinoma: a multicentre, single-group, open-label, phase 2 trial. *Lancet Oncol.* 2016;17(10):1374−1385.

49. El-Khoueiry AB, Sangro B, Yau T, et al. Nivolumab in patients with advanced hepatocellular carcinoma (CheckMate 040): an open-label, non-comparative, phase 1/2 dose escalation and expansion trial. *Lancet.* 2017;389(10088):2492−2502.

50. Fuchs CS, Doi T, Jang RW, et al. Safety and efficacy of pembrolizumab monotherapy in patients with previously treated advanced gastric and gastroesophageal junction cancer: phase 2 clinical KEYNOTE-059 trial. *JAMA Oncol.* 2018;4.

51. Sun C, Mezzadra R, Schumacher TN. Regulation and function of the PD-L1 checkpoint. *Immunity.* 2018; 48(3):434−452.

52. Weichselbaum RR, Liang H, Deng L, Fu YX. Radiotherapy and immunotherapy: a beneficial liaison? *Nat Rev Clin Oncol.* 2017;14(6):365−379.

53. Galluzzi L, Buque A, Kepp O, Zitvogel L, Kroemer G. Immunological effects of conventional chemotherapy and targeted anticancer agents. *Cancer Cell.* 2015;28(6):690−714.

54. Demaria S, Golden EB, Formenti SC. Role of local radiation therapy in cancer immunotherapy. *JAMA Oncol.* 2015;1(9):1325−1332.

55. Barker HE, Paget JT, Khan AA, Harrington KJ. The tumour microenvironment after radiotherapy: mechanisms of resistance and recurrence. *Nat Rev Cancer.* 2015;15(7): 409−425.

56. Weber JS. Current perspectives on immunotherapy. *Semin Oncol.* 2014;41(suppl 5):S14−S29.

57. Junttila MR, de Sauvage FJ. Influence of tumour microenvironment heterogeneity on therapeutic response. *Nature.* 2013;501(7467):346−354.

58. Gadducci A, Guerrieri ME, Greco C. Tissue biomarkers as prognostic variables of cervical cancer. *Crit Rev Oncol Hematol.* 2013;86(2):104−129.

59. Topalian SL, Hodi FS, Brahmer JR, et al. Safety, activity, and immune correlates of anti-PD-1 antibody in cancer. *N Engl J Med.* 2012;366(26):2443−2454.

60. Fridman WH, Pages F, Sautes-Fridman C, Galon J. The immune contexture in human tumours: impact on clinical outcome. *Nat Rev Cancer.* 2012;12(4):298−306.

61. Brahmer JR, Tykodi SS, Chow LQ, et al. Safety and activity of anti-PD-L1 antibody in patients with advanced cancer. *N Engl J Med.* 2012;366(26):2455−2465.

62. Llosa NJ, Cruise M, Tam A, et al. The vigorous immune microenvironment of microsatellite instable colon cancer is balanced by multiple counter-inhibitory checkpoints. *Cancer Discov.* 2015;5(1):43−51.

63. Kroemer G, Galluzzi L, Zitvogel L, Fridman WH. Colorectal cancer: the first neoplasia found to be under immunosurveillance and the last one to respond to immunotherapy? *Oncoimmunology.* 2015;4(7):e1058597.

64. Patel SA, Minn AJ. Combination cancer therapy with immune checkpoint blockade: mechanisms and strategies. *Immunity.* 2018;48(3):417−433.

65. Pitt JM, Vetizou M, Daillere R, et al. Resistance mechanisms to immune-checkpoint blockade in cancer: tumor-intrinsic and -extrinsic factors. *Immunity.* 2016; 44(6):1255−1269.

66. Gatalica Z, Snyder C, Maney T, et al. Programmed cell death 1 (PD-1) and its ligand (PD-L1) in common cancers and their correlation with molecular cancer type. *Cancer Epidemiol Biomarkers Prev.* 2014;23(12):2965−2970.

67. Tse BW, Collins A, Oehler MK, Zippelius A, Heinzelmann-Schwarz VA. Antibody-based immunotherapy for ovarian cancer: where are we at? *Ann Oncol.* 2014;25(2):322−331.

68. Hamanishi J, Mandai M, Ikeda T, et al. Safety and antitumor activity of anti-PD-1 antibody, nivolumab, in patients with platinum-resistant ovarian cancer. *J Clin Oncol.* 2015;33(34):4015−4022.

69. Galon J, Costes A, Sanchez-Cabo F, et al. Type, density, and location of immune cells within human colorectal tumors predict clinical outcome. *Science.* 2006;313(5795): 1960−1964.

70. Galon J, Fridman WH, Pages F. The adaptive immunologic microenvironment in colorectal cancer: a novel perspective. *Cancer Res.* 2007;67(5):1883−1886.

71. Zhang L, Conejo-Garcia JR, Katsaros D, et al. Intratumoral T cells, recurrence, and survival in epithelial ovarian cancer. *N Engl J Med.* 2003;348(3):203−213.

72. Sato E, Olson SH, Ahn J, et al. Intraepithelial CD8+ tumor-infiltrating lymphocytes and a high CD8+/regulatory T cell ratio are associated with favorable prognosis in ovarian cancer. *Proc Natl Acad Sci U S A.* 2005;102(51): 18538−18543.

73. Nishimura H, Nose M, Hiai H, Minato N, Honjo T. Development of lupus-like autoimmune diseases by disruption of the PD-1 gene encoding an ITIM motif-carrying immunoreceptor. *Immunity.* 1999;11(2):141−151.

74. Nishimura H, Okazaki T, Tanaka Y, et al. Autoimmune dilated cardiomyopathy in PD-1 receptor-deficient mice. *Science.* 2001;291(5502):319−322.

75. Ansari MJ, Salama AD, Chitnis T, et al. The programmed death-1 (PD-1) pathway regulates autoimmune diabetes in nonobese diabetic (NOD) mice. *J Exp Med.* 2003; 198(1):63−69.

76. Wang J, Yoshida T, Nakaki F, Hiai H, Okazaki T, Honjo T. Establishment of NOD-Pdcd1-/- mice as an efficient animal model of type I diabetes. *Proc Natl Acad Sci U S A.* 2005;102(33):11823−11828.

77. Guleria I, Khosroshahi A, Ansari MJ, et al. A critical role for the programmed death ligand 1 in fetomaternal tolerance. *J Exp Med.* 2005;202(2):231−237.

78. Agata Y, Kawasaki A, Nishimura H, et al. Expression of the PD-1 antigen on the surface of stimulated mouse T and B lymphocytes. *Int Immunol.* 1996;8(5):765−772.

79. Honda T, Egen JG, Lammermann T, Kastenmuller W, Torabi-Parizi P, Germain RN. Tuning of antigen sensitivity by T cell receptor-dependent negative feedback controls T cell effector function in inflamed tissues. *Immunity.* 2014;40(2):235−247.

80. Perkins D, Wang Z, Donovan C, et al. Regulation of CTLA-4 expression during T cell activation. *J Immunol.* 1996;156(11):4154−4159.

81. Finn PW, He H, Wang Y, et al. Synergistic induction of CTLA-4 expression by costimulation with TCR plus CD28 signals mediated by increased transcription and messenger ribonucleic acid stability. *J Immunol.* 1997; 158(9):4074−4081.

82. Sansom DM. CD28, CTLA-4 and their ligands: who does what and to whom? *Immunology.* 2000;101(2):169−177.

83. Harper K, Balzano C, Rouvier E, Mattéi MG, Luciani MF, Golstein P. CTLA-4 and CD28 activated lymphocyte molecules are closely related in both mouse and human as to sequence, message expression, gene structure, and chromosomal location. *J Immunol.* 1991; 147(3):1037.

84. Leung HT, Bradshaw J, Cleaveland JS, Linsley PS. Cytotoxic T lymphocyte-associated molecule-4, a high avidity receptor for CD80 and CD86, contains an intracellular localization motif in its cytoplasmic tail. *J Biol Chem.* 1995;270(42):25107−25114.

85. Linsley PS, Bradshaw J, Greene J, Peach R, Bennett KL, Mittler RS. Intracellular trafficking of CTLA-4 and focal localization towards sites of TCR engagement. *Immunity.* 1996;4(6):535−543.

86. Bachmann MF, Köhler G, Ecabert B, Mak TW, Kopf M. Cutting edge: lymphoproliferative disease in the absence of CTLA-4 is not T cell autonomous. *J Immunol.* 1999; 163(3):1128.

87. Walker LSK. EFIS lecture: understanding the CTLA-4 checkpoint in the maintenance of immune homeostasis. *Immunol Lett.* 2017;184:43−50.

88. Qureshi OS, Zheng Y, Nakamura K, et al. Transendocytosis of CD80 and CD86: a molecular basis for the cell-extrinsic function of CTLA-4. *Science.* 2011; 332(6029):600.

89. Du X, Tang F, Liu M, et al. A reappraisal of CTLA-4 checkpoint blockade in cancer immunotherapy. *Cell Res.* 2018;28.

90. Ishida Y, Agata Y, Shibahara K, Honjo T. Induced expression of PD-1, a novel member of the immunoglobulin gene superfamily, upon programmed cell death. *EMBO J.* 1992;11(11):3887−3895.

91. Yearley JH, Gibson C, Yu N, et al. PD-L2 expression in human tumors: relevance to anti-PD-1 therapy in cancer. *Clin Cancer Res.* 2017;23(12):3158−3167.

92. Zhang X, Schwartz JC, Guo X, et al. Structural and functional analysis of the costimulatory receptor programmed death-1. *Immunity.* 2004;20(3):337−347.

93. Dong H, Zhu G, Tamada K, Chen L. B7-H1, a third member of the B7 family, co-stimulates T-cell proliferation and interleukin-10 secretion. *Nat Med.* 1999;5(12): 1365−1369.

94. Keir ME, Butte MJ, Freeman GJ, Sharpe AH. PD-1 and its ligands in tolerance and immunity. *Annu Rev Immunol.* 2008;26:677−704.

95. Lin DY, Tanaka Y, Iwasaki M, et al. The PD-1/PD-L1 complex resembles the antigen-binding Fv domains of antibodies and T cell receptors. *Proc Natl Acad Sci U S A.* 2008;105(8):3011−3016.

96. Gauen LK, Zhu Y, Letourneur F, et al. Interactions of p59fyn and ZAP-70 with T-cell receptor activation motifs: defining the nature of a signalling motif. *Mol Cell Biol.* 1994;14(6):3729−3741.

97. Straus DB, Weiss A. Genetic evidence for the involvement of the lck tyrosine kinase in signal transduction through the T cell antigen receptor. *Cell.* 1992;70(4):585−593.

98. Zak KM, Kitel R, Przetocka S, et al. Structure of the complex of human programmed death 1, PD-1, and its ligand PD-L1. *Structure.* 2015;23(12):2341−2348.

99. Chemnitz JM, Parry RV, Nichols KE, June CH, Riley JL. SHP-1 and SHP-2 associate with immunoreceptor tyrosine-based switch motif of programmed death 1 upon primary human T cell stimulation, but only receptor ligation prevents T cell activation. *J Immunol.* 2004; 173(2):945−954.

100. Sheppard KA, Fitz LJ, Lee JM, et al. PD-1 inhibits T-cell receptor induced phosphorylation of the ZAP70/CD3zeta signalosome and downstream signaling to PKCtheta. *FEBS Lett.* 2004;574(1−3):37−41.

101. Ugi S, Maegawa H, Olefsky JM, Shigeta Y, Kashiwagi A. Src homology 2 domains of protein tyrosine phosphatase are associated in vitro with both the insulin receptor and insulin receptor substrate-1 via different phosphotyrosine motifs. *FEBS Lett.* 1994;340(3):216−220.

102. Hui E, Cheung J, Zhu J, et al. T cell costimulatory receptor CD28 is a primary target for PD-1-mediated inhibition. *Science.* 2017;355(6332):1428−1433.

103. Kamphorst AO, Wieland A, Nasti T, et al. Rescue of exhausted CD8 T cells by PD-1-targeted therapies is CD28-dependent. *Science.* 2017;355(6332):1423−1427.

104. Butte MJ, Keir ME, Phamduy TB, Sharpe AH, Freeman GJ. Programmed death-1 ligand 1 interacts specifically with the B7-1 costimulatory molecule to inhibit T cell responses. *Immunity.* 2007;27(1):111−122.

105. Chang TT, Jabs C, Sobel RA, Kuchroo VK, Sharpe AH. Studies in B7-deficient mice reveal a critical role for B7 costimulation in both induction and effector phases of experimental autoimmune encephalomyelitis. *J Exp Med.* 1999;190(5):733−740.

106. Curiel TJ, Wei S, Dong H, et al. Blockade of B7-H1 improves myeloid dendritic cell-mediated antitumor immunity. *Nat Med.* 2003;9(5):562−567.

107. Freeman GJ, Long AJ, Iwai Y, et al. Engagement of the PD-1 immunoinhibitory receptor by a novel B7 family member leads to negative regulation of lymphocyte activation. *J Exp Med.* 2000;192(7):1027−1034.

108. Keir ME, Liang SC, Guleria I, et al. Tissue expression of PD-L1 mediates peripheral T cell tolerance. *J Exp Med.* 2006;203(4):883−895.

109. Latchman YE, Liang SC, Wu Y, et al. PD-L1-deficient mice show that PD-L1 on T cells, antigen-presenting cells, and host tissues negatively regulates T cells. *Proc Natl Acad Sci U S A.* 2004;101(29):10691−10696.

110. Benson Jr DM, Bakan CE, Mishra A, et al. The PD-1/PD-L1 axis modulates the natural killer cell versus multiple myeloma effect: a therapeutic target for CT-011, a novel monoclonal anti-PD-1 antibody. *Blood.* 2010;116(13): 2286−2294.

111. Terme M, Ullrich E, Aymeric L, et al. IL-18 induces PD-1-dependent immunosuppression in cancer. *Cancer Res.* 2011;71(16):5393−5399.

112. Zhao L, Yu H, Yi S, et al. The tumor suppressor miR-138-5p targets PD-L1 in colorectal cancer. *Oncotarget.* 2016; 7(29):45370−45384.

113. Gordon SR, Maute RL, Dulken BW, et al. PD-1 expression by tumour-associated macrophages inhibits phagocytosis and tumour immunity. *Nature.* 2017;545(7655):495−499.

114. Azuma T, Yao S, Zhu G, Flies AS, Flies SJ, Chen L. B7-H1 is a ubiquitous antiapoptotic receptor on cancer cells. *Blood.* 2008;111(7):3635−3643.

115. Gato-Canas M, Zuazo M, Arasanz H, et al. PDL1 signals through conserved sequence motifs to overcome interferon-mediated cytotoxicity. *Cell Rep.* 2017;20(8): 1818−1829.

116. Chang CH, Qiu J, O'Sullivan D, et al. Metabolic competition in the tumor microenvironment is a driver of cancer progression. *Cell.* 2015;162(6):1229−1241.

117. Yu X, Harden K, Gonzalez LC, et al. The surface protein TIGIT suppresses T cell activation by promoting the generation of mature immunoregulatory dendritic cells. *Nat Immunol.* 2009;10(1):48−57.

118. Stanietsky N, Simic H, Arapovic J, et al. The interaction of TIGIT with PVR and PVRL2 inhibits human NK cell cytotoxicity. *Proc Natl Acad Sci U S A.* 2009;106(42): 17858−17863.

119. Casado JG, Pawelec G, Morgado S, et al. Expression of adhesion molecules and ligands for activating and costimulatory receptors involved in cell-mediated cytotoxicity in a large panel of human melanoma cell lines. *Cancer Immunol Immunother.* 2009;58(9):1517−1526.

120. Johnston RJ, Yu X, Grogan JL. The checkpoint inhibitor TIGIT limits antitumor and antiviral CD8(+) T cell responses. *Oncoimmunology.* 2015;4(9):e1036214.

121. Anderson AC, Joller N, Kuchroo VK. Lag-3, Tim-3, and TIGIT: co-inhibitory receptors with specialized functions in immune regulation. *Immunity.* 2016;44(5):989−1004.

122. Wang F, He W, Zhou H, et al. The Tim-3 ligand galectin-9 negatively regulates CD8+ alloreactive T cell and prolongs survival of skin graft. *Cell Immunol.* 2007; 250(1−2):68−74.

123. Zhu C, Anderson AC, Schubart A, et al. The Tim-3 ligand galectin-9 negatively regulates T helper type 1 immunity. *Nat Immunol.* 2005;6(12):1245−1252.

124. Banerjee H, Kane LP. Immune regulation by Tim-3. *F1000Res.* 2018;7:316.

125. Das M, Zhu C, Kuchroo VK. Tim-3 and its role in regulating anti-tumor immunity. *Immunol Rev.* 2017;276(1): 97−111.

126. Szender JB, Papanicolau-Sengos A, Eng KH, et al. NY-ESO-1 expression predicts an aggressive phenotype of ovarian cancer. *Gynecol Oncol.* 2017;145(3):420−425.

127. Ferris RL, Lu B, Kane LP. Too much of a good thing? Tim-3 and TCR signaling in T cell exhaustion. *J Immunol.* 2014;193(4):1525–1530.
128. Marin-Acevedo JA, Dholaria B, Soyano AE, Knutson KL, Chumsri S, Lou Y. Next generation of immune checkpoint therapy in cancer: new developments and challenges. *J Hematol Oncol.* 2018;11(1):39.
129. Workman CJ, Dugger KJ, Vignali DA. Cutting edge: molecular analysis of the negative regulatory function of lymphocyte activation gene-3. *J Immunol.* 2002; 169(10):5392–5395.
130. Goldberg MV, Drake CG. LAG-3 in cancer immunotherapy. *Curr Top Microbiol Immunol.* 2011;344:269–278.
131. He Y, Rivard CJ, Rozeboom L, et al. Lymphocyte-activation gene-3, an important immune checkpoint in cancer. *Cancer Sci.* 2016;107(9):1193–1197.
132. Sierro S, Romero P, Speiser DE. The CD4-like molecule LAG-3, biology and therapeutic applications. *Expert Opin Ther Targets.* 2011;15(1):91–101.
133. Deng J, Le Mercier I, Kuta A, Noelle RJ. A new VISTA on combination therapy for negative checkpoint regulator blockade. *J Immunother Cancer.* 2016;4:86.
134. Nowak EC, Lines JL, Varn FS, et al. Immunoregulatory functions of VISTA. *Immunol Rev.* 2017;276(1):66–79.
135. Xu W, Hieu T, Malarkannan S, Wang L. The structure, expression, and multifaceted role of immune-checkpoint protein VISTA as a critical regulator of anti-tumor immunity, autoimmunity, and inflammation. *Cell Mol Immunol.* 2018;14:1–9.
136. Lines JL, Pantazi E, Mak J, et al. VISTA is an immune checkpoint molecule for human T cells. *Cancer Res.* 2014;74(7):1924–1932.
137. Le Mercier I, Chen W, Lines JL, et al. VISTA regulates the development of protective antitumor immunity. *Cancer Res.* 2014;74(7):1933–1944.
138. Lines JL, Sempere LF, Broughton T, Wang L, Noelle R. VISTA is a novel broad-spectrum negative checkpoint regulator for cancer immunotherapy. *Cancer Immunol Res.* 2014;2(6):510–517.
139. Lo B, Abdel-Motal UM. Lessons from CTLA-4 deficiency and checkpoint inhibition. *Curr Opin Immunol.* 2017; 49:14–19.
140. Scalapino KJ, Daikh DI. CTLA-4: a key regulatory point in the control of autoimmune disease. *Immunol Rev.* 2008; 223:143–155.
141. Wing K, Yamaguchi T, Sakaguchi S. Cell-autonomous and -non-autonomous roles of CTLA-4 in immune regulation. *Trends Immunol.* 2011;32(9):428–433.
142. Gros A, Robbins PF, Yao X, et al. PD-1 identifies the patient-specific CD8(+) tumor-reactive repertoire infiltrating human tumors. *J Clin Invest.* 2014;124(5):2246–2259.
143. Gros A, Parkhurst MR, Tran E, et al. Prospective identification of neoantigen-specific lymphocytes in the peripheral blood of melanoma patients. *Nat Med.* 2016;22(4): 433–438.
144. Sun Z, Fourcade J, Pagliano O, et al. IL10 and PD-1 cooperate to limit the activity of tumor-specific CD8+ T cells. *Cancer Res.* 2015;75(8):1635–1644.
145. Park BV, Freeman ZT, Ghasemzadeh A, et al. TGFbeta1-mediated SMAD3 enhances PD-1 expression on antigen-specific T cells in cancer. *Cancer Discov.* 2016; 6(12):1366–1381.
146. Roemer MG, Advani RH, Ligon AH, et al. PD-L1 and PD-L2 genetic alterations define classical Hodgkin lymphoma and predict outcome. *J Clin Oncol.* 2016;34(23): 2690–2697.
147. Armand P, Shipp MA, Ribrag V, et al. Programmed death-1 blockade with pembrolizumab in patients with classical Hodgkin lymphoma after brentuximab vedotin failure. *J Clin Oncol.* 2016;34(31):3733–3739.
148. Younes A, Santoro A, Shipp M, et al. Nivolumab for classical Hodgkin's lymphoma after failure of both autologous stem-cell transplantation and brentuximab vedotin: a multicentre, multicohort, single-arm phase 2 trial. *Lancet Oncol.* 2016;17(9):1283–1294.
149. Ikeda S, Okamoto T, Okano S, et al. PD-L1 is upregulated by simultaneous amplification of the PD-L1 and JAK2 genes in non–small cell lung cancer. *J Thorac Oncol.* 2016;11(1):62–71.
150. George J, Saito M, Tsuta K, et al. Genomic amplification of CD274 (PD-L1) in small-cell lung cancer. *Clin Cancer Res.* 2017;23(5):1220–1226.
151. Straub M, Drecoll E, Pfarr N, et al. CD274/PD-L1 gene amplification and PD-L1 protein expression are common events in squamous cell carcinoma of the oral cavity. *Oncotarget.* 2016;7(11):12024–12034.
152. Song M, Chen D, Lu B, et al. PTEN loss increases PD-L1 protein expression and affects the correlation between PD-L1 expression and clinical parameters in colorectal cancer. *PLoS One.* 2013;8(6):e65821.
153. Zhang X, Zeng Y, Qu Q, et al. PD-L1 induced by IFN-gamma from tumor-associated macrophages via the JAK/STAT3 and PI3K/AKT signaling pathways promoted progression of lung cancer. *Int J Clin Oncol.* 2017;22(6): 1026–1033.
154. Atefi M, Avramis E, Lassen A, et al. Effects of MAPK and PI3K pathways on PD-L1 expression in melanoma. *Clin Cancer Res.* 2014;20(13):3446–3457.
155. Lastwika KJ, Wilson 3rd W, Li QK, et al. Control of PD-L1 expression by oncogenic activation of the AKT-mTOR pathway in non-small cell lung cancer. *Cancer Res.* 2016;76(2):227–238.
156. Parsa AT, Waldron JS, Panner A, et al. Loss of tumor suppressor PTEN function increases B7-H1 expression and immunoresistance in glioma. *Nat Med.* 2007;13(1): 84–88.
157. Xu C, Fillmore CM, Koyama S, et al. Loss of Lkb1 and Pten leads to lung squamous cell carcinoma with elevated PD-L1 expression. *Cancer Cell.* 2014;25(5): 590–604.
158. Liu J, Hamrouni A, Wolowiec D, et al. Plasma cells from multiple myeloma patients express B7-H1 (PD-L1) and increase expression after stimulation with IFN-{gamma} and TLR ligands via a MyD88-, TRAF6-, and MEK-dependent pathway. *Blood.* 2007; 110(1):296–304.

159. Loi S, Dushyanthen S, Beavis PA, et al. RAS/MAPK activation is associated with reduced tumor-infiltrating lymphocytes in triple-negative breast cancer: therapeutic cooperation between MEK and PD-1/PD-L1 immune checkpoint inhibitors. *Clin Cancer Res.* 2016;22(6):1499–1509.

160. Jiang X, Zhou J, Giobbie-Hurder A, Wargo J, Hodi FS. The activation of MAPK in melanoma cells resistant to BRAF inhibition promotes PD-L1 expression that is reversible by MEK and PI3K inhibition. *Clin Cancer Res.* 2013;19(3):598–609.

161. Sumimoto H, Takano A, Teramoto K, Daigo Y. RAS-mitogen-activated protein kinase signal is required for enhanced PD-L1 expression in human lung cancers. *PLoS One.* 2016;11(11):e0166626.

162. Zhang X, Wrzeszczynska MH, Horvath CM, Darnell Jr JE. Interacting regions in Stat3 and c-Jun that participate in cooperative transcriptional activation. *Mol Cell Biol.* 1999;19(10):7138–7146.

163. Karakhanova S, Meisel S, Ring S, Mahnke K, Enk AH. ERK/p38 MAP-kinases and PI3K are involved in the differential regulation of B7-H1 expression in DC subsets. *Eur J Immunol.* 2010;40(1):254–266.

164. Qian Y, Deng J, Geng L, et al. TLR4 signaling induces B7-H1 expression through MAPK pathways in bladder cancer cells. *Cancer Invest.* 2008;26(8):816–821.

165. Yamamoto R, Nishikori M, Tashima M, et al. B7-H1 expression is regulated by MEK/ERK signaling pathway in anaplastic large cell lymphoma and Hodgkin lymphoma. *Cancer Sci.* 2009;100(11):2093–2100.

166. Chen N, Fang W, Lin Z, et al. KRAS mutation-induced upregulation of PD-L1 mediates immune escape in human lung adenocarcinoma. *Cancer Immunol Immunother.* 2017;66(9):1175–1187.

167. Coelho MA, de Carne Trecesson S, Rana S, et al. Oncogenic RAS signaling promotes tumor immunoresistance by stabilizing PD-L1 mRNA. *Immunity.* 2017;47(6):1083–1099.e1086.

168. Akbay EA, Koyama S, Carretero J, et al. Activation of the PD-1 pathway contributes to immune escape in EGFR-driven lung tumors. *Cancer Discov.* 2013;3(12):1355–1363.

169. Concha-Benavente F, Srivastava RM, Trivedi S, et al. Identification of the cell-intrinsic and -extrinsic pathways downstream of EGFR and IFNgamma that induce PD-L1 expression in head and neck cancer. *Cancer Res.* 2016;76(5):1031–1043.

170. Lin K, Cheng J, Yang T, Li Y, Zhu B. EGFR-TKI downregulates PD-L1 in EGFR mutant NSCLC through inhibiting NF-kappaB. *Biochem Biophys Res Commun.* 2015;463(1–2):95–101.

171. Marzec M, Zhang Q, Goradia A, et al. Oncogenic kinase NPM/ALK induces through STAT3 expression of immunosuppressive protein CD274 (PD-L1, B7-H1). *Proc Natl Acad Sci U S A.* 2008;105(52):20852–20857.

172. Brown JM, Wilson WR. Exploiting tumour hypoxia in cancer treatment. *Nat Rev Cancer.* 2004;4:437.

173. Barsoum IB, Smallwood CA, Siemens DR, Graham CH. A mechanism of hypoxia-mediated escape from adaptive immunity in cancer cells. *Cancer Res.* 2014;74(3):665.

174. Messai Y, Gad S, Noman MZ, et al. Renal cell carcinoma programmed death-ligand 1, a new direct target of hypoxia-inducible factor-2 alpha, is regulated by *von Hippel–Lindau* gene mutation status. *Eur Urol.* 2016;70(4):623–632.

175. Guo C, Hu F, Yi H, et al. Myeloid-derived suppressor cells have a proinflammatory role in the pathogenesis of autoimmune arthritis. *Ann Rheum Dis.* 2016;75(1):278–285.

176. Koh HS, Chang CY, Jeon S-B, et al. The HIF-1/glial TIM-3 axis controls inflammation-associated brain damage under hypoxia. *Nat Commun.* 2015;6:6340.

177. Noman MZ, Desantis G, Janji B, et al. PD-L1 is a novel direct target of HIF-1α, and its blockade under hypoxia enhanced MDSC-mediated T cell activation. *J Exp Med.* 2014;211(5):781.

178. Buettner R, Mora LB, Jove R. Activated STAT signaling in human tumors provides novel molecular targets for therapeutic intervention. *Clin Cancer Res.* 2002;8(4):945–954.

179. Atsaves V, Tsesmetzis N, Chioureas D, et al. PD-L1 is commonly expressed and transcriptionally regulated by STAT3 and MYC in ALK-negative anaplastic large-cell lymphoma. *Leukemia.* 2017;31(7):1633–1637.

180. Bu LL, Yu GT, Wu L, et al. STAT3 induces immunosuppression by upregulating PD-1/PD-L1 in HNSCC. *J Dent Res.* 2017;96(9):1027–1034.

181. Bi XW, Wang H, Zhang WW, et al. PD-L1 is upregulated by EBV-driven LMP1 through NF-kappaB pathway and correlates with poor prognosis in natural killer/T-cell lymphoma. *J Hematol Oncol.* 2016;9(1):109.

182. Gowrishankar K, Gunatilake D, Gallagher SJ, Tiffen J, Rizos H, Hersey P. Inducible but not constitutive expression of PD-L1 in human melanoma cells is dependent on activation of NF-kappaB. *PLoS One.* 2015;10(4):e0123410.

183. Huang G, Wen Q, Zhao Y, Gao Q, Bai Y. NF-kappaB plays a key role in inducing CD274 expression in human monocytes after lipopolysaccharide treatment. *PLoS One.* 2013;8(4):e61602.

184. Bouillez A, Rajabi H, Jin C, et al. MUC1-C integrates PD-L1 induction with repression of immune effectors in non-small-cell lung cancer. *Oncogene.* 2017;36(28):4037–4046.

185. Xue J, Chen C, Qi M, et al. Type Igamma phosphatidylinositol phosphate kinase regulates PD-L1 expression by activating NF-kappaB. *Oncotarget.* 2017;8(26):42214–42427.

186. Dong H, Strome SE, Salomao DR, et al. Tumor-associated B7-H1 promotes T-cell apoptosis: a potential mechanism of immune evasion. *Nat Med.* 2002;8(8):793–800.

187. Brown JA, Dorfman DM, Ma FR, et al. Blockade of programmed death-1 ligands on dendritic cells enhances T cell activation and cytokine production. *J Immunol.* 2003;170(3):1257–1266.

188. de Kleijn S, Langereis JD, Leentjens J, et al. IFN-gamma-stimulated neutrophils suppress lymphocyte proliferation through expression of PD-L1. *PLoS One.* 2013;8(8): e72249.

189. Kryczek I, Wei S, Gong W, et al. Cutting edge: IFN-gamma enables APC to promote memory Th17 and abate Th1 cell development. *J Immunol.* 2008;181(9):5842–5846.

190. Mazanet MM, Hughes CC. B7-H1 is expressed by human endothelial cells and suppresses T cell cytokine synthesis. *J Immunol.* 2002;169(7):3581–3588.

191. Nakazawa A, Dotan I, Brimnes J, et al. The expression and function of costimulatory molecules B7H and B7-H1 on colonic epithelial cells. *Gastroenterology.* 2004;126(5): 1347–1357.

192. Schoop R, Wahl P, Le Hir M, Heemann U, Wang M, Wuthrich RP. Suppressed T-cell activation by IFN-gamma-induced expression of PD-L1 on renal tubular epithelial cells. *Nephrol Dial Transpl.* 2004;19(11): 2713–2720.

193. Wintterle S, Schreiner B, Mitsdoerffer M, et al. Expression of the B7-related molecule B7-H1 by glioma cells: a potential mechanism of immune paralysis. *Cancer Res.* 2003;63(21):7462–7467.

194. Lee SJ, Jang BC, Lee SW, et al. Interferon regulatory factor-1 is prerequisite to the constitutive expression and IFN-gamma-induced upregulation of B7-H1 (CD274). *FEBS Lett.* 2006;580(3):755–762.

195. Eppihimer MJ, Gunn J, Freeman GJ, et al. Expression and regulation of the PD-L1 immunoinhibitory molecule on microvascular endothelial cells. *Microcirculation.* 2002; 9(2):133–145.

196. Garcia-Diaz A, Shin DS, Moreno BH, et al. Interferon receptor signaling pathways regulating PD-L1 and PD-L2 expression. *Cell Rep.* 2017;19(6):1189–1201.

197. Schreiner B, Mitsdoerffer M, Kieseier BC, et al. Interferon-beta enhances monocyte and dendritic cell expression of B7-H1 (PD-L1), a strong inhibitor of autologous T-cell activation: relevance for the immune modulatory effect in multiple sclerosis. *J Neuroimmunol.* 2004;155(1–2): 172–182.

198. Kondo A, Yamashita T, Tamura H, et al. Interferon-gamma and tumor necrosis factor-alpha induce an immunoinhibitory molecule, B7-H1, via nuclear factor-kappaB activation in blasts in myelodysplastic syndromes. *Blood.* 2010; 116(7):1124–1131.

199. Ou JN, Wiedeman AE, Stevens AM. TNF-alpha and TGF-beta counter-regulate PD-L1 expression on monocytes in systemic lupus erythematosus. *Sci Rep.* 2012;2:295.

200. Zhao Q, Xiao X, Wu Y, et al. Interleukin-17-educated monocytes suppress cytotoxic T-cell function through B7-H1 in hepatocellular carcinoma patients. *Eur J Immunol.* 2011;41(8):2314–2322.

201. Quandt D, Jasinski-Bergner S, Muller U, Schulze B, Seliger B. Synergistic effects of IL-4 and TNFalpha on the induction of B7-H1 in renal cell carcinoma cells inhibiting allogeneic T cell proliferation. *J Transl Med.* 2014;12:151.

202. Lim SO, Li CW, Xia W, et al. Deubiquitination and stabilization of PD-L1 by CSN5. *Cancer Cell.* 2016;30(6): 925–939.

203. Wang X, Yang L, Huang F, et al. Inflammatory cytokines IL-17 and TNF-alpha up-regulate PD-L1 expression in human prostate and colon cancer cells. *Immunol Lett.* 2017; 184:7–14.

204. Wong JL, Obermajer N, Odunsi K, Edwards RP, Kalinski P. Synergistic COX2 induction by IFNgamma and TNFalpha self-limits type-1 immunity in the human tumor microenvironment. *Cancer Immunol Res.* 2016; 4(4):303–311.

205. Kil SH, Estephan R, Sanchez J, et al. PD-L1 is regulated by interferon gamma and interleukin 6 through STAT1 and STAT3 signaling in cutaneous T-cell lymphoma. *Blood.* 2017;130(suppl 1):1458.

206. Karakhanova S, Bedke T, Enk AH, Mahnke K. IL-27 renders DC immunosuppressive by induction of B7-H1. *J Leukoc Biol.* 2011;89(6):837–845.

207. Matta BM, Raimondi G, Rosborough BR, Sumpter TL, Thomson AW. IL-27 production and STAT3-dependent upregulation of B7-H1 mediate immune regulatory functions of liver plasmacytoid dendritic cells. *J Immunol.* 2012;188(11):5227–5237.

208. Carbotti G, Barisione G, Airoldi I, et al. IL-27 induces the expression of IDO and PD-L1 in human cancer cells. *Oncotarget.* 2015;6(41):43267–43280.

209. Loke P, Allison JP. PD-L1 and PD-L2 are differentially regulated by Th1 and Th2 cells. *Proc Natl Acad Sci U S A.* 2003;100(9):5336–5341.

210. Mezzadra R, Sun C, Jae LT, et al. Identification of CMTM6 and CMTM4 as PD-L1 protein regulators. *Nature.* 2017; 549(7670):106–110.

211. Pulko V, Liu X, Krco CJ, et al. TLR3-stimulated dendritic cells up-regulate B7-H1 expression and influence the magnitude of CD8 T cell responses to tumor vaccination. *J Immunol.* 2009;183(6):3634–3641.

212. Cole JE, Navin TJ, Cross AJ, et al. Unexpected protective role for Toll-like receptor 3 in the arterial wall. *Proc Natl Acad Sci U S A.* 2011;108(6):2372–2377.

213. Boes M, Meyer-Wentrup F. TLR3 triggering regulates PD-L1 (CD274) expression in human neuroblastoma cells. *Cancer Lett.* 2015;361(1):49–56.

214. Fridman WH, Galon J, Pages F, Tartour E, Sautes-Fridman C, Kroemer G. Prognostic and predictive impact of intra- and peritumoral immune infiltrates. *Cancer Res.* 2011;71(17):5601–5605.

215. Goc J, Germain C, Vo-Bourgais TK, et al. Dendritic cells in tumor-associated tertiary lymphoid structures signal a Th1 cytotoxic immune contexture and license the positive prognostic value of infiltrating CD8+ T cells. *Cancer Res.* 2014;74(3):705–715.

216. Formica V, Cereda V, di Bari MG, et al. Peripheral CD45RO, PD-1, and TLR4 expression in metastatic colorectal cancer patients treated with bevacizumab, fluorouracil, and irinotecan (FOLFIRI-B). *Med Oncol.* 2013;30(4):743.

217. Yamada N, Oizumi S, Kikuchi E, et al. CD8+ tumor-infiltrating lymphocytes predict favorable prognosis in malignant pleural mesothelioma after resection. *Cancer Immunol Immunother.* 2010;59(10):1543–1549.

218. Anraku M, Cunningham KS, Yun Z, et al. Impact of tumor-infiltrating T cells on survival in patients with malignant pleural mesothelioma. *J Thorac Cardiovasc Surg.* 2008;135(4):823–829.

219. Pages F, Berger A, Camus M, et al. Effector memory T cells, early metastasis, and survival in colorectal cancer. *N Engl J Med.* 2005;353(25):2654–2666.

220. Naito Y, Saito K, Shiiba K, et al. CD8+ T cells infiltrated within cancer cell nests as a prognostic factor in human colorectal cancer. *Cancer Res.* 1998;58(16):3491–3494.

221. Hennequin A, Derangere V, Boidot R, et al. Tumor infiltration by Tbet+ effector T cells and CD20+ B cells is associated with survival in gastric cancer patients. *Oncoimmunology.* 2016;5(2):e1054598.

222. Speetjens FM, Zeestraten EC, Kuppen PJ, Melief CJ, van der Burg SH. Colorectal cancer vaccines in clinical trials. *Expert Rev Vaccin.* 2011;10(6):899–921.

223. de Weger VA, Turksma AW, Voorham QJ, et al. Clinical effects of adjuvant active specific immunotherapy differ between patients with microsatellite-stable and microsatellite-instable colon cancer. *Clin Cancer Res.* 2012;18(3):882–889.

224. Koido S, Ohkusa T, Homma S, et al. Immunotherapy for colorectal cancer. *World J Gastroenterol.* 2013;19(46): 8531–8542.

225. Ji RR, Chasalow SD, Wang L, et al. An immune-active tumor microenvironment favors clinical response to ipilimumab. *Cancer Immunol Immunother.* 2012;61(7): 1019–1031.

226. Phillips SM, Banerjea A, Feakins R, Li SR, Bustin SA, Dorudi S. Tumour-infiltrating lymphocytes in colorectal cancer with microsatellite instability are activated and cytotoxic. *Br J Surg.* 2004;91(4):469–475.

227. Albuquerque C, Baltazar C, Filipe B, et al. Colorectal cancers show distinct mutation spectra in members of the canonical WNT signaling pathway according to their anatomical location and type of genetic instability. *Genes Chromosomes Cancer.* 2010;49(8):746–759.

228. Kim MS, Kim SS, Ahn CH, Yoo NJ, Lee SH. Frameshift mutations of Wnt pathway genes AXIN2 and TCF7L2 in gastric carcinomas with high microsatellite instability. *Hum Pathol.* 2009;40(1):58–64.

229. Martensson A, Oberg A, Jung A, Cederquist K, Stenling R, Palmqvist R. Beta-catenin expression in relation to genetic instability and prognosis in colorectal cancer. *Oncol Rep.* 2007;17(2):447–452.

230. Nazemalhosseini Mojarad E, Kashfi SM, Mirtalebi H, et al. Prognostic significance of nuclear beta-catenin expression in patients with colorectal cancer from Iran. *Iran Red Crescent Med J.* 2015;17(7):e22324.

231. Ortega P, Moran A, de Juan C, et al. Differential Wnt pathway gene expression and E-cadherin truncation in sporadic colorectal cancers with and without microsatellite instability. *Clin Cancer Res.* 2008;14(4):995–1001.

232. Rawson JB, Manno M, Mrkonjic M, et al. Promoter methylation of Wnt antagonists DKK1 and SFRP1 is associated with opposing tumor subtypes in two large populations of colorectal cancer patients. *Carcinogenesis.* 2011; 32(5):741–747.

233. Rawson JB, Mrkonjic M, Daftary D, et al. Promoter methylation of Wnt5a is associated with microsatellite instability and BRAF V600E mutation in two large populations of colorectal cancer patients. *Br J Cancer.* 2011; 104(12):1906–1912.

234. Silva AL, Dawson SN, Arends MJ, et al. Boosting Wnt activity during colorectal cancer progression through selective hypermethylation of Wnt signaling antagonists. *BMC Cancer.* 2014;14:891.

235. Sonay TB, Koletou M, Wagner A. A survey of tandem repeat instabilities and associated gene expression changes in 35 colorectal cancers. *BMC Genomics.* 2015; 16(1):702.

236. Spranger S, Bao R, Gajewski TF. Melanoma-intrinsic beta-catenin signalling prevents anti-tumour immunity. *Nature.* 2015;523(7559):231–235.

237. Castellone MD, Teramoto H, Williams BO, Druey KM, Gutkind JS. Prostaglandin E2 promotes colon cancer cell growth through a Gs-axin-beta-catenin signaling axis. *Science.* 2005;310(5753):1504–1510.

238. Goessling W, North TE, Loewer S, et al. Genetic interaction of PGE$_2$ and Wnt signaling regulates developmental specification of stem cells and regeneration. *Cell.* 2009; 136(6):1136–1147.

239. Li HJ, Reinhardt F, Herschman HR, Weinberg RA. Cancer-stimulated mesenchymal stem cells create a carcinoma stem cell niche via prostaglandin E2 signaling. *Cancer Discov.* 2012;2(9):840–855.

240. Shao J, Jung C, Liu C, Sheng H. Prostaglandin E2 stimulates the beta-catenin/T cell factor-dependent transcription in colon cancer. *J Biol Chem.* 2005;280(28): 26565–26572.

241. Spranger S, Gajewski TF. A new paradigm for tumor immune escape: beta-catenin-driven immune exclusion. *J Immunother Cancer.* 2015;3:43.

242. Yarchoan M, Hopkins A, Jaffee EM. Tumor mutational burden and response rate to PD-1 inhibition. *N Engl J Med.* 2017;377(25):2500–2501.

243. Rizvi NA, Hellmann MD, Snyder A, et al. Mutational landscape determines sensitivity to PD-1 blockade in non–small cell lung cancer. *Science.* 2015;348(6230): 124–128.

244. Panda A, Betigeri A, Subramanian K, et al. Identifying a clinically applicable mutational burden threshold as a potential biomarker of response to immune checkpoint therapy in solid tumors. *JCO Precis Oncol.* 2017;1:1–13.

245. Kalluri R. The biology and function of fibroblasts in cancer. *Nat Rev Cancer.* 2016;16(9):582–598.

246. Harper J, Sainson RC. Regulation of the anti-tumour immune response by cancer-associated fibroblasts. *Semin Cancer Biol.* 2014;25:69–77.

247. Hill RP. The changing paradigm of tumour response to irradiation. *Br J Radiol.* 2017;90(1069):20160474.

248. Sato T, Terai M, Tamura Y, Alexeev V, Mastrangelo MJ, Selvan SR. Interleukin 10 in the tumor microenvironment: a target for anticancer immunotherapy. *Immunol Res.* 2011;51(2−3):170−182.

249. Sarvaria A, Madrigal JA, Saudemont A. B cell regulation in cancer and anti-tumor immunity. *Cell Mol Immunol.* 2017;14.

250. Hiraoka N, Onozato K, Kosuge T, Hirohashi S. Prevalence of FOXP3+ regulatory T cells increases during the progression of pancreatic ductal adenocarcinoma and its premalignant lesions. *Clin Cancer Res.* 2006;12(18): 5423−5434.

251. Guillerey C, Huntington ND, Smyth MJ. Targeting natural killer cells in cancer immunotherapy. *Nat Immunol.* 2016;17(9):1025−1036.

252. Vivier E, Ugolini S, Blaise D, Chabannon C, Brossay L. Targeting natural killer cells and natural killer T cells in cancer. *Nat Rev Immunol.* 2012;12(4):239−252.

253. Whiteside TL, Herberman RB. The role of natural killer cells in immune surveillance of cancer. *Curr Opin Immunol.* 1995;7(5):704−710.

253a. Fu B, Tian Z, Wei H. Subsets of human natural killer cells and their regulatory effects. *Immunology.* Apr 2014; 141(4):483−489.

254. Kroeger DR, Milne K, Nelson BH. Tumor-infiltrating plasma cells are associated with tertiary lymphoid structures, cytolytic T-cell responses, and superior prognosis in ovarian cancer. *Clin Cancer Res.* 2016;22(12): 3005−3015.

255. Joshi NS, Akama-Garren EH, Lu Y, et al. Regulatory T cells in tumor-associated tertiary lymphoid structures suppress anti-tumor T cell responses. *Immunity.* 2015;43(3): 579−590.

256. Kim KH, Kim TM, Go H, et al. Clinical significance of tumor-infiltrating FOXP3+ T cells in patients with ocular adnexal mucosa-associated lymphoid tissue lymphoma. *Cancer Sci.* 2011;102(11):1972−1976.

257. Alam I, Frahad K, Griffiths PA, Hurley M. Simultaneous gastrointestinal stromal tumor and mucosa-associated lymphoid tissue lymphoma of the stomach. *J Clin Oncol.* 2007;25(9):1136−1138.

258. Schrama D, thor Straten P, Fischer WH, et al. Targeting of lymphotoxin-alpha to the tumor elicits an efficient immune response associated with induction of peripheral lymphoid-like tissue. *Immunity.* 2001;14(2):111−121.

259. Musha H, Ohtani H, Mizoi T, et al. Selective infiltration of CCR5(+)CXCR3(+) T lymphocytes in human colorectal carcinoma. *Int J Cancer.* 2005;116(6):949−956.

260. Kunz M, Toksoy A, Goebeler M, Engelhardt E, Brocker E, Gillitzer R. Strong expression of the lymphoattractant C-X-C chemokine Mig is associated with heavy infiltration of T cells in human malignant melanoma. *J Pathology.* 1999;189(4):552−558.

261. Ohtani H, Jin Z, Takegawa S, Nakayama T, Yoshie O. Abundant expression of CXCL9 (MIG) by stromal cells that include dendritic cells and accumulation of CXCR3+ T cells in lymphocyte-rich gastric carcinoma. *J Pathology.* 2009;217(1):21−31.

262. Muthuswamy R, Berk E, Junecko BF, et al. NF-kappaB hyperactivation in tumor tissues allows tumor-selective reprogramming of the chemokine microenvironment to enhance the recruitment of cytolytic T effector cells. *Cancer Res.* 2012;72(15):3735−3743.

263. Watchmaker PB, Berk E, Muthuswamy R, et al. Independent regulation of chemokine responsiveness and cytolytic function versus CD8+ T cell expansion by dendritic cells. *J Immunol.* 2010;184(2):591−597.

264. Muthuswamy R, Urban J, Lee JJ, Reinhart TA, Bartlett D, Kalinski P. Ability of mature dendritic cells to interact with regulatory T cells is imprinted during maturation. *Cancer Res.* 2008;68(14):5972−5978.

265. Fujita M, Zhu X, Ueda R, et al. Effective immunotherapy against murine gliomas using type 1 polarizing dendritic cells−significant roles of CXCL10. *Cancer Res.* 2009; 69(4):1587−1595.

266. Zhu X, Fallert-Junecko BA, Fujita M, et al. Poly-ICLC promotes the infiltration of effector T cells into intracranial gliomas via induction of CXCL10 in IFN-alpha and IFN-gamma dependent manners. *Cancer Immunol Immunother.* 2010;59(9):1401−1409.

267. Muthuswamy R, Wang L, Pitteroff J, Gingrich JR, Kalinski P. Combination of IFNalpha and poly-I: C reprograms bladder cancer microenvironment for enhanced CTL attraction. *J Immunother Cancer.* 2015;3:6.

268. Muthuswamy R, Corman JM, Dahl K, Chatta GS, Kalinski P. Functional reprogramming of human prostate cancer to promote local attraction of effector CD8(+) T cells. *Prostate.* 2016;76(12):1095−1105.

269. Demaria O, De Gassart A, Coso S, et al. STING activation of tumor endothelial cells initiates spontaneous and therapeutic antitumor immunity. *Proc Natl Acad Sci U S A.* 2015;112.

270. Vasaturo A, Halilovic A, Bol KF, et al. T-cell landscape in a primary melanoma predicts the survival of patients with metastatic disease after their treatment with dendritic cell vaccines. *Cancer Res.* 2016;76(12):3496−3506.

271. Fong L, Carroll P, Weinberg V, et al. Activated lymphocyte recruitment into the tumor microenvironment following preoperative sipuleucel-T for localized prostate cancer. *J Natl Cancer Inst.* 2014;106(11).

272. Siegel RL, Miller KD, Jemal A. Cancer statistics, 2017. *CA Cancer J Clin.* 2017;67(1):7−30.

CHAPTER 2

Immune Checkpoints: Melanoma and Other Skin Cancers

SYLVIA LEE, MD • SHAILENDER BHATIA, MD

MELANOMA

INTRODUCTION

The recent unprecedented success of the immune checkpoint inhibitors (ICIs), which are now transforming treatment paradigms and outcomes in multiple cancer types, is owed to no other cancer more than melanoma. In a relatively short span of 5 years, from the U.S. Food and Drug Administration (FDA) approval of ipilimumab in 2011 to the more recent approval of nivolumab plus ipilimumab combination therapy in 2016, we have seen the diagnosis of metastatic melanoma transformed from being a virtual "death sentence" to being a chronic disease, where there is now a realistic chance for long-term survival and where "cure" may not be just a researcher's fantasy anymore.

Melanoma is the fifth most common cancer in the United States, with a rapidly rising incidence.[1] Because it often affects younger patients, metastatic melanoma has been associated with a higher loss in productive life years per patient than each of the other four major cancers (breast, prostate, colorectal, and lung).[2] For many decades, metastatic melanoma was a frustrating disease for clinicians and researchers alike with only two FDA-approved treatments—dacarbazine in 1975 and interleukin-2 (IL-2) in 1998—and no therapies that had ever succeeded in demonstrating an improvement in overall survival (OS) in a randomized phase III trial.

However, melanoma has also long been recognized as one of the most immunogenic of all cancers. Intermittent successes with a variety of immunotherapies in melanoma provided proof of concept for immune modulation as a viable strategy to pursue against cancer and sustained the enthusiasm of dedicated immunologists and immunotherapists for decades. Having proven itself as a fertile testing ground for immune-based strategies, melanoma is now positioned at the forefront of the widespread effort to develop and understand the immune checkpoint therapies. It has been the first beneficiary of this new class of therapies while providing invaluable lessons for the rest of oncology along the way.

BACKGROUND

Melanoma has long been considered the archetypal "immunogenic" cancer. Spontaneous regressions of cancer had been reported frequently in melanoma.[3] On histologic examination of primary melanoma tumors, partial tumor regression can be found in greater than 25% of the tumors.[4] The areas of spontaneous tumor regression have been found to be enriched with T-cell subsets, supporting immune-mediated mechanisms.[5] Approximately 5% of melanoma patients are diagnosed without a known primary lesion, designated "melanoma of unknown primary", presumably owing to an immune-mediated regression of their primary lesion. These patients have better OS than matched patients with a known primary lesion, possibly owing to having a more active immune surveillance of their tumor.[6,7]

Therapeutic development of high-dose interleukin-2 (HD IL-2), a cytokine that stimulates T-cell proliferation and function, in melanoma provided proof of concept that successful modulation of the immune system could induce systemic and durable tumor regressions.[8,9] Although the objective response rates (ORR) of 10%–15% with HD IL-2 were not too impressive and toxicities were considerable, the small subset (5%–6%) of patients with durable complete responses (CRs) captured the attention of the cancer immunologists. The long-term follow-up indicated that these responses were sustained 10 years and beyond in a disease that was otherwise fatal in 6–9 months.

The curative potential of T-cells was further demonstrated in melanoma with the development of T-cell therapy using autologous tumor-infiltrating lymphocytes (TIL), expanded ex vivo from a patient's tumor and reinfused following a lymphodepleting chemotherapy regimen, and followed with HD IL-2.[10] Trials conducted in the 1990s and 2000s demonstrated response rates over 50% and durable response rates of 20%; however, several barriers prevented this therapy from becoming a mainstream treatment option, including the need for surgical resection of a tumor for TIL generation, the practical and financial challenges of producing a single-patient product, and the limited availability of TIL therapy at only a handful of academic centers.[11]

Because the early successes of immunotherapy in melanoma could not reliably be translated in other cancer types (with the exception of HD IL-2 for renal cell carcinoma), melanoma and the earlier generation of tumor immunologists were exiled to their own island for many decades. Immunotherapy successes in melanoma were considered to be irrelevant to the rest of the cancer world partly because other tumors were not believed to be immunogenic. In the setting of numerous disappointing studies of interferon and multiple negative cancer vaccine trials, few oncology researchers believed that an immune-based strategy would ever prove effective against most cancers.

The development of antibodies to block cytotoxic T-lymphocyte–associated protein-4 (CTLA-4), a negative regulator of T-cell activation, was a pivotal turning point in cancer immunology—and melanoma provided the platform needed to usher in this new wave of immunotherapy. In a landmark phase III trial in 2010, ipilimumab became the first therapy ever to demonstrate an improved OS in a randomized phase III trial for metastatic melanoma.[12]

On the heels of the success with CTLA-4 blockade, a massive effort emerged to target another T-cell immune checkpoint, the programmed cell death protein 1 (PD-1) and its ligand (PD-L1). Only a few months after ipilimumab became the first ICI to be FDA approved, two back-to-back studies were reported in the prestigious *New England Journal of Medicine* (NEJM) communicating the remarkably surprising phase I results from two monoclonal antibodies to PD-1 and PD-L1.[13,14] This was perhaps the most pivotal point in the immune checkpoint era because these studies demonstrated activity of immunotherapy in not only melanoma but in several other tumor types as well. At this moment, melanoma gained a new relevance to the cancer world. No longer thought of as the outlier, or as the only immunogenic tumor, melanoma became a leader in immunotherapy's rapid ascent, forging the way in

elucidating toxicities and management, outcomes and resistance, unique response patterns, and ultimately what was possible in this new frontier of cancer therapy.

IPILIMUMAB (ANTI–CTLA-4 ANTIBODY)

First discovered in 1987, CTLA-4 is present on the surface of T-cells and plays a role in the negative regulation of T-cell activation, in part by outcompeting CD28 for the B7 ligand on antigen-presenting cells (APCs) and thus disrupting the T-cell activation signal.[15] Antibodies that block CTLA-4 were first tested in mouse tumor models and demonstrated tumor regressions, which led to the clinical development of two fully human immunoglobulin monoclonal antibodies, ipilimumab and tremelimumab.[16]

In 2010, a pivotal phase III trial with ipilimumab was heralded as the first phase III clinical trial to have demonstrated an OS benefit in melanoma, which ultimately led to the FDA approval of ipilimumab for advanced melanoma in March 2011.[12] In this study, previously treated metastatic melanoma patients were randomized to ipilimumab plus a glycoprotein 100 (gp100) peptide vaccine, ipilimumab alone or gp100 alone. The results demonstrated significantly improved OS with ipilimumab groups as compared with gp100 monotherapy (median OS of 10 vs. 6.4 months, respectively). Ipilimumab was administered intravenously (IV) at a dose of 3 mg/kg every 3 weeks for up to four doses without any maintenance dosing; however, patients were eligible for reinduction therapy (with four more doses) at the time of progressive disease (PD) after initial benefit. The best ORR in the ipilimumab monotherapy group was 11% (CR-1.5%, partial response [PR]-9.5%), and the disease control rate (DCR), defined as proportion of patients with objective response or stable disease (SD), was 28%. Although the ORR and CR rates were low, responses were mostly durable with 60% of the responders maintaining the response beyond 2 years. Although 60% of patients on ipilimumab monotherapy experienced immune-related adverse events (irAEs), severe (grade 3 or higher) irAEs were seen in only 15% of patients and included diarrhea/colitis (8%), endocrinopathy (2%), dermatologic toxicity (<2%), and hepatic toxicity (<1%). Most irAEs resolved by 6–8 weeks with appropriate immunosuppressive treatment (mostly glucocorticoids), although residual symptoms (e.g., vitiligo, endocrinopathy symptoms, rectal pain) were sometimes present in long-term survivors.

A second randomized phase III trial that compared ipilimumab (10 mg/kg) plus dacarbazine versus dacarbazine alone in patients with previously untreated metastatic melanoma also showed longer median OS with ipilimumab plus dacarbazine (11.2 months) versus dacarbazine alone (9.1 months) and higher 3-year survival of 21% versus 12%, respectively.[17] Interestingly, tremelimumab had not demonstrated an OS benefit in a prior phase III pivotal trial, which may have largely been due to the choice of the comparator group (dacarbazine) in that trial and perhaps due to suboptimal dosing and scheduling; however, it is now being further investigated in combination strategies and other tumor types.[18]

However, it was not the modest response rates and improvement in OS, measured in months, in these aforementioned trials that captured the attention of the field. It was the "tail" on the survival curve that indicated a substantial proportion of these patients becoming long-term survivors and staying alive 5–10 years after treatment. In a period void of other effective melanoma treatments, the observations that the responses were remarkably durable and the OS curve plateaued were the first signals that the strategy of immune checkpoint blockade could lead the way to the Holy Grail of cancer therapy—cure for metastatic cancer. A meta-analysis of pooled OS data from ipilimumab trials, which includes data from 1861 melanoma patients, highlights the potential for long-term survival in a subset of patients. This report listed a 3-year OS rate of 22% with a plateau in the pooled Kaplan–Meier curve beginning at approximately 3 years after initiation of therapy and extending through follow-up of as long as 10 years.[19]

Ipilimumab Dosing

Ipilimumab was approved at 3 mg/kg in the metastatic setting based on the initial phase III trial in previously treated melanoma patients.[12] There is evidence from two randomized trials that the 10 mg/kg dose level achieves a higher response rate and slightly better OS than the 3 mg/kg dosing but carries a higher rate for toxicities.

A phase II multiinstitutional trial randomized 217 previously treated, advanced melanoma patients between 0.3, 3, and 10 mg/kg IV every 3 weeks for four cycles, followed by maintenance every 3 months.[20] The best ORR was 11.1% for 10 mg/kg, 4.2% for 3 mg/kg, and 0% for 0.3 mg/kg. The study was not designed to look at OS; however, there were nonsignificant differences in OS at 1 year, 18 and 24 months, favoring the 10 mg/kg group, despite a third of the patients in the lower two dosing groups crossing over to the 10 mg/kg group. Grade 3–4 irAEs were reported

for 25% (mostly diarrhea) of the 10 mg/kg group, 7% of the 3 mg/kg group, and 0% for the 0.3 mg/kg group.

More recently, a double-blinded, multicenter phase III trial randomized 727 advanced melanoma patients to ipilimumab at 10 mg/kg versus 3 mg/kg. None had received prior immune checkpoint therapy to either CTLA-4 or PD-1/PD-L1. The study observed a higher 3-year OS of 31.2% versus 23.2% and median OS of 15.7 versus 11.5 months, favoring the 10 mg/kg arm.[21] Not surprisingly, the incidence of grade 3–5 adverse events (AEs) was also higher at 37% for the 10 mg/kg dose, versus 18% with the 3 mg/kg dose.

Since the start of this trial in 2012, ipilimumab has been supplanted by PD-1 therapy or combination PD-1/CTLA-4 in the first-line setting, and thus the impact of these findings is somewhat muted. It is not known whether the increase in efficacy of the higher 10 mg/kg dosing will be significant in the PD-1 refractory population; however, these findings do support further investigation of the role of the higher dose of ipilimumab in certain situations, such as patients who either do not respond to standard dose ipilimumab but have minimal toxicity, or in patients with tumor characteristics or biomarkers suggesting a lower chance for response.

Unconventional Response Patterns

Early studies with ipilimumab quickly revealed atypical patterns of responses that were very different from the traditional patterns observed with chemotherapy. Three types of novel response patterns were initially observed with ipilimumab (and can also be seen with PD-1 blockade therapy):

1. *Delayed, slow responses.* Responses can occur late, often not until 12–16 weeks into the therapy, sometimes occurring slowly across 6–12 months, well after treatment had been completed.[12,17,22] This may reflect the complex downstream actions of ipilimumab-induced T-cell activation to lead to an antitumor response. Tumor regression with pembrolizumab, as well as ipilimumab plus nivolumab combined therapy, appears to have an earlier onset than ipilimumab, with most responses identified at 9–12 weeks.[23–25]

2. *Pseudoprogression.* Patients can experience a response after an initial increase in total tumor burden or a response after the development of new lesions. Pseudoprogression has been attributed to the infiltration of tumors by immune cells causing transient inflammatory swelling of tumors that could be mistaken for disease progression on imaging or examination versus just a delayed onset of

the antitumor immune response that allows unchecked progression of the tumor mass early on.

3. *Prolonged OS in nonresponders.* With traditional cytotoxic chemotherapy, an objective response, whether complete or partial, has been used to indicate the antitumor activity of the treatment. SD per RECIST was generally not considered a "success" because it typically is not sustained and does not reflect a meaningful clinical benefit. However, the first phase III ipilimumab study demonstrated an interesting discordance with ORR of only 11% but an OS curve that plateaued at 20%. This demonstrated the inadequacy of the traditional definition of response to capture the clinical efficacy of ipilimumab because there were patients who were considered nonresponders but still experienced long-term survival after treatment. In a follow-up analysis of patients with 4-year survival after ipilimumab, 25% of these patients had a best response of PD as defined by World Health Organization (WHO) criteria.[26]

These unique patterns of delayed response, pseudoprogression, and prolonged survival in patients with SD or PD led to the development of alternative response criteria to capture the clinical efficacy of the immune checkpoints. The immune-related response criteria (irRC) were proposed in 2009 and allowed new lesions to be included in an overall assessment of tumor burden rather than being an automatic determinant of PD.[27] The definition for "PR" was also modified to a ≥50% decrease in tumor burden compared with the RECIST definition of ≥30% decrease. These criteria were found to correlate better with OS than conventional antitumor response assessment criteria (RECIST[28] or WHO[29]) and allowed for continuation of immune therapy despite mild increase of existing lesions or appearance of isolated new lesions as long as the total tumor burden is not significantly increased.

These initial observations in melanoma have shaped the use of the immune checkpoints in other cancers, and it is not unreasonable for practitioners to continue treatment beyond mild radiographic progression. The phenomenon of pseudoprogression appears to be somewhat more common in melanoma than other tumor types. With ipilimumab, these atypical patterns have been reported in up to 10% of melanoma patients.[27] These patterns have also been observed in PD-1 therapy, and in KEYNOTE-001, 7% of melanoma patients receiving pembrolizumab demonstrated pseudoprogression.[30] In contrast, only 1 (1.5%) in 65 bladder cancer patients and 1 in 60 head and neck cancer patients (1.7%) were noted to

have pseudoprogression.[31,32] Similarly, a renal cell trial reported a 1.8% incidence of pseudoprogression (3 of 168 patients).[32,33] As more cancer types receive FDA approval for the immune checkpoints, the challenge of determining who should continue treatment beyond progression will be increasingly important and likely specific to each disease type and individualized to the patient's clinical situation.

PD-1 BLOCKADE

While CTLA-4 plays a role in the initial stages of T-cell activation in the lymph nodes, the PD-1 pathway regulates previously activated T-cells, primarily in the peripheral tissues, in later stages of the immune response. PD-1 was identified in the 1990s on activated T-cells and binds to PD-L1 and PD-L2, which are expressed on the surface of many different tissue types in the tumor microenvironment including many cancer cells and immune cells. This interaction has several immunosuppressive effects, including inhibiting T-cell activation pathways, promoting peripheral T effector cell exhaustion and promoting the conversion of T effector cells to T regulatory cells.[34,35] Recent years have witnessed several (as many as eight) different anti–PD-1 and anti–PD-L1 antibodies in simultaneous, competitive development in numerous cancer types.

In September 2014, pembrolizumab became the first PD-1 antibody to be approved by the U.S. FDA for patients with metastatic melanoma who had previously been treated with ipilimumab (and if *BRAF*-mutated, with BRAF-inhibitors). This approval was based on the results of a randomized open-label trial (KEYNOTE-001) comparing the efficacy and safety of two doses of pembrolizumab (2 mg/kg and 10 mg/kg administered IV every 3 weeks) in melanoma patients who were considered refractory to ipilimumab treatment.[24] Treatment with pembrolizumab (2 mg/kg dose) in this trial was associated with an ORR of 26%, an estimated progression-free survival (PFS) at 24 weeks of 45%, and an estimated 1-year OS of 58%. The majority (88%) of responders were alive and progression-free at the time of analysis with at least 6 months of follow-up. Treatment was tolerated well with drug-related grade 3−4 AEs in only 12% of patients. Only 3% of patients discontinued treatment owing to AEs. Safety data were consistent with other reported trials of PD-1 blockade,[14,23,36] although this trial report did not comment on the safety of pembrolizumab in those patients who may have had prior irAEs with ipilimumab. There were no significant differences in safety and efficacy endpoints between the two dose levels. These data led to the FDA approval of pembrolizumab at the 2 mg/kg every 2 weeks dose. In a phase III trial (CHECKMATE-037) comparing nivolumab with chemotherapy (either dacarbazine or carboplatin plus paclitaxel) in ipilimumab-treated melanoma patients, nivolumab demonstrated antitumor activity; specifically, nivolumab was associated with higher ORR (32% vs. 11%) and lower rate of grade 3−4 AEs (9% vs. 31%) as compared with chemotherapy.[37]

These early successes supported further investigation of PD-1 blockade in the front-line setting. In a phase III trial that compared nivolumab with dacarbazine in previously untreated patients with metastatic melanoma without a *BRAF* mutation, nivolumab was associated with significantly better 1-year OS rate (73% vs. 42%), median PFS (5.1 months vs. 2.2 months), and ORR (40% vs. 14%) than dacarbazine.[38]

Anti−PD-1 Versus anti−CTLA-4

Soon after the FDA approval of pembrolizumab for ipilimumab-treated melanoma, the favorability of PD-1 therapy in the first-line setting was also confirmed. The KEYNOTE-006 study randomized 834 patients to either pembrolizumab at one of two dosing schedules, 10 mg/kg every 2 weeks (n = 279) or 10 mg/kg every 3 weeks (n = 277) for up to 2 years, or to ipilimumab at 3 mg/kg every 3 weeks for four doses (n = 278).[39,40] In this head-to-head comparison, pembrolizumab showed superior efficacy in 2-year OS of 55% (identical for both pembrolizumab schedules) versus 43% for ipilimumab, despite 30% of the ipilimumab arm "crossing over" to receive subsequent PD-1 therapy. There was also an advantage in 24-month PFS of 29% versus 14% and ORR of 36.5% versus 13%. Grade 3−4 toxicities were slightly lower at 17% versus 20% for the pembrolizumab arms and ipilimumab arm, respectively. Longer follow-up is needed to determine whether the long-term OS curves for PD-1 will remain higher than the 20% 10-year OS benchmark set by ipilimumab.

The increased efficacy of PD-1 therapy over anti−CTLA-4 in the front-line setting was further validated by CHECKMATE-067, which randomized untreated melanoma patients to nivolumab monotherapy, ipilimumab monotherapy, and the combination of nivolumab and ipilimumab. When comparing the two monotherapy arms, nivolumab outperformed ipilimumab with not only a higher median OS of 38 versus 20 months but also improved tolerability with treatment-related grade 3−4 AEs at 16% versus 27% for nivolumab and ipilimumab, respectively. This study is further described in the next section.[41,42]

Anti−PD-1 drugs quickly became favored in the clinical setting over ipilimumab owing to their higher response rates in individual trials and better tolerability. Moreover, ipilimumab was associated with slow onset of responses, which could be problematic in patients with bulky tumors or rapidly progressing disease; the anti−PD-1 drugs appeared to work more quickly and offered faster disease control for symptomatic patients.

Combination Nivolumab Plus Ipilimumab

The early observations that patients can respond to PD-1 blockade after progression on CTLA-4 blockade and vice versa supported the understanding of PD-1 and CTLA-4 inhibition as two distinct therapeutic approaches with unique mechanisms of action. The distinct sites of action and the complementary roles of CTLA-4 and PD-1 in the regulation of adaptive immune responses fueled the interest in combination strategies.

It became apparent early on that the combination of PD-1 and CTLA-4 blockade could achieve higher antitumor activity but at the price of increased toxicity. These early findings were confirmed by a randomized phase II trial and then more extensively by the CHECKMATE-067 phase III trial, which randomized 945 previously untreated patients to nivolumab and ipilimumab, nivolumab monotherapy, and ipilimumab monotherapy.[41] The ORR was 58%, 44%, and 19%, and the median PFS was 11.5, 6.9, and 2.9 months, and 2-year OS was 64%, 59%, and 46% for the combination, nivolumab, and ipilimumab, respectively.[43] In an updated analysis, the 3-year OS was 58%, 52%, and 34%, respectively.[42] Median OS was 19.9 months for ipilimumab, 37.6 months for nivolumab, and not yet reached for the combination arm. Grade 3−4 treatment-related AEs were 55% in the combination group compared with 16.3% for nivolumab and 27.3% for ipilimumab.

Nivolumab Plus Ipilimumab Dosing

The standard dosing used in melanoma for the nivolumab and ipilimumab combination consists of an induction phase of ipilimumab 3 mg/kg and nivolumab 1 mg/kg q 3 weeks for four doses followed by maintenance phase of nivolumab 3 mg/kg q 2 weeks. This was based on findings from dose-escalation phase I study that demonstrated this was the maximum dose with an acceptable level of AEs.[25] This regimen also demonstrated clinical activity that did not appear inferior to the higher dosing regimens, although the study was not powered to compare these.

However, owing to the substantial toxicities seen in the clinic setting, there has been renewed interest in exploring alternative dosing regimens that could be better tolerated. In non–small cell lung cancer (NSCLC) (CHECKMATE-012), an alternate regimen of nivolumab 3 mg/kg every 2 weeks concurrently with ipilimumab 1 mg/kg every 6 or 12 weeks regimen was studied after the standard melanoma regimen proved to be too poorly tolerated in the lung cancer population with a 51% incidence of grade 3–4 AEs and three deaths. The reduction in the ipilimumab dose and frequency led to an improvement in tolerability of the combination regimen while maintaining clinical efficacy. Interestingly, the every-12-week frequency of the concurrent ipilimumab 1 mg/kg actually demonstrated a higher response rate than the every-6-week frequency of 47% compared with 38%, attributed to differences in patient populations and small sample size (n = 78); however, this does suggest that a lower dose of ipilimumab may be optimal for synergy with nivolumab. There are several trials underway in melanoma investigating a combination strategy using ipilimumab at lower doses and frequencies in combination with pembrolizumab (NCT02089685, NCT02656706).

Sequential therapy
The early observations that patients can respond to PD-1 blockade after progression on anti–CTLA-4 antibodies and vice versa supported the understanding of PD-1 and CTLA-4 inhibition as two distinct therapeutic approaches with unique mechanisms of action. Owing to their higher response rates and improved tolerability, anti–PD-1 antibodies became favored over CTLA-4 blockade in the clinical setting as the front-line

treatment option; however, the OS superiority of sequencing PD-1 therapy before CTLA-4 blockade was supported by CHECKMATE-064, an open-label, randomized phase II study of treatment-naïve patients that assigned patients to nivolumab every 2 weeks for 12 weeks followed by ipilimumab every 3 weeks for 12 weeks versus ipilimumab followed by nivolumab for the same duration.[44] Both schedules were followed with nivolumab until disease progression or unacceptable toxicity. The nivolumab followed by ipilimumab cohort demonstrated a superior ORR at every time point, including an ORR of 41% versus 20% at week 25, and the 12-month OS was superior for the nivolumab to ipilimumab sequence at 76% versus 54%. The median OS was 14.7 months for the ipilimumab to nivolumab group but had not yet been reached for the nivolumab to ipilimumab group with a median follow-up of 19.8 months. Grade 3–5 toxicities were also slightly higher with the nivolumab to ipilimumab sequence at 50% versus 43%.

A retrospective analysis evaluated responses to ipilimumab monotherapy and ipilimumab plus nivolumab combination in patients after progression on anti–PD-1 monotherapy.[45] The ORR was 16% for the ipilimumab group (n = 47) and 21% for the combination group (n = 37). The 1-year OS was 54% and 55%, respectively. Although a direct comparison is limited by the retrospective, nonrandomized nature of the study, it suggests that ipilimumab monotherapy in the second-line may perform as well as combination nivolumab–ipilimumab therapy in a PD-1 progressing population.

SPECIAL CONSIDERATIONS WITH THE USE OF IMMUNE CHECKPOINT INHIBITOR

IMMUNE-RELATED ADVERSE EVENTS
The details of irAEs associated with the ICIs and their management are discussed in another chapter in this book, but a brief summary is included below. The initial approval of ipilimumab included a Risk Evaluation and Mitigation Strategy (REMS) to help guide the management of these novel irAEs. The very broad spectrum of potential toxicities combined with the low incidence of each is particularly challenging as the use of PD-1 inhibitors becomes increasingly widespread in the community. Although there was more of a deliberate effort to provide oncology practitioners with REMS training at the time of ipilimumab approval for melanoma, this was not replicated with the approval of PD-1 therapy or, more importantly, with the approval of nivolumab–ipilimumab combination therapy. As a consequence,

many community oncologists and emergency room physicians have not been adequately trained to consider the wide variety of possible toxicities when evaluating a patient with vague symptoms such as fatigue or headache. Early diagnosis of these immune-related toxicities and prompt initiation of treatment, typically with high-dose steroids, can lead to better outcomes. Therefore, as PD-1 therapy becomes more prevalent in melanoma and other tumor types, it will be critical to develop more concerted efforts to provide education in toxicity recognition and management for clinicians as well as patients.

Ipilimumab
The arrival of ipilimumab to the clinical arena was accompanied by a myriad of novel, unexpected, and

sometimes life-threatening toxicities. It was apparent early on that the T-cell activation induced by ipilimumab was potent enough to break immune tolerance to self, leading to T-cell–mediated inflammation and injury against specific tissues. The phase III study using 3 mg/kg dose of ipilimumab reported 60% frequency of any grade immune-related events and 10%–15% of grade 3–4 irAEs. The most common toxicity was diarrhea (37% for any grade; 6.3% for grade 3–4). There were also endocrinopathies (4.8%), including hypothyroidism, hypopituitarism, hypophysitis, and adrenal insufficiency. There were 12 (2.3%) treatment-related deaths, mostly due to not only colitis-related complications but also Guillain–Barre syndrome and liver failure. In most cases, the toxicities are reversible with treatment cessation alone or with the initiation of steroids. However additional therapies are occasionally needed for steroid-refractory toxicities, such as infliximab. Endocrinopathies tend to be irreversible but can be easily treated with lifelong hormone replacement (e.g., hydrocortisone for adrenal insufficiency, levothyroxine for hypothyroidism).

PD-1 Blockade

The types of toxicities that can occur with anti–PD-1 agents are generally the same as those seen with anti–CTLA-4 but at a much lower frequency and severity. The toxicity profile is less dominated by diarrhea and colitis in PD-1 therapy. Less common endocrinopathies such as hypophysitis and type 1 diabetes and rare pathologies such as Guillain–Barre syndrome, myasthenia gravis, and sarcoidlike illnesses have been observed in PD-1 therapy, similarly to CTLA-4. There does appear to be some tumorspecificity of the toxicities. As one might expect, melanoma seems to carry a higher incidence of skin-specific toxicities and vitiligo but less pneumonitis than what is observed in lung cancer.[14]

Nivolumab Plus Ipilimumab

Despite promising higher response rates, the nivolumab and ipilimumab combination regimen has not become the automatic first-line choice for melanoma patients owing to the substantial increase in toxicities. In CHECKMATE-067, the incidence of grade 3 or 4 toxicities was 55% compared with 16% for nivolumab monotherapy and 27% for ipilimumab (3 mg/kg dose) monotherapy.[41] The toxicity profile was not unique compared with either monotherapy, but the incidence of almost every toxicity was higher. The dominant toxicity was diarrhea at 44% (any grade) and 9% (grade 3 or higher) compared with 33% and 6%, respectively, for ipilimumab. The most pronounced toxicity change due to the combination of nivolumab and ipilimumab was a roughly fourfold increase in liver toxicity at 15%–18% (any grade) and 6%–8% (grade 3 or higher) compared with either monotherapy, which had an incidence of 3.5%–3.9% for any grade and an incidence of 0.6%–1.6% for grade 3 or higher AEs. Most toxicities, except the endocrinopathies, resolved with steroids as seen in the monotherapy studies.

A subsequent analysis of health-related quality of life (HRQoL) for CHECKMATE-067 was recently reported in which patients from both the nivolumab and ipilimumab combination group and patients from the nivolumab group underwent HRQoL assessments at weeks 1 and 5 per 6-week cycle for the first 6 months and then once every 6 weeks.[46] Despite the higher occurence of grade 3 or higher AEs for the combination group, there were no clinically meaningful differences in the HRQoL reported among the randomized population and among subgroup analysis based on BRAF status, PR or CR, treatment-related grade 3 or higher AEs, and patients who discontinued treatment for any reason and due to an AE.

Toxicity and Response

Several studies have demonstrated that patients who stop treatment early owing to toxicity appear to have the same chance of responding to the immune checkpoints as patients who remain on treatment.[47–49] It has also been found in several studies that the use of immunosuppressive therapy, primarily steroids, for the management of irAEs does not appear to mitigate the clinical responses in either the rate or duration of response.[50] These findings have helped assuage, to some degree, concerns about starting corticosteroids in patients with irAEs that could potentially compromise the efficacy of the immune checkpoints.

Early observations with anti–CTLA-4 have also fueled speculation that the development of certain immune-related toxicities may serve as a marker for immune activation and possibly even a predictive marker for response. One analysis of 234 melanoma and renal cell cancer patients treated with ipilimumab at the National Cancer Institute found that the 21% of patients who developed enterocolitis went on to have a response rate of 36% (melanoma) and 35% (renal cell carcinoma) compared with 11% and 2%, respectively, of the patients who did not develop enterocolitis.[51] A separate analysis of 139 patients who received ipilimumab found that the development of an immune-related AE was associated with a greater probability of a response ($P = .0004$) and also noted that all three patients with a CR experienced more severe irAEs.[52] Similarly, a randomized, blinded, phase II study evaluated the use of prophylactic budesonide with ipilimumab observed a higher DCR in patients with grade 3−4 irAEs (DCR of 46%−59%) compared with patients with grade 1−2 irAEs (DCR of 26%−27%).[53] Even in the adjuvant setting, an association was observed between significant irAEs with improved relapse-free survival.[54] However, results have been inconclusive, and a larger analysis of 855 melanoma patients found no association between any irAEs with response to ipilimumab.[55]

PD-1−based therapy has been similarly evaluated. A retrospective analysis of 576 melanoma patients treated with anti−PD-1 monotherapy, pooled from four studies, found the ORR was significantly higher in patients who had irAEs compared with patients who did not.[50] In a post hoc analysis of CHECKMATE-067, patients who did not complete all four doses of nivolumab and ipilimumab induction owing to toxicity had a 58% ORR compared with a 50% response rate for patients who completed treatment.[56] However, the group that completed induction treatment had higher risk features such as elevated Lactate Dehydrogenase (LDH) and higher proportion of M1c disease, which limits the interpretation of these data.

DURATION OF TREATMENT

Ipilimumab, the only commercially available anti−CTLA-4 inhibitor, is given for only four doses in the metastatic setting. Only 60% of patients were able to complete all four doses in the initial phase III trial owing to the increasing frequency and severity of toxicities that occur with each subsequent dose. However, many patients can tolerate PD-1 inhibitors every 2 or 3 weeks with minimal symptoms for many years. There are currently no clear guidelines for how long patients with metastatic melanoma should be continued on PD-1 blockade. Given the durable responses experienced by many patients on PD-1 blockade, as well as the observation with ipilimumab of responses lasting 10 years after their last actual treatment, there has been uncertainty over what the ideal duration of PD-1 treatment should be in responding patients. This is becoming an increasingly relevant issue owing to the high costs associated with these drugs and also the potential for delayed toxicities with continued administration that has to be weighed against the benefits of prolonged administration after achieving the maximal response. In a recent analysis of KEYNOTE-006, in which pembrolizumab was stopped at 2 years, there

was an ongoing response of 91% at 9.7 months' median follow-up.[40] The ongoing responses were seen not only in patients with CR (PFS rate of 95%) but also in partial responders (PFS 91%) and even patients with SD (PFS of 83%). Longer follow-up from this trial and others will be informative in determining the ideal duration of treatment, which will also be relevant to the burgeoning health care costs from the use of expensive cancer therapies, the so called "financial toxicity" of cancer treatment. Another important consideration for future investigation is using intermittent pulses or reduced frequency of administration in the maintenance setting after achieving the maximal response from the initial induction therapy.

THE USE OF IMMUNE CHECKPOINT INHIBITORS IN SPECIFIC POPULATIONS
Melanoma With Brain Metastases

Melanoma is one of the cancers with the highest potential to metastasize to the brain and accounts for 10% of all patients with brain metastases, behind only lung cancer and breast cancer.[57] Approximately 50% of stage IV melanoma patients are diagnosed with brain metastases, but autopsy reports indicate the prevalence may be as high as 75%.[58] Melanoma metastases also tend to be more vascular and therefore brain metastases are more likely to become hemorrhagic for melanoma compared with other cancers. The management of brain metastases in melanoma is further challenged by the relative resistance of melanoma to radiation therapy (RT), one of the mainstays in the treatment of brain metastases in other cancers. Historically, the prognosis for melanoma patients with brain metastases has been poor with a median survival of 3−4 months.[59]

Fortunately, both ipilimumab and PD-1 inhibitors, given as single agents, have demonstrated activity in the brain. In a phase II trial of ipilimumab in melanoma patients with brain metastases, there was a 24% response rate seen in asymptomatic patients who were not on concurrent steroids and 10% response rate in symptomatic patients who required a stable dose of steroids.[60] There was also a 2-year survival rate of 26%, demonstrating the possibility of long-term survival in a patient group with an otherwise poor prognosis. Similarly, pembrolizumab demonstrated a 22% response rate in 18 melanoma patients with brain metastases in a phase II study.[61]

As seen with extracranial sites of melanoma, the combination of nivolumab and ipilimumab also demonstrates greater efficacy in the brain compared with monotherapy. The CHECKMATE-204 phase II study treated 75 patients with nivolumab plus ipilimumab and observed a 55% response rate in the brain, including a 21% CR rate, and a 6-month PFS of 67%.[62] The safety profile was similar to the experience in patients without brain metastases receiving combination nivolumab and ipilimumab. The randomized phase II ABC (anti−PD-1 brain collaboration) trial assigned patients with asymptomatic brain metastases to nivolumab and ipilimumab combination (n = 25) versus nivolumab monotherapy (n = 25).[63] The combination arm demonstrated a 44% intracranial response rate compared with 20% for monotherapy, intracranial response of 16% versus 12%, and 6-month OS of 76% versus 59%. Treatment-related grade 3 or higher toxicities were 68% versus 40%.

These impressive data on the efficacy of ICIs in addressing intracranial brain metastases, especially with a previously unseen durability of responses, are poised to change the traditional management of these patients, which was mostly centered around surgery and/or RT.

Mucosal Melanoma

Melanoma can arise from mucosal linings in the head and neck, anorectal, and vulvovaginal regions. These mucosal melanomas carry a worse prognosis than cutaneous melanoma, in part, owing to a different biology and also likely owing to a delay in diagnosis. They do not arise in the setting of UV light damage and therefore have a lower mutation burden compared with cutaneous melanoma, which is theoretically associated with a lower immunogenicity.[64] Nevertheless, responses have been observed in mucosal melanoma to both anti−CTLA-4 and anti−PD-1 approaches, although at lower frequencies.

In a retrospective analysis of ipilimumab in 33 mucosal melanoma patients, there was a 24% response rate, with one CR, one PR, and six SD, using irRC.[65] In a pooled analysis of six studies with nivolumab and nivolumab−ipilimumab combination, 86 mucosal melanoma patients and 665 cutaneous melanoma patients were compared. For nivolumab monotherapy, the ORR was 23% versus 41% and the median PFS was 3 versus 6.2 months for mucosal melanoma and cutaneous melanoma, respectively.[66] For the combination therapy, the ORR was 37% versus 60% and the median PFS was 5.9 versus 11.7 months for mucosal and cutaneous melanoma, respectively. Similar results were reported from a retrospective analysis performed on 35 mucosal melanoma patients treated with nivolumab or pembrolizumab at seven institutions, which demonstrated a 23% ORR and 3.9 month median PFS.[67] Although these data were gathered retrospectively, they provide convincing evidence of activity from the immune checkpoints in mucosal melanoma and provide justification for the use of these agents in a similar manner to cutaneous melanoma.

Ocular (Uveal) Melanoma

Approximately 3%−5% of melanomas arise in the eye, almost always from the uvea.[68] Uveal melanomas are unique from cutaneous melanomas in that they harbor few genetic mutations, and up to 96% of cases are found to have GNAQ/GNA11 mutations specifically, which have downstream effects on the MAP kinase pathway and others. Sun exposure—the culprit for the rich mutational burden of cutaneous melanoma—has been inconsistently associated with uveal melanoma. One case-control analysis found there was an association with sunbathing and time outdoors as well as geographic latitude; however, a more recent meta-analysis did not find this association, although welding without eye protection was determined to be a risk factor.

Ocular melanomas appear to be the least responsive to immune checkpoint blockade, of all melanoma subtypes. Less data are available because ocular melanoma is not only rare but also usually excluded from immunotherapy trials. In a phase II study of ipilimumab in 53 uveal melanoma patients, there were no PRs or CRs.[69] Sixteen patients had SD. In a multicenter retrospective study of 56 patients treated with pembrolizumab, nivolumab, or atezolizumab, there were only two PRs (3.6%) and five patients (9%) with SD for ≥6 months.[70]

Although the low mutational burden likely is a factor in the relative immune resistance of ocular melanoma, another consideration is the unique environment of "immune privilege" that exists in the eye, where primary uveal melanomas develop. Immune responses are generally suppressed in the eye to protect nonregenerating ocular tissues from damage by inflammation.[71] It has been proposed that intraocular tumor growth with the expression of melanoma differentiation antigens in the eye may induce a systemic tolerance to these antigens, which allows the sustained evasion of the adaptive immune system even after uveal melanomas metastasize and escape the immunologic sanctuary of the eye.[72] This may be one of the differences that account for why mucosal melanoma shows superior responses to immune checkpoint inhibition than ocular melanoma even though they share in common a low mutational burden compared with cutaneous melanoma.

IMMUNE CHECKPOINT INHIBITORS FOR ADJUVANT THERAPY

Stage III melanoma carries a high risk for relapse, and even after curative-intent surgical resection, the 5-year OS is only 63%, and the 5-year recurrence rate is as high as 68% for stage IIIB and 89% for stage IIIC.[73,74] Before the development of the ICIs, interferon alfa was the only option for adjuvant therapy and was notoriously unpopular for its high toxicity profile and questionable benefit. With this low benchmark to beat, ipilimumab was granted FDA approval in 2015 for stage III patients with >1 mm of nodal involvement, based on early results from EORTC 18071 demonstrating a median relapse-free survival (RFS) benefit (26.1 vs. 17.1 months), before the data had even matured to indicate a difference in OS. This trial was a randomized phase III trial that assigned patients who had undergone a complete resection of stage III melanoma to ipilimumab 10 mg/kg versus placebo every 3 weeks for four doses and then every 3 months for up to 3 years. In 2016, a post hoc analysis confirmed there was a 5-year OS benefit of 65.4% in the ipilimumab group compared with 54.4% in the placebo group and a 5-year RFS of 40.8% versus 30.3%, respectively.[75] The toxicities with high-dose ipilimumab were as expected. Grade 3–4 AEs occurred in 54.1% of the ipilimumab arm compared with 26.2% of the placebo arm, and five patients (1.1%) died from irAEs.

Recent studies have investigated the role of PD-1 antibodies in the adjuvant setting. A phase III study randomized 900 melanoma patients with stage IIIB, IIIC, and IV disease that had been completely resected to 1 year of either nivolumab or high-dose ipilimumab.[76] The 18-month RFS was 66.4% versus 52.7% for the nivolumab and ipilimumab arms, respectively. As expected, the nivolumab arm also had decreased grade 3–4 treatment-related toxicities of 14% versus 46%. Given the promising results and favorable toxicity profile, the FDA has recently approved nivolumab for adjuvant therapy of stage III melanoma, and the National Comprehensive Cancer Network (NCCN) guidelines have already modified its recommendation to prioritize nivolumab over ipilimumab in the adjuvant setting. A study of adjuvant pembrolizumab is underway in Europe, while CHECKMATE-915 is examining nivolumab plus ipilimumab combination versus ipilimumab or nivolumab monotherapy for adjuvant therapy (NCT03068455).

The emerging data from these adjuvant studies have eroded the long-held skepticism surrounding the efficacy of immune checkpoint blockade in the adjuvant setting, based on the theoretical concern that micrometastatic tumor cells would not provide a well-organized tumor microenvironment for the immune checkpoint molecules to act. However, this is yet another example of the immune checkpoints continuing to surprise us and demonstrate the limits of our current understanding of tumor immunology.

BIOMARKERS FOR IMMUNE CHECKPOINT INHIBITOR RESPONSE

The rapid emergence of the immune checkpoint field has been accompanied by a huge amount of interest in identifying biomarkers that could predict which patients are likely to respond or not respond to different ICIs, which patients would benefit from more aggressive combination strategies, and also who should be treated with immune checkpoint therapies as frontline treatment, especially for melanoma patients with driver mutations in genes such as *BRAF* or *KIT*, who have other nonimmune treatment options. Even though there are no reliable biomarkers currently available to be used for clinical decision-making in melanoma patients, there are several important leads.

PD-L1 Expression

PD-L1 expression has been shown to be somewhat predictive of a response in melanoma. Data from numerous studies have repeatedly demonstrated that the higher the level of membranous PD-L1 expression in melanoma cells, the higher the chance for a response to PD-1/PD-L1 blockade. However, there are extensive examples of treatment responses to PD-1 antibodies in PD-L1–negative patients, typically in the 8%–20% range but as high as 41% in CHECKMATE-067, thus rendering PD-L1 expression as an unreliable means to distinguish which melanoma patients should get PD-1 therapy.[41,77] The observation of responses in PD-L1–negative patients may be due to the inherent limitations of a single biopsy to capture the dynamic changes in PD-L1 expression or heterogeneity in expression.

Interestingly, PD-L1 status appears to be less predictive for a response to nivolumab–ipilimumab combination therapy. PD-L1–positive patients demonstrated a 46% response rate while PD-L1–negative patients demonstrated a 41% response rate, indicating that patients can respond similarly well to combination nivolumab–ipilimumab regardless of PD-L1 status.[25] In this manner, PD-L1 expression could be used to justify a more well-tolerated PD-1 monotherapy in PD-L1–positive patients while a more intense combination strategy could be reserved for patients who are PD-L1 negative and have a lower chance of responding to PD-L1 monotherapy. However, more mature OS data are needed from these studies before reliable conclusions can be made on whether PD-L1 expression could be applied in this way.

Mutational Load

From an early point, it was widely theorized that the superior immunogenicity of melanoma compared with other cancers was due to its high mutational load from repeated UV light damage, resulting in neoantigens that are able to stimulate a more effective antitumor immune response. It is noteworthy that the top five cancers with the highest burden of somatic mutations across human tumor types are melanoma, squamous cell carcinoma of the lung, adenocarcinoma of the lung, bladder cancer, and small cell lung cancer, which corresponds largely with the specific tumor types that have demonstrated the most promising responses to PD-1 blockade.[78] In two separate studies with melanoma patients, whole exome sequencing on their pretreatment tumors demonstrated a significant correlation between overall mutational load and neoantigen load with their clinical benefit to anti−CTLA-4 blockade; however, this alone was not sufficient to predict a response.[79,80] The correlation of neoantigen burden to clinical efficacy of PD-1 inhibition has been established as well, in melanoma and other tumors.[81,82]

Tumor Microenvironment

Multiple groups have characterized distinct gene expression signatures that can be used to categorize melanoma into a "hot" or "inflamed" tumor type that has a high likelihood of responding to immune checkpoint therapies versus a "cold" or "noninflamed" type that tends to be resistant to immunotherapies. Notably, the inflamed/noninflamed phenotypes are independent of the neoantigen load, indicating that these gene signatures capture additional distinctions contributing to immune checkpoint response.[83]

The inflamed tumors have a robust infiltration of CD8+ T-cells, which strongly correlate with a response to immune checkpoint blockade.[84] Functional studies indicate these tumor-infiltrating T-cells secrete interferon-γ (IFN-γ) that can induce PD-L1 expression in tumor cells, suggesting that PD-L1 expression in tumors cells may be an indirect marker of CD8+ T-cells infiltrating the tumor microenvironment.[85] Further characterization of these T-cells indicate a partially exhausted phenotype with high expression of both PD-1 and CTLA-4, which is predictive of response to

anti−PD-1 therapy.[86] Because anti−CTLA-4 has been shown to increase the infiltrating tumor cells, it is proposed that patients with tumors found to have a low number of CTLA-4+PD-L1+ TILs may benefit from a combination approach rather than PD-1 monotherapy. IFN-γ signaling genes, which play a role in antigen presentation, chemokine expression, and cytotoxic activity, have been identified as part of the inflamed gene signature that predicts a response to immune checkpoint blockade.[87,88]

Gut Microbiota

In recent years, there has been growing fascination in the role of the gut microbiome in the response of melanoma to immunotherapy. Mouse studies initially demonstrated that modulation of the gut microbiome could influence antitumor immunity and the response to immune checkpoint blockade, via enhanced dendritic cell function and priming of CD8+T-cells leading to increased tumor infiltration.[89,90] In a recent analysis of oral and gut microbiome samples from 112 melanoma patients, there was a significant association between increased diversity and composition of the patient's gut microbiome to the response rates and PFS to PD-1 therapy.[91] Of note, all bacterial strains were not equally beneficial, and the gut microbiome of responders was enriched for the Clostridiales order (specifically the *Faecalibacterium* genus), while nonresponders carried higher levels of the Bacteroidales order. There were associations found between the diversity and abundance of specific bacteria with CD8+ T-cell tumor infiltrates and metabolic gene signatures of responders and nonresponders. An intriguing analysis of 249 cancer patients (with advanced NSCLC, renal cell carcinoma, or urothelial carcinoma) treated with anti−PD-1 therapy found that the group of 69 patients who took antibiotics 2 months before or 1 month after their first dose of PD-1 therapy experienced a significantly shorter OS and PFS than patients not treated with antibiotics.[92] These findings were confirmed in validation cohort of 239 advanced NSCLC patients. Metagenomics of patient stool samples at diagnosis revealed correlations between clinical responses to ICIs and the relative abundance of *Akkermansia muciniphila*.

Based on these several intriguing studies that suggest the gut microbiome as influencing response to immune checkpoint blockade, there are upcoming human trials to examine whether fecal transplants can improve responses to PD-1 therapy.

MECHANISMS OF RESISTANCE

Long-term follow-up for the IL-2, TIL, and anti−CTLA-4 studies have shown durable responses in melanoma that can translate into lifelong remissions or "cures".[10,93] Although the development of PD-1 agents is still relatively recent and more mature survival data lag behind, nivolumab has now demonstrated a 35% OS at both the 4-year and 5-year mark, suggesting the start of a plateau in its OS curve as well. Thus, in the melanoma field, the ultimate gauge for the true clinical efficacy of a treatment has become durable response. However, this high bar remains elusive for most melanoma patients who either do not respond to ICIs (**primary resistance**) or progress after an initial response to PD-1 or CTLA-4 immune checkpoint therapy (**acquired resistance**). Thus, there are ongoing extensive efforts aimed at understanding why only a minority of melanoma patients derive long-term benefit from immune checkpoint therapy and what mechanisms lead to primary and acquired resistance. There is substantial overlap in the mechanisms that contribute to primary and acquired resistance, in part because the immune checkpoints work by enhancing endogenous immune responses that may have already been in play at different points in the tumor's lifespan and thus have already been subjected to the same immune editing adaptations and escape mechanisms that occur in response to treatment.

A comprehensive discussion of the resistance mechanisms to ICIs is included in another chapter of this book, but we list below some of the resistance mechanisms specific for melanoma:

1. *Deficiency of immunogenic tumor antigen target*: The presence of a tumor target that can be recognized by endogenous T-cells is a necessary first component of any antitumor immune response that can be unleashed by an immune checkpoint strategy. Tumors with lower mutational burden generally tend to have a lower chance of response to immune checkpoint blockade. This potential mechanism of primary resistance was first implied by the long-observed correlation between high mutational burden of a cancer type (e.g., melanoma, NSCLC, bladder cancer) and its responsiveness to PD-1 therapy. The high somatic mutation rate has a higher propensity to generate a diversity of neo-antigens that can, in turn, stimulate a reactive T-cell population.[94,95] In melanoma, this phenomenon not only has been demonstrated within cutaneous melanoma but is also illustrated by differences in response rates to the immune checkpoints between the melanoma subtypes. The lower response rates to

anti−CTLA-4 and anti−PD-1 in mucosal and ocular melanoma as compared with cutaneous melanomas may partially be explained by their lower mutational burdens.[65,66,69,70,96] An exception to this correlation is acral melanoma, which has a lower mutational burden but may have a similar response as cutaneous melanomas, although data are quite limited and mostly retrospective.[67]

2. *Downregulation of antigen presentation*: When tumors do possess an immunogenic antigen that is capable of eliciting an active T-cell response, there are several mechanisms by which melanoma tumors can then downregulate the expression of that immunogenic antigen. β-2-microglobulin, a component in the MHC class I molecule, plays an important role in antigen presentation for T-cell recognition. Defects in β-2-microglobulin and the impact on MHC function have been implicated in impaired antitumor T-cell responses to both anti−CTLA-4 and anti−PD-1 in several melanoma studies.[97−99] Recent analysis of tumor biopsies from melanoma patients who initially responded and then progressed on PD-1 therapy identified an acquired deletion in β-2-microglobulin, resulting in a loss of surface expression of MHC class I.[100]

3. *Immunosuppressive tumor microenvironment*: At the time of initial diagnosis and resection, the degree of T-cell infiltrates found in the primary melanoma tumor is routinely included in the histologic assessment as one of the prognostic features. At diagnosis, some melanoma tumors appear to have established a protective fortress that prevents T-cell infiltration. These tumors are void of lymphocytes and tend to carry a worse prognosis with a lower chance of responding to immune checkpoint therapy.[101] Several groups have found differences between melanoma patient tumors in the expression of chemokines responsible for CD8+T-cell recruitment, as well as the recruitment of immunosuppressive cells such as myeloid-derived suppressor cells and regulatory T-cells. Increases in proangiogenic signaling through upregulated vascular endothelial growth factor (VEGF) expression by loss of PTEN has also been identified in patients who acquire resistance.[102,103] A transcriptional signature, termed innate anti−PD-1 resistance (IPRES), has been recently characterized in resistant melanoma tumors and includes genes involved in mesenchymal transition, cell adhesion, extracellular matrix remodeling, and angiogenesis, which are thought to contribute to the tumor's ability to make itself impenetrable to T-cells.[104] Investigation into the use

of VEGF inhibitors with immune checkpoint blockade is underway and described below.

1. *Impairment in T-cell function*: One of the most essential tools used by T-cells against tumor cells is IFN-γ, a cytokine that has antiproliferative and proapoptotic effects on tumor cells and also upregulates tumor antigen presentation molecules. The immune effector functions of IFN-γ are mediated by the Janus kinase (JAK)-STAT pathway. In a recent analysis of matched pretreatment and postprogression biopsies in four melanoma patients who initially responded for a median of 1.8 years on continuous pembrolizumab and then developed resistance, two of the four patients had acquired loss-of-function mutations in JAK1 and JAK2. Additional studies have implicated the role of JAK1 and JAK2 in the development of both primary and acquired resistance to PD-1 blockade, as well as primary resistance to anti−CTLA-4.[100,105,106] There is also increasing evidence of the upregulation of additional immune checkpoints (e.g., T-cell immunoglobulin and mucin domain 3 [TIM-3], LAG-3) that leads to T-cell exhaustion and dysfunction seen in both primary and acquired resistance.[107,108]

A thorough understanding of the mechanisms is obviously critical to identifying predictive biomarkers, developing the next generation of immunotherapies for melanoma patients, and realizing the full promise of immunotherapy towards long-term disease control.

NOVEL IMMUNE CHECKPOINT INHIBITORS AND COMBINATIONS IN DEVELOPMENT

With the remarkable successes of anti−PD-1 and anti−CTLA-4, it is easy to forget that the majority of melanoma patients actually do not experience a response to the immune checkpoints. Approximately 50%−60% of treatment-naïve melanoma patients will demonstrate primary resistance to PD-1 therapy, while approximately 80% will have primary resistance to first-line CTLA-4 therapy.[42] The majority of PD-1 trials demonstrate a response rate of approximately 30%−40%. Thus, there is great interest in finding combination strategies with novel agents that can increase the portion of melanoma patients responding to immune checkpoint therapy without causing the substantial toxicity observed with the CTLA-4/PD-1 combination. Although there are many agents under various stages of investigation, we focus here on the following novel agents and strategies that have garnered more clinical research attention and early therapeutic signal in melanoma.

Lymphocyte Activation Gene 3

Lymphocyte activation gene 3 (LAG3) protein is a cell surface molecule that binds class II MHC.[109] LAG3 is expressed on activated CD8+T-cells and other immune cells and enhances regulatory T-cell activity and negatively regulates cellular proliferation and activation and T-cell homeostasis. A preliminary report of an anti−LAG-3 antibody (BMS-986016) and nivolumab in 31 evaluable melanoma patients following progression on or after prior PD-1 blockade indicated a 16% ORR and 45% DCR, supporting a potential strategy of combining these agents for PD-1 refractory patients.[110]

T-Cell Immunoglobulin and Mucin Domain 3

TIM-3 is another inhibitory receptor that is upregulated on dysfunctional and exhausted tumor-reactive T-cells that have decreased survival and impaired ability to produce cytokines such as IL-2 and IFN-γ.[108] There are two TIM-3 antagonistic monoclonal antibodies that are currently in first-in-human phase I trials, both in combination with anti−PD-1 therapy (NCT02608268, NCT02817633) and these results are highly anticipated.

Indoleamine 2,3-dioxygenase

Indoleamine 2,3-dioxygenase 1 (IDO1) is a tryptophan-catabolizing enzyme involved in T-cell suppression and upregulated in many cancers. IDO inhibitors have shown minimal responses as a monotherapy, but when combined with immune checkpoint blockade, there has been encouraging activity.[111] A phase I trial with IDO inhibitor epacadostat and ipilimumab demonstrated a 31% ORR in 32 immunotherapy-naïve patients.[112] A phase II trial combining another IDO inhibitor indoximod with pembrolizumab in 60 patients with advanced melanoma reported an ORR of 52% and a CR rate of 8%.[113] With the caveats of comparing independent trials, both of these studies demonstrated a substantially higher response rate with a combination than the ORR historically observed with either ipilimumab or pembrolizumab monotherapy, suggesting IDO inhibition may provide a truly synergistic approach with immune checkpoint blockade.

OX40

OX40 is a member of the tumor necrosis factor receptor family that gets expressed after activation of CD4 and CD8 T-cells and can enhance T-cell proliferation, memory, and antitumor activity.[114] Its ligand, OX40L, can be found on APC and activated CD4 T-cells, and when there is insufficient OX40L expression, T-cell survival is very poor. A phase I study of an agonistic OX40 antibody demonstrated tumor shrinkage in at least one lesion in 12 of 30 patients with solid tumors including melanoma, although none met RECIST criteria for PR. There are at least seven OX40 antibodies in development, and additional trials are underway testing OX40 antibodies with ICIs. A preliminary report of a phase Ib study of OX40 agonist and anti–PD-L1 described the combination to be well tolerated with objective responses observed.[115]

Angiogenesis Inhibition

There is a growing body of work demonstrating an important role of angiogenesis in the tumor microenvironment and factors limiting the infiltration of tumor-reactive T-cells.[116] As a result, there has been increased interest in combinatorial strategies with anti-VEGF agents and immunotherapy. The most well-known VEGF inhibitor, bevacizumab, was explored in combination with ipilimumab in a phase I melanoma trial and demonstrated high CD8+T-cell infiltration and a median OS of 25 months, which compared impressively with the historical control of 10-month survival of ipilimumab monotherapy, despite the caveats of making intertrial comparisons.[117] This strategy has been further validated by similar findings combining bevacizumab with anti–PD-L1 in renal cell carcinoma.[118]

Combinations of Immune Checkpoint Inhibitors with Other Immunotherapy Agents

Talimogene laherparepvec (T-VEC) is an oncolytic virus comprised of an attenuated herpes simplex virus that expresses Granulocyte and Macrophage Colony Stimulating Factor (GM-CSF). Approved in the United States as an intralesional therapy, it offers a 16% response rate but has little activity as monotherapy beyond the injection sites. However, this agent has shown early promise in a combination strategy with anti–CTLA-4. A phase Ib trial combining T-VEC with ipilimumab in 19 unresectable stage IIIB–IV melanoma patients demonstrated an

ORR of 50% by irRC, including four CRs, five PRs, as well as four SDs. Three of the nine responders had stage IV M1b/c disease; the other six responders had stage IIIB–IVM1a disease. Responses were seen in 50% of both visceral and uninjected nonvisceral lesions.

In the phase Ib component of MASTERKEY-265, a combination approach of T-VEC with pembrolizumab was tested in 21 patients with unresectable stage IIIB/IV melanoma and demonstrated similarly promising results with a 57% confirmed ORR (unconfirmed ORR of 67%) and 24% confirmed CR rate with a 71% DCR.[119] The phase III component of this trial, which randomizes T-VEC plus pembrolizumab versus pembrolizumab monotherapy is currently underway (NCT02263508).

CONCLUSION

Despite the potential for excellent outcomes in melanoma, the field has a long way to go. Most melanoma patients still face the disappointment of eventual relapse or do not respond initially. Increasing the numbers of melanoma patients who can benefit in a lasting way from the immune checkpoints will rely on a better understanding of the complex mechanisms of resistance and how these can be targeted.

In many ways, melanoma has served the oncology world as the canary in the coal mine—lowered into the dark depths of the unknown and pulled back to see what happens. The earliest melanoma patients brought to light not only the remarkable successes of the immune checkpoint antibodies but also the unconventional patterns of response and the unique toxicities of immune checkpoint blockade. To this day, melanoma cohorts on phase I trials continue to inform us which novel immune combinations are promising for future development in melanoma and other cancers. Most of all, the remarkable sensitivity of melanoma to immune checkpoint blockade has shifted our mindset of "what is possible" in oncology, with an increasing sense of optimism that the durable responses in melanoma are within reach for the rest of the cancer world.

MERKEL CELL CARCINOMA

INTRODUCTION

Merkel cell carcinoma (MCC) is an aggressive neuroendocrine skin cancer with a case fatality rate that is three times that of malignant melanoma (46% vs. 15%, respectively).[120] MCC is an uncommon cancer with an estimated 2500 cases/year in the Unites States.[121] The reported incidence is constantly increasing since

the initial description by Toker et al. in 1972, and the health impact of MCC is growing rapidly with the proportional increase in the aging population.[121,122] This increasing incidence is not only due to heightened awareness and improved detection following availability of a specific immunohistochemical marker (cytokeratin-20)[123] but also likely due to the higher prevalence of known risk factors for MCC: T-cell immune suppression and Caucasian over 50 years of age with extensive prior sun exposure.[121,122]

MCC is an aggressive cancer with prognosis dependent on the stage at presentation. Stages I and II represent low-risk and high-risk primary disease, respectively, while stages III and IV represent the presence of nodal and distant metastases, respectively. The reported 5-year relative survival for patients with local, nodal, and metastatic disease is 64%, 39%, and 18%, respectively.[120] Although surgery and/or RT may be curative for patients with locoregional MCC without distant metastases, relapses are common and often difficult to treat. There is no established adjuvant therapy after definitive management. For patients with distant metastatic disease not amendable to surgery or radiation, until recently, systemic chemotherapy was the only treatment option beside best supportive care. The reported ORR with either mono- or polychemotherapy regimens is high, in some reports up to 60 percent.[124,125] However, these responses are usually short-lived and the impact on survival is unclear and thought to be modest at best. Moreover, the chemotherapy regimens are associated with significant toxicity and may not be suitable for many MCC patients who usually tend to be older with multiple comorbidities.

Fortunately, rapid strides have recently been made in our understanding of the biology of MCC that have provided a strong rationale for investigation of immunotherapies in this aggressive disease.[126,127] These initial investigations have been extremely fruitful leading to remarkable advances in therapies for metastatic MCC in a relatively short period of time. Below, we review the immunology of MCC and the recent advances in MCC treatment with a special focus on the outstanding success of ICIs. We also discuss the current unmet needs of MCC patients and the future directions for MCC research.

Immunology of Merkel Cell Cancer

Epidemiologic data had long suggested a strong link between MCC and the immune system. Individuals with T-cell dysfunction (solid organ transplant recipients, HIV-infected patients with acquired immune deficiency syndrome [AIDS], or chronic lymphocytic leukemia patients) are at 5- to 15-fold increased risk of developing MCC.[128] MCC tumors sometimes regress following improvement in immune function. Additionally, there are several reported cases of complete spontaneous regression in the MCC literature (a far greater number than expected for its rarity).[129–131] These epidemiologic data had raised the possibility of an infectious etiology for MCC. Indeed, the discovery of the Merkel cell polyomavirus (MCPyV) in 2008 provided the missing link between MCC and its strong association with the immune system.[132] This strong association was independently confirmed in an unbiased gene expression analysis of MCC tumors that revealed overexpression of immune response genes in tumors with favorable prognoses.[133] Intratumoral (but not peritumoral) infiltration of CD8+ lymphocytes was found to be an independent predictor of improved survival among MCC patients in a cohort of 156 MCC cases; patients with robust CD8+ intratumoral infiltration had 100% MCC-specific survival as compared with 60% survival among patients with sparse or no CD8+ T-cells intratumoral infiltration.[133] It should be noted, however, that a substantial number of cases in this series did not express the MCPyV-derived oncoproteins on an mRNA level. Indeed, approximately 20% of MCC cases in the United States and Europe, as well as almost 70% of cases in Australia lack detectable tumor-associated MCPyV DNA or oncoproteins. Strikingly, the mutational burden of virus-negative MCC is even higher than that of melanoma and has a signature suggestive of UV-induced mutations.[134,135] These genetic changes that accumulate over several decades likely lead to generation and expression of novel proteins and epitopes and, subsequently, neoantigen-directed immune responses.[134] Thus, these observations readily explain the important role of cellular immune responses in the natural history of both in MCPyV- and UV-associated MCC.[127]

Since the discovery of the prognostic impact of CD8+ TILs, our understanding of the host–virus immune interactions in MCC pathogenesis has increased rapidly with new insights into both humoral and cellular immunity in MCC patients.[126,127] In patients with MCPyV+ tumors, there is now ample evidence for ongoing expression of viral proteins in tumor cells and their recognition by the adaptive (humoral as well as cellular) arm of the immune system.[132,136–139] MCPyV T-antigen–specific antibodies correlate with tumor burden in MCC patients, and this observation has led to the development of a clinically validated assay (*AMERK*) for surveillance of high-risk patients with MCPyV+ MCC tumors.[140,141] MCPyV-specific T-cells have been isolated from the peripheral blood or tumors of affected patients and are even being investigated for therapy after ex vivo expansion and adoptive transfer.[139,142,143]

Despite this persistent expression of immunogenic proteins, whether it be viral antigens in MCPyV+ tumors or UV-induced neoantigens in MCPyV- tumors, MCCs that become clinically evident are able to evade host immune responses. Our understanding of the host–virus immune interactions in MCC pathogenesis and the immune evasion mechanisms used by the MCC tumors continue to evolve rapidly. The progression from the immune equilibrium to the immune escape phase may occur owing to changes in tumor cell population that may acquire new immune evasive characteristics or owing to changes in the host immune system that may get suppressed either generally or more selectively toward the tumor cells. Both of these broad mechanistic categories appear relevant to MCC.[126,127] The tumor cell characteristics include mechanisms such as downregulation of antigen presentation (such as MHC-I loss) to become "less visible" to the immune system[144,145] or decreased susceptibility to immune control mechanisms to become "more resistant" to the effects of the cytotoxic immune cells. The host immune features include systemic immune suppression, either therapeutically or due to comorbid immune suppressive diseases, or more commonly due to immunosenescence, an erosion of the immune response with aging. MCC tumor cells also establish a local immune suppressive tumor microenvironment (TME) via production of immunosuppressive cytokines or via recruitment of immunosuppressive cells, such as CD4+CD25+ regulatory T-cells (Tregs) or myeloid-derived suppressor cells.[146] In response to chronic antigen exposure, antigen-specific CD8+ T-cells in the MCC TME often develop an exhausted phenotype with poor effector function, sustained expression of inhibitory receptors (such as PD-1, TIM-3), and a transcriptional state distinct from that of functional effector or memory T-cells.[138]

IMMUNOTHERAPY OF MERKEL CELL CARCINOMA

The aforementioned data have provided a strong rationale for using immunotherapy to treat MCC.[126,127] These immunotherapy efforts have focused on a multitude of approaches aiming to render cancer cells more visible to the immune cells, reinvigorate existing immune responses, generate new ones, or simply use the viral targets for selective delivery of cancer therapeutics to tumors. Several early phase trials of immunotherapy approaches, including intratumoral IL-12 injection,[147] intratumoral injection of the TLR4 agonist G100,[148] and adoptive T-cell therapy,[142,143] have all provided preliminary evidence of the potential efficacy of a variety of immune-based approaches in MCC. However, the most remarkable successes have been with the ICIs, which are discussed in detail below.

Immune Checkpoint Inhibitors

PD-L1 is expressed on tumor and immune cells in both MCPyV+ and MCPyV- MCC tumors[149] provided the rationale for investigating checkpoint inhibitors targeting PD-1 or PD-L1 in MCC. The presence of PD-1 and PD-L1 in the MCC TME reflects the result of chronic antigen presentation of processed viral proteins and UV-induced neoantigens. Consequently, anti–PD-1 and anti–PD-L1 antibodies have been investigated as first-line and as second-line or later therapy in patients with advanced-stage MCC.

Pembrolizumab is a humanized IgG4 anti–PD-1 monoclonal antibody and is being investigated for first-line systemic treatment of immunocompetent patients with advanced MCC in a phase II clinical trial (www.clinicaltrials.gov; NCT02267603). The first report of this trial included 25 evaluable patients with unresectable stage IIIB or stage IV MCC, out of whom 16% (n = 4) had a CR and 40% (n = 10) had a PR, resulting in an ORR of 56% (14/25).[150] Although the ORR is not strikingly different from what would have been expected from front-line chemotherapy, the responses are remarkably more durable than those expected from chemotherapy. Of the 14 confirmed responses, 12 (86%) were ongoing at last follow-up with the median follow-up being close to 8 months. Response to pembrolizumab did not correlate significantly with PD-L1 expression, a biomarker that has been evaluated extensively in several trials of PD-1 pathway blockade. Importantly, responses were seen in both MCPyV+ and MCPyV− tumors consistent with immunogenicity of both subtypes. Twenty-six patients were included in the safety analysis, and treatment was generally well tolerated, with 77% (n = 20) of patients reporting an AE of any grade, of which 15% (n = 4) were grade 3 or 4. AEs were consistent with prior reports in other cancer types and were managed well through the discontinuation of pembrolizumab and, if necessary, glucocorticoid treatment. The results also led to the listing of pembrolizumab as a therapeutic option in the 2017 US National Comprehensive Cancer Network (NCCN) guidelines. An expansion cohort of 24 patients was added to confirm these initial results, and the results on these 50 patients total are eagerly awaited.

Concurrently with the aforementioned study, another phase II study (NCT02155647) was investigating avelumab in immunocompetent patients with metastatic MCC who had previously received one or more lines of cytotoxic chemotherapy.[151] Avelumab is a human IgG1 anti–PD-L1 monoclonal antibody that also has a wild-type IgG1 Fc region that may, in addition to blocking PD-1/PD-L1 interactions, activate NK cell–mediated antibody-dependent cell-mediated cytotoxicity. In this much larger pivotal phase II trial, 88 patients with chemotherapy refractory distant metastatic (stage IV) disease were treated, out of whom 9% (n = 8) had a CR and 23% (n = 20) had a PR, resulting in an ORR of 32%.[151] Responses were impressively durable with the proportion of responses with a duration of at least 6 months being 92%. Similar to the pembrolizumab study, responses to avelumab occurred quickly (generally at the time of the first scan at 6 weeks) and occurred irrespective of PD-L1 expression or MCPyV status of the MCC tumors. Avelumab was well tolerated, with 70% (n = 62) of patients reporting an AE, but only 5% (n = 4) were grade 3, and there were no grade 4 events. Only fatigue (n = 21, 24%) and infusion-related reaction (n = 15, 17%) occurred in more than 10% of patients. Based on the impressive results from this phase II study, avelumab received approval by the US FDA, Swissmedic, and the European Medical Association (EMA) in 2017 for treatment of metastatic MCC, regardless of prior chemotherapy administration. This trial has recently expanded to include MCC patients who are treatment naïve to systemic therapy in the metastatic setting. Preliminary results of the first 39 patients enrolled in part B were presented at the 2017 annual European Society of Medical Oncology (ESMO) meeting. At the time of the data cutoff, the ORR with first-line avelumab was 62%, with 14% of patients experiencing a CR and 48% of patients experiencing a PR.[152] Sixty-seven percent of patients experienced a PFS rate of 3 months.

Yet another ongoing study (NCT02488759) is investigating nivolumab, an anti–PD-1 antibody, in patients with virus-associated cancers including MCC. Patients with metastatic MCC are enrolled regardless of MCPyV status or prior chemotherapy. Preliminary results were presented at the 2017 annual American Association of Cancer Research (AACR) meeting. ORR in 22 enrolled patients was an impressive 64%.[153] The majority (75%) of the responses occurred by ~week 8. Responses were durable with 75% of the responses ongoing at a median follow-up time of ~12 months. Similar to the aforementioned studies, responses were noted regardless of the PD-L1 expression or MCPyV status. The trial is still ongoing and has added another cohort investigating the combination of nivolumab plus low-dose ipilimumab (1 mg/kg) in metastatic MCC patients. This trial is also investigating the neoadjuvant use of nivolumab (two doses total) in locoregional MCC before surgery (+/− RT).

The impressive and concordant results from these aforementioned trials using three different drugs blocking the PD-1/PD-L1 interaction have offered powerful new options to the clinicians for managing advanced MCC. All of these ICIs have been remarkably well tolerated with low rates of grade 3 or higher treatment-related AEs and no treatment-related deaths. The response rates are the best in treatment-naïve patients and appear to be lower in patients with prior chemotherapy exposure, likely owing to the immune suppression associated with chemotherapy. The responses occur quickly and at a frequency similar to that expected with front-line chemotherapy but are much more durable and can be assumed to lead to a meaningful improvement in OS with reasonably good quality of life (QoL) and perhaps even a chance at "cure" for an otherwise terminal disease. Additionally, these studies suggest that in both MCPyV+ and MCPyV− tumors, a large proportion of patients have MCC-specific T-cells that can be reactivated to provide clinically beneficial antitumor activity. Taken together, these data suggest that PD-1−/PD-L1−based immunotherapy should be considered as the new standard-of-care for first-line treatment for patients with metastatic MCC, regardless of MCPyV status, unless there are contraindications to using ICIs. This is reflected in the recent listing of avelumab, pembrolizumab, and nivolumab as the preferred treatment options for metastatic MCC in the 2018 US NCCN guidelines, although avelumab is currently the only FDA- and EMA-approved therapy for metastatic MCC.

Unmet Needs and Future Directions

The durable responses to PD-1−/PD-L1−blocking antibodies confirm the importance of immune mechanisms in MCC pathogenesis. However, not all patients respond to immunotherapy and some develop secondary resistance. Thus, a key question remains as to what tumor or host characteristics might be used to predict response and/or resistance. In addition to finding predictive biomarkers, there is a dire unmet need for finding effective therapies in ~50% of immune-competent patients who do not respond to PD-1/PD-L1 blockade. Mechanistic studies to understand both intrinsic and acquired mechanisms of resistance are critical to uncover new rational therapies to overcome these. Given the heterogeneity of MCC tumors and individual variations in host immune systems, it is unlikely that one single approach will be effective in all patients. Rather, a combination of various strategies and personalization to the unique biologic characteristics of MCC tumors in individual patients will be required.

Facilitated by the ongoing excitement for cancer immunotherapy, several trials of novel immunotherapeutic approaches (both innate and adaptive) are already ongoing in patients with advanced MCC. An innate immunotherapy approach is using allogeneic irradiated activated NK-92 cells (an NK cell line derived from a patient with larger granulocytic leukemia) in combination with an IL-15 agonist in MCC patients who may have received prior PD-1 blockade (NCT02465957). Another innate immunotherapy approach is studying intratumoral administration of TTI-621, a recombinant fusion protein targeting CD47 that regulates phagocytosis in patients with injectable MCC lesions (NCT02890368). Trials are underway to evaluate the oncolytic virus T-VEC administered intratumorally, both as a monotherapy approach and in combination with radiotherapy (NCT02819843) or with anti–PD-1 (nivolumab) treatment in patients with advanced MCC (NCT02978625). The profound success with checkpoint inhibitors has also increased interest in clinical studies using combinations of other therapies with the ICIs. A triple-combination study of tremelimumab (an anti–CTLA-4 antibody), durvalumab (an anti–PD-L1 antibody), and TLR3 agonist poly-ICLC in advanced MCC (NCT02643303) is testing the hypothesis that the TLR3 agonist will influence the tumor microenvironment and potentiate the activity of the ICIs. A study to investigate the localized upregulation of antigen expression (using radiation or interferon) plus adoptive immunotherapy (MCPyV T-antigen–specific T-cells) with avelumab is also ongoing (NCT02584829). Efforts are also underway to test the safety and efficacy of several ICIs (ipilimumab, nivolumab, and avelumab) in the adjuvant setting in patients with locoregional MCC amenable to definitive therapy with surgery +/− RT (NCT02196961 and NCT03271372). It is indeed an exciting time for investigation of novel targeted and/or immune therapies in this fascinating malignancy.

CONCLUSION

An improved understanding of the biology and immunology of MCC revolutionized the therapeutic possibilities in advanced MCC. The immune system appears to be playing a major role in MCC biology irrespective of their virus- or UV-associated carcinogenesis. A new era in the systemic therapy of metastatic MCC has begun with the recent successes of immune checkpoint blockade. Promising new immunotherapy and molecularly targeted therapy approaches are in development. The possibility of further improvement in patient outcomes is exciting and the dream of curing advanced MCC patients is poised to become a reality for more patients!

Other Nonmelanoma Skin Cancers (Cutaneous Squamous Cell Carcinoma and Basal Cell Carcinoma)

Nonmelanoma skin cancer (NMSC) represents one of the most common cancers representing one-third of all malignancies.[154] The most common cancers that constitute NMSC are basal cell carcinoma (BCC) and cutaneous squamous cell carcinoma (CSCC). These two cancers roughly account for 80% and 20% of NMSC, respectively, with only ∼1% of NMSC consisting of other skin cancers, including MCC.[155–157] The rate of metastatic spread between these two types of skin cancers is also markedly different. Metastatic CSCC accounts for 20% of skin cancer deaths, whereas metastatic BCC is rarely diagnosed.

Use of Immune Checkpoint Inhibitors for Nonmelanoma Skin Cancer

The majority of NMSCs develop as a result of excessive sun exposure and have a high mutational load from repeated UV light damage. This is theorized to result in neoantigens that should be able to stimulate a more effective antitumor immune response and be responsive to PD-1 blockade.[78–82] In one study, among 40 BCC specimens, 9/40 (22%) demonstrated PD-L1 expression on tumor cells and 33/40 (82%) demonstrated PD-L1 expression on TIL and associated macrophages.[158] However, unlike melanoma and MCC, there are limited data on the use of ICIs for CSCC and BCC.

Cutaneous Squamous Cell carcinoma

One case series included four heavily pretreated patients with advanced unresectable or metastatic CSCC treated with anti–PD-1 antibodies (two with pembrolizumab and two with nivolumab). Two patients had a PR and two had SD, with PFS being 4 months in all four patients.[159]

In the dose-escalation portion of the phase I study of cemiplimab (REGN2810), an anti–PD-1 antibody, a patient with metastatic CSCC experienced a durable (19+ months) radiologic CR. This led to expansion cohorts testing the safety and efficacy of cemiplimab in patients with distantly metastatic as well as locally advanced CSCC. Preliminary reports of this trial revealed an impressive ORR of 52% (12/23; ninePR, three CR) and DCR (ORR + SD) of 70% (16/23, including four SD), respectively.[160] A pivotal trial of cemiplimab for patients with advanced CSCC is enrolling patients (clinicaltrials.gov; NCT02383212).

Basal Cell Carcinoma

The data on use of ICIs for metastatic BCC are limited to case reports at this time. A patient with metastatic PD-L1 (+) BCC, whose disease had previously progressed through hedgehog pathway–directed therapy, experienced a durable PR to pembrolizumab, ongoing at 14 months after initiation of therapy.[158] Another patient with lung metastases from BCC who had progressed after receiving vismodegib for 5 months received cemiplimab (REGN2810) and experienced a PR ongoing at 12+ months.[161] Interestingly, immunohistochemical analysis of PD-L1 expression in a BCC metastasis was negative in tumor cells and infiltrating immune cells.

Trials are underway with pembrolizumab (NCT02690948) and cemiplimab (NCT03132636) in patients with metastatic BCC that is progressing after the use of hedgehog inhibitors, and data are eagerly awaited.

CONCLUSION

Preliminary results from clinical trials and case reports suggest potential clinical benefit from the use of PD-1 blockade in patients with advanced CSCC and BCC. Clinical trials are underway to further define the safety and efficacy of ICIs in these NMSCs.

DISCLOSURE STATEMENT

SL reports research funding to her institutions (Fred Hutchinson Cancer Research Center and University of Washington) from Juno, MedImmune, and Altor. SB reports research funding to his institution (University of Washington) from Merck, BMS, EMD-Serono, OncoSec, ImmuneDesign, and NantKwest. SB has received honoraria for participation in advisory boards for EMD-Serono and Genentech.

REFERENCES

1. Siegel RL, Miller KD, Jemal A. Cancer statistics, 2016. *CA Cancer J Clin.* 2016;66(1):7−30.
2. Ekwueme DU, Guy Jr GP, Li C, Rim SH, Parelkar P, Chen SC. The health burden and economic costs of cutaneous melanoma mortality by race/ethnicity-United States, 2000 to 2006. *J Am Acad Dermatol.* 2011;65(5 suppl 1):S133−S143.
3. Printz C. Spontaneous regression of melanoma may offer insight into cancer immunology. *J Natl Cancer Inst.* 2001; 93(14):1047−1048.
4. Gray A, Grushchak S, Mudaliar K, Kliethermes S, Carey K, Hutchens KA. The microenvironment in primary cutaneous melanoma with associated spontaneous tumor regression: evaluation for T-regulatory cells and the presence of an immunosuppressive microenvironment. *Melanoma Res.* 2017;27(2):104−109.
5. Halliday GM, Patel A, Hunt MJ, Tefany FJ, Barnetson RS. Spontaneous regression of human melanoma/nonmelanoma skin cancer: association with infiltrating CD^{4+} T cells. *World J Surg.* 1995;19(3):352−358.
6. Chang AE, Karnell LH, Menck HR. The National cancer data Base report on cutaneous and noncutaneous melanoma: a summary of 84,836 cases from the past decade. The American College of Surgeons Commission on cancer and the American cancer Society. *Cancer.* 1998;83(8):1664−1678.
7. Lee CC, Faries MB, Wanek LA, Morton DL. Improved survival for stage IV melanoma from an unknown primary site. *J Clin Oncol.* 2009;27(21):3489−3495.
8. Rosenberg SA, Lotze MT, Muul LM, et al. Observations on the systemic administration of autologous lymphokine-activated killer cells and recombinant interleukin-2 to patients with metastatic cancer. *N Engl J Med.* 1985; 313(23):1485−1492.
9. Rosenberg SA, Yang JC, White DE, Steinberg SM. Durability of complete responses in patients with metastatic cancer treated with high-dose interleukin-2: identification of the antigens mediating response. *Ann Surg.* 1998;228(3):307−319.
10. Rosenberg SA, Yang JC, Sherry RM, et al. Durable complete responses in heavily pretreated patients with metastatic melanoma using T-cell transfer immunotherapy. *Clin Cancer Res.* 2011;17(13):4550−4557.
11. Lee S, Margolin K. Tumor-infiltrating lymphocytes in melanoma. *Curr Oncol Rep.* 2012;14(5):468−474.
12. Hodi FS, O'Day SJ, McDermott DF, et al. Improved survival with ipilimumab in patients with metastatic melanoma. *N Engl J Med.* 2010;363(8):711−723.
13. Brahmer JR, Tykodi SS, Chow LQ, et al. Safety and activity of anti-PD-L1 antibody in patients with advanced cancer. *N Engl J Med.* 2012;366(26):2455−2465.
14. Topalian SL, Hodi FS, Brahmer JR, et al. Safety, activity, and immune correlates of anti-PD-1 antibody in cancer. *N Engl J Med.* 2012;366(26):2443−2454.
15. Krummel MF, Allison JP. CD28 and CTLA-4 have opposing effects on the response of T cells to stimulation. *J Exp Med.* 1995;182(2):459−465.
16. Leach DR, Krummel MF, Allison JP. Enhancement of antitumor immunity by CTLA-4 blockade. *Science.* 1996;271(5256):1734−1736.
17. Robert C, Thomas L, Bondarenko I, et al. Ipilimumab plus dacarbazine for previously untreated metastatic melanoma. *N Engl J Med.* 2011;364(26):2517−2526.

18. Ribas A, Kefford R, Marshall MA, et al. Phase III randomized clinical trial comparing tremelimumab with standard-of-care chemotherapy in patients with advanced melanoma. *J Clin Oncol.* 2013;31(5):616−622.

19. Schadendorf D, Hodi FS, Robert C, et al. Pooled analysis of long-term survival data from phase II and phase III trials of ipilimumab in unresectable or metastatic melanoma. *J Clin Oncol.* 2015;33(17):1889−1894.

20. Wolchok JD, Neyns B, Linette G, et al. Ipilimumab monotherapy in patients with pretreated advanced melanoma: a randomised, double-blind, multicentre, phase 2, dose-ranging study. *Lancet Oncol.* 2010;11(2):155−164.

21. Ascierto PA, Del Vecchio M, Robert C, et al. Ipilimumab 10 mg/kg versus ipilimumab 3 mg/kg in patients with unresectable or metastatic melanoma: a randomised, double-blind, multicentre, phase 3 trial. *Lancet Oncol.* 2017;18(5):611−622.

22. Saenger YM, Wolchok JD. The heterogeneity of the kinetics of response to ipilimumab in metastatic melanoma: patient cases. *Cancer Immun.* 2008;8:1.

23. Hamid O, Robert C, Daud A, et al. Safety and tumor responses with lambrolizumab (anti-PD-1) in melanoma. *N Engl J Med.* 2013;369(2):134−144.

24. Robert C, Ribas A, Wolchok JD, et al. Anti-programmed-death-receptor-1 treatment with pembrolizumab in ipilimumab-refractory advanced melanoma: a randomised dose-comparison cohort of a phase 1 trial. *Lancet.* 2014;384(9948):1109−1117.

25. Wolchok JD, Kluger H, Callahan MK, et al. Nivolumab plus ipilimumab in advanced melanoma. *N Engl J Med.* 2013;369(2):122−133.

26. Wolchok JD, Weber JS, Maio M, et al. Four-year survival rates for patients with metastatic melanoma who received ipilimumab in phase II clinical trials. *Ann Oncol.* 2013;24(8):2174−2180.

27. Wolchok JD, Hoos A, O'Day S, et al. Guidelines for the evaluation of immune therapy activity in solid tumors: immune-related response criteria. *Clin Cancer Res.* 2009;15(23):7412−7420.

28. Eisenhauer EA, Therasse P, Bogaerts J, et al. New response evaluation criteria in solid tumours: revised RECIST guideline (version 1.1). *Eur J Cancer.* 2009;45(2):228−247.

29. James K, Eisenhauer E, Christian M, et al. Measuring response in solid tumors: unidimensional versus bidimensional measurement. *J Natl Cancer Inst.* 1999;91(6):523−528.

30. Hodi FS, Hwu WJ, Kefford R, et al. Evaluation of immune-related response criteria and RECIST v1.1 in patients with advanced melanoma treated with pembrolizumab. *J Clin Oncol.* 2016;34(13):1510−1517.

31. Seiwert TY, Burtness B, Mehra R, et al. Safety and clinical activity of pembrolizumab for treatment of recurrent or metastatic squamous cell carcinoma of the head and neck (KEYNOTE-012): an open-label, multicentre, phase 1b trial. *Lancet Oncol.* 2016;17(7):956−965.

32. Powles T, Eder JP, Fine GD, et al. MPDL3280A (anti-PD-L1) treatment leads to clinical activity in metastatic bladder cancer. *Nature.* 2014;515(7528):558−562.

33. Motzer RJ, Rini BI, McDermott DF, et al. Nivolumab for metastatic renal cell carcinoma: results of a randomized phase II trial. *J Clin Oncol.* 2015;33(13):1430−1437.

34. Francisco LM, Salinas VH, Brown KE, et al. PD-L1 regulates the development, maintenance, and function of induced regulatory T cells. *J Exp Med.* 2009;206(13):3015−3029.

35. Freeman GJ, Long AJ, Iwai Y, et al. Engagement of the PD-1 immunoinhibitory receptor by a novel B7 family member leads to negative regulation of lymphocyte activation. *J Exp Med.* 2000;192(7):1027−1034.

36. Brahmer JR, Drake CG, Wollner I, et al. Phase I study of single-agent anti-programmed death-1 (MDX-1106) in refractory solid tumors: safety, clinical activity, pharmacodynamics, and immunologic correlates. *J Clin Oncol.* 2010;28(19):3167−3175.

37. Weber JS, D'Angelo SP, Minor D, et al. Nivolumab versus chemotherapy in patients with advanced melanoma who progressed after anti-CTLA-4 treatment (CheckMate 037): a randomised, controlled, open-label, phase 3 trial. *Lancet Oncol.* 2015;16(4):375−384.

38. Robert C, Long GV, Brady B, et al. Nivolumab in previously untreated melanoma without BRAF mutation. *N Engl J Med.* 2014;372(4):320−330.

39. Robert C, Schachter J, Long GV, et al. Pembrolizumab versus ipilimumab in advanced melanoma. *N Engl J Med.* 2015;372(26):2521−2532.

40. Schachter J, Ribas A, Long GV, et al. Pembrolizumab versus ipilimumab for advanced melanoma: final overall survival results of a multicentre, randomised, open-label phase 3 study (KEYNOTE-006). *Lancet.* 2017;390(10105):1853−1862.

41. Larkin J, Chiarion-Sileni V, Gonzalez R, et al. Combined nivolumab and ipilimumab or monotherapy in untreated melanoma. *N Engl J Med.* 2015;373(1):23−34.

42. Wolchok JD, Chiarion-Sileni V, Gonzalez R, et al. Overall survival with combined nivolumab and ipilimumab in advanced melanoma. *N Engl J Med.* 2017;377(14):1345−1356.

43. Larkin JC-SV, Gonzalez R, et al. Overall survival results from a phaes III trial of nivolumab combined with ipilimumab in treatment-naive patients with advanced melanoma (CheckMate 067). In: *Paper Presented at: AACR Annual Meeting.* April 3, 2017.

44. Weber JS, Gibney G, Sullivan RJ, et al. Sequential administration of nivolumab and ipilimumab with a planned switch in patients with advanced melanoma (CheckMate 064): an open-label, randomised, phase 2 trial. *Lancet Oncol.* 2016;17(7):943−955.

45. Zimmer L, Apuri S, Eroglu Z, et al. Ipilimumab alone or in combination with nivolumab after progression on anti-PD-1 therapy in advanced melanoma. *Eur J Cancer.* 2017;75:47−55.

46. Schadendorf D, Larkin J, Wolchok J, et al. Health-related quality of life results from the phase III CheckMate 067 study. *Eur J Cancer*. 2017;82:80−91.

47. Hodi FS, Postow MA, Chesney JA, et al. Overall survival in patients with advanced melanoma (MEL) who discontinued treatment with nivolumab (NIVO) plus ipilimumab (IPI) due to toxicity in a phase II trial (CheckMate 069). *J Clin Oncol*. 2016;34(15 suppl):9518.

48. Hodi FS, Chesney J, Pavlick AC, et al. Combined nivolumab and ipilimumab versus ipilimumab alone in patients with advanced melanoma: 2-year overall survival outcomes in a multicentre, randomised, controlled, phase 2 trial. *Lancet Oncol*. 2016;17(11):1558−1568.

49. Postow MA, Chesney J, Pavlick AC, et al. Nivolumab and ipilimumab versus ipilimumab in untreated melanoma. *N Engl J Med*. 2015;372(21):2006−2017.

50. Weber JS, Hodi FS, Wolchok JD, et al. Safety profile of nivolumab monotherapy: a pooled analysis of patients with advanced melanoma. *J Clin Oncol*. 2017;35(7):785−792.

51. Beck KE, Blansfield JA, Tran KQ, et al. Enterocolitis in patients with cancer after antibody blockade of cytotoxic T-lymphocyte−associated antigen 4. *J Clin Oncol*. 2006;24(15):2283−2289.

52. Downey SG, Klapper JA, Smith FO, et al. Prognostic factors related to clinical response in patients with metastatic melanoma treated by CTL-associated antigen-4 blockade. *Clin Cancer Res*. 2007;13(22):6681−6688.

53. Weber J, Thompson JA, Hamid O, et al. A randomized, double-blind, placebo-controlled, phase II study comparing the tolerability and efficacy of ipilimumab administered with or without prophylactic budesonide in patients with unresectable stage III or IV melanoma. *Clin Cancer Res*. 2009;15(17):5591−5598.

54. Sarnaik AA, Yu B, Yu D, et al. Extended dose ipilimumab with a peptide vaccine: immune correlates associated with clinical benefit in patients with resected high-risk stage IIIc/IV melanoma. *Clin Cancer Res*. 2011;17(4):896−906.

55. Ascierto PA, Simeone E, Sileni VC, et al. Clinical experience with ipilimumab 3 mg/kg: real-world efficacy and safety data from an expanded access programme cohort. *J Transl Med*. 2014;12:116.

56. Schadendorf D, Wolchok JD, Hodi FS, et al. Efficacy and safety outcomes in patients with advanced melanoma who discontinued treatment with nivolumab and ipilimumab because of adverse events: a pooled analysis of randomized phase II and III trials. *J Clin Oncol*. 2017;35(34):3807−3814.

57. Johnson JD, Young B. Demographics of brain metastasis. *Neurosurg Clin N Am*. 1996;7(3):337−344.

58. Amer MH, Al-Sarraf M, Baker LH, Vaitkevicius VK. Malignant melanoma and central nervous system metastases: incidence, diagnosis, treatment and survival. *Cancer*. 1978;42(2):660−668.

59. Fife KM, Colman MH, Stevens GN, et al. Determinants of outcome in melanoma patients with cerebral metastases. *J Clin Oncol*. 2004;22(7):1293−1300.

60. Margolin K, Ernstoff MS, Hamid O, et al. Ipilimumab in patients with melanoma and brain metastases: an open-label, phase 2 trial. *Lancet Oncol*. 2012;13(5):459−465.

61. Goldberg SB, Gettinger SN, Mahajan A, et al. Pembrolizumab for patients with melanoma or non-small-cell lung cancer and untreated brain metastases: early analysis of a non-randomised, open-label, phase 2 trial. *Lancet Oncol*. 2016;17(7):976−983.

62. Tawbi HAFP, Algazi AP, et al. Efficacy and safety of nivolumab plus ipilimumab in patients with melanoma metastatic to the brain: results of the phase II study checkmate 204. In: *Paper Presented at: 2017 American Society of Clinical Oncology Annual Meeting*. 2017.

63. Long GVAV, Menzies AM, et al. A randomized phase II study of nivolumab or nivolumab combined with ipilimumab in patients with melanoma brain metastases: the Anti-PD1 Collaboration (ABC). In: *Paper Presented at: 2017 American Society of Clinical Oncology Annual Meeting*. 2017.

64. Chabanon RM, Pedrero M, Lefebvre C, Marabelle A, Soria J-C, Postel-Vinay S. Mutational landscape and sensitivity to immune checkpoint blockers. *Clin Cancer Res*. 2016;22(17):4309−4321.

65. Postow MA, Luke JJ, Bluth MJ, et al. Ipilimumab for patients with advanced mucosal melanoma. *Oncologist*. 2013;18(6):726−732.

66. D'Angelo SP, Larkin J, Sosman JA, et al. Efficacy and safety of nivolumab alone or in combination with ipilimumab in patients with mucosal melanoma: a pooled analysis. *J Clin Oncol*. 2017;35(2):226−235.

67. Shoushtari AN, Munhoz RR, Kuk D, et al. The efficacy of anti-PD-1 agents in acral and mucosal melanoma. *Cancer*. 2016;122(21):3354−3362.

68. Krantz BA, Dave N, Komatsubara KM, Marr BP, Carvajal RD. Uveal melanoma: epidemiology, etiology, and treatment of primary disease. *Clin Ophthalmol*. 2017;11:279−289.

69. Zimmer L, Vaubel J, Mohr P, et al. Phase II DeCOG-study of ipilimumab in pretreated and treatment-naive patients with metastatic uveal melanoma. *PLoS One*. 2015;10(3):e0118564.

70. Algazi AP, Tsai KK, Shoushtari AN, et al. Clinical outcomes in metastatic uveal melanoma treated with PD-1 and PD-L1 antibodies. *Cancer*. 2016;122(21):3344−3353.

71. Niederkorn JY. Ocular immune privilege and ocular melanoma: parallel universes or immunological plagiarism? *Front Immunol*. 2012;3:148.

72. Kaplan HJ, Streilein JW. Immune response to immunization via the anterior chamber of the eye. I. F. lymphocyte-induced immune deviation. *J Immunol*. 1977;118(3):809−814.

73. Balch CM, Gershenwald JE, Soong SJ, et al. Multivariate analysis of prognostic factors among 2,313 patients with stage III melanoma: comparison of nodal micrometastases versus macrometastases. *J Clin Oncol*. 2010;28(14):2452−2459.

74. Romano E, Scordo M, Dusza SW, Coit DG, Chapman PB. Site and timing of first relapse in stage III melanoma patients: implications for follow-up guidelines. *J Clin Oncol.* 2010;28(18):3042–3047.

75. Eggermont AMM, Chiarion-Sileni V, Grob J-J, et al. Prolonged survival in stage III melanoma with ipilimumab adjuvant therapy. *N Engl J Med.* 2016;375(19):1845–1855.

76. Weber J, Mandala M, Del Vecchio M, et al. Adjuvant nivolumab versus ipilimumab in resected stage III or IV melanoma. *N Engl J Med.* 2017;377(19):1824–1835.

77. Daud AI, Wolchok JD, Robert C, et al. Programmed death-ligand 1 expression and response to the anti-programmed death 1 antibody pembrolizumab in melanoma. *J Clin Oncol.* 2016;34(34):4102–4109.

78. Alexandrov LB, Nik-Zainal S, Wedge DC, et al. Signatures of mutational processes in human cancer. *Nature.* 2013;500(7463):415–421.

79. Snyder A, Makarov V, Merghoub T, et al. Genetic basis for clinical response to CTLA-4 blockade in melanoma. *N Engl J Med.* 2014;371(23):2189–2199.

80. Van Allen EM, Miao D, Schilling B, et al. Genomic correlates of response to CTLA-4 blockade in metastatic melanoma. *Science.* 2015;350(6257):207–211.

81. McGranahan N, Furness AJ, Rosenthal R, et al. Clonal neoantigens elicit T cell immunoreactivity and sensitivity to immune checkpoint blockade. *Science.* 2016;351(6280):1463–1469.

82. Rizvi NA, Hellmann MD, Snyder A, et al. Cancer immunology. Mutational landscape determines sensitivity to PD-1 blockade in non-small cell lung cancer. *Science.* 2015;348(6230):124–128.

83. Spranger S, Luke JJ, Bao R, et al. Density of immunogenic antigens does not explain the presence or absence of the T-cell-inflamed tumor microenvironment in melanoma. *Proc Natl Acad Sci U S A.* 2016;113(48):E7759–E7768.

84. Daud AI, Loo K, Pauli ML, et al. Tumor immune profiling predicts response to anti-PD-1 therapy in human melanoma. *J Clin Invest.* 2016;126(9):3447–3452.

85. Tumeh PC, Harview CL, Yearley JH, et al. PD-1 blockade induces responses by inhibiting adaptive immune resistance. *Nature.* 2014;515(7528):568–571.

86. Loo K, Tsai KK, Mahuron K, et al. Partially exhausted tumor-infiltrating lymphocytes predict response to combination immunotherapy. *JCI Insight.* 2017;2(14).

87. Ribas ARC, Hodi FS, et al. Association of response to programmed death receptor 1 (PD-1) blockade with pembrolizumab (MK-3475) with an interferon-inflammatory immune gene signature. *J Clin Oncol.* 2015;(suppl):33; abstr3001.

88. Ayers M, Lunceford J, Nebozhyn M, et al. IFN–related mRNA profile predicts clinical response to PD-1 blockade. *J Clin Invest.* 2017;127(8):2930–2940.

89. Sivan A, Corrales L, Hubert N, et al. Commensal Bifidobacterium promotes antitumor immunity and facilitates anti-PD-L1 efficacy. *Science.* 2015;350(6264):1084–1089.

90. Vetizou M, Pitt JM, Daillere R, et al. Anticancer immunotherapy by CTLA-4 blockade relies on the gut microbiota. *Science.* 2015;350(6264):1079–1084.

91. Gopalakrishnan V, Spencer CN, Nezi L, et al. Gut microbiome modulates response to anti-PD-1 immunotherapy in melanoma patients. *Science.* 2018;359(6371):97–103.

92. Routy B, Le Chatelier E, Derosa L, et al. Gut microbiome influences efficacy of PD-1-based immunotherapy against epithelial tumors. *Science.* 2018;359(6371):91–97.

93. Gollob JA, Mier JW, Veenstra K, et al. Phase I trial of twice-weekly intravenous interleukin 12 in patients with metastatic renal cell cancer or malignant melanoma: ability to maintain IFN- induction is associated with clinical response. *Clin Cancer Res.* 2000;6(5):1678–1692.

94. Nv Rooij, MMv Buuren, Philips D, et al. Tumor exome analysis reveals neoantigen-specific T-cell reactivity in an ipilimumab-responsive melanoma. *J Clin Oncol.* 2013;31(32):e439–e442.

95. Schumacher TN, Schreiber RD. Neoantigens in cancer immunotherapy. *Science.* 2015;348(6230):69–74.

96. Hayward NK, Wilmott JS, Waddell N, et al. Whole-genome landscapes of major melanoma subtypes. *Nature.* 2017;545:175.

97. Restifo NP, Marincola FM, Kawakami Y, Taubenberger J, Yannelli JR, Rosenberg SA. Loss of functional beta 2-microglobulin in metastatic melanomas from five patients receiving immunotherapy. *J Natl Cancer Inst.* 1996;88(2):100–108.

98. del Campo AB, Kyte JA, Carretero J, et al. Immune escape of cancer cells with beta2-microglobulin loss over the course of metastatic melanoma. *Int J Cancer.* 2014;134(1):102–113.

99. Roh W, Chen PL, Reuben A, et al. Integrated molecular analysis of tumor biopsies on sequential CTLA-4 and PD-1 blockade reveals markers of response and resistance. *Sci Transl Med.* 2017;9(379).

100. Zaretsky JM, Garcia-Diaz A, Shin DS, et al. Mutations associated with acquired resistance to PD-1 blockade in melanoma. *N Engl J Med.* 2016;375(9):819–829.

101. Fridman WH, Pagès F, Sautès-Fridman C, Galon J. The immune contexture in human tumours: impact on clinical outcome. *Nat Rev Cancer.* 2012;12:298.

102. Peng W, Chen JQ, Liu C, et al. Loss of PTEN promotes resistance to T cell-mediated immunotherapy. *Cancer Discov.* 2016;6(2):202–216.

103. Gajewski TF, Schreiber H, Fu YX. Innate and adaptive immune cells in the tumor microenvironment. *Nat Immunol.* 2013;14(10):1014–1022.

104. Hugo W, Zaretsky JM, Sun L, et al. Genomic and transcriptomic features of response to anti-PD-1 therapy in metastatic melanoma. *Cell.* 2016;165(1):35–44.

105. Shin DS, Zaretsky JM, Escuin-Ordinas H, et al. Primary resistance to PD-1 blockade mediated by JAK1/2 mutations. *Cancer Discov.* 2017;7(2):188–201.

106. Gao J, Shi LZ, Zhao H, et al. Loss of IFN- pathway genes in tumor cells as a mechanism of resistance to anti-CTLA-4 therapy. *Cell.* 2016;167(2):397–404. e399.

107. Koyama S, Akbay EA, Li YY, et al. Adaptive resistance to therapeutic PD-1 blockade is associated with upregulation of alternative immune checkpoints. *Nat Commun.* 2016;7:10501.

108. Sakuishi K, Apetoh L, Sullivan JM, Blazar BR, Kuchroo VK, Anderson AC. Targeting Tim-3 and PD-1 pathways to reverse T cell exhaustion and restore anti-tumor immunity. *J Exp Med.* 2010;207(10): 2187−2194.

109. Grosso JF, Goldberg MV, Getnet D, et al. Functionally distinct LAG-3 and PD-1 subsets on activated and chronically stimulated CD8 T cells. *J Immunol.* 2009;182(11): 6659−6669.

110. Ascierto PA, Melero I, Bhatia S, et al. Initial efficacy of anti-lymphocyte activation gene-3 (anti−LAG-3; BMS-986016) in combination with nivolumab (nivo) in pts with melanoma (MEL) previously treated with anti−PD-1/PD-L1 therapy. *J Clin Oncol.* 2017;35(15 suppl):9520.

111. Beatty GL, O'Dwyer PJ, Clark J, et al. First-in-human phase I study of the oral inhibitor of indoleamine 2,3-dioxygenase-1 epacadostat (INCB024360) in patients with advanced solid malignancies. *Clin Cancer Res.* 2017;23(13):3269−3276.

112. Gibney GTHO, Lutzky J, et al. Updated results from a phase 1/2 study of epacadostat (INCB024360) in combination with ipilimumab in patients with metastatic melanoma. In: *Paper Presented at: ECCO-esmo.* 2015.

113. Zakharia YMR, Shaheen M, et al. Interim analysis of the phase 2 clinical trial of the Ido pathway inhibitor indoximod in combination with pembrolizumab for patients with advanced melanoma. In: *Paper Presented at: 2017 AACR Annual Meeting.* 2017.

114. Gough MJ, Ruby CE, Redmond WL, Dhungel B, Brown A, Weinberg AD. OX40 agonist therapy enhances CD8 infiltration and decreases immune suppression in the tumor. *Cancer Res.* 2008;68(13):5206−5215.

115. Infante JR, Hansen AR, Pishvaian MJ, et al. A phase Ib dose escalation study of the OX40 agonist MOXR0916 and the PD-L1 inhibitor atezolizumab in patients with advanced solid tumors. *J Clin Oncol.* 2016;34(15 suppl):101.

116. Ott PA, Hodi FS, Buchbinder EI. Inhibition of immune checkpoints and vascular endothelial growth factor as combination therapy for metastatic melanoma: an overview of rationale, preclinical evidence, and initial clinical data. *Front Oncol.* 2015;5(202).

117. Hodi FS, Lawrence D, Lezcano C, et al. Bevacizumab plus ipilimumab in patients with metastatic melanoma. *Cancer Immunol Res.* 2014;2(7):632−642.

118. Wallin JJ, Bendell JC, Funke R, et al. Atezolizumab in combination with bevacizumab enhances antigen-specific T-cell migration in metastatic renal cell carcinoma. *Nat Commun.* 2016;7:12624.

119. Long GV, Dummer R, Ribas A, et al. Efficacy analysis of MASTERKEY-265 phase 1b study of talimogene laherparepvec (T-VEC) and pembrolizumab (pembro) for unresectable stage IIIB-IV melanoma. In: *Paper Presented at: 2016 American Society of Clinical Oncology (ASCO) Annual Meeting.* 2016.

120. Lemos BD, Storer BE, Iyer JG, et al. Pathologic nodal evaluation improves prognostic accuracy in Merkel cell carcinoma: analysis of 5823 cases as the basis of the first consensus staging system. *J Am Acad Dermatol.* 2010; 63(5):751−761.

121. Paulson KG, Park SY, Vandeven NA, et al. Merkel cell carcinoma: current United States incidence and projected increases based on changing demographics. *J Am Acad Dermatol.* 2018;78(3):457−463.e2.

122. Albores-Saavedra J, Batich K, Chable-Montero F, Sagy N, Schwartz AM, Henson DE. Merkel cell carcinoma demographics, morphology, and survival based on 3870 cases: a population based study. *J Cutan Pathol.* 2010;37(1): 20−27.

123. Moll R, Lowe A, Laufer J, Franke WW. Cytokeratin 20 in human carcinomas. A new histodiagnostic marker detected by monoclonal antibodies. *Am J Pathol.* 1992; 140(2):427−447.

124. Iyer JG, Blom A, Doumani R, et al. Response rates and durability of chemotherapy among 62 patients with metastatic Merkel cell carcinoma. *Cancer Med.* 2016;5(9): 2294−2301.

125. Becker JC, Lorenz E, Ugurel S, et al. Evaluation of real-world treatment outcomes in patients with distant metastatic Merkel cell carcinoma following second-line chemotherapy in Europe. *Oncotarget.* 2017;8(45): 79731−79741.

126. Bhatia S, Afanasiev O, Nghiem P. Immunobiology of Merkel cell carcinoma: implications for immunotherapy of a polyomavirus-associated cancer. *Curr Oncol Rep.* 2011;13(6):488−497.

127. Schadendorf D, Nghiem P, Bhatia S, et al. Immune evasion mechanisms and immune checkpoint inhibition in advanced merkel cell carcinoma. *Oncoimmunology.* 2017;6(10):e1338237.

128. Penn I, First MR. Merkel's cell carcinoma in organ recipients: report of 41 cases. *Transplantation.* 1999;68(11): 1717−1721.

129. Karkos PD, Sastry A, Hampal S, Al-Jafari M. Spontaneous regression of Merkel cell carcinoma of the nose. *Head Neck.* 2010;32(3):411−414.

130. Kubo H, Matsushita S, Fukushige T, Kanzaki T, Kanekura T. Spontaneous regression of recurrent and metastatic Merkel cell carcinoma. *J Dermatol.* 2007;34(11):773−777.

131. Wooff JC, Trites JR, Walsh NM, Bullock MJ. Complete spontaneous regression of metastatic Merkel cell carcinoma: a case report and review of the literature. *Am J Dermatopathol.* 2010;32(6):614−617.

132. Feng H, Shuda M, Chang Y, Moore PS. Clonal integration of a polyomavirus in human Merkel cell carcinoma. *Science.* 2008;319(5866):1096−1100.

133. Paulson KG, Iyer JG, Tegeder AR, et al. Transcriptome-wide studies of merkel cell carcinoma and validation of intratumoral CD^{8+} lymphocyte invasion as an independent predictor of survival. *J Clin Oncol.* 2011;29(12): 1539−1546.

134. Goh G, Walradt T, Markarov V, et al. Mutational landscape of MCPyV-positive and MCPyV-negative Merkel cell carcinomas with implications for immunotherapy. *Oncotarget*. 2016;7(3):3403—3415.

135. Wong SQ, Waldeck K, Vergara IA, et al. UV-associated mutations underlie the etiology of MCV-negative Merkel cell carcinomas. *Cancer Res*. 2015;75(24):5228—5234.

136. Houben R, Shuda M, Weinkam R, et al. Merkel cell polyomavirus-infected Merkel cell carcinoma cells require expression of viral T antigens. *J Virol*. 2010; 84(14):7064—7072.

137. Shuda M, Arora R, Kwun HJ, et al. Human Merkel cell polyomavirus infection I. MCV T antigen expression in Merkel cell carcinoma, lymphoid tissues and lymphoid tumors. *Int J Cancer*. 2009;125(6):1243—1249.

138. Afanasiev OK, Yelistratova L, Miller N, et al. Merkel polyomavirus-specific T cells fluctuate with merkel cell carcinoma burden and express therapeutically targetable PD-1 and Tim-3 exhaustion markers. *Clin Cancer Res*. 2013;19(19):5351—5360.

139. Iyer JG, Afanasiev OK, McClurkan C, et al. Merkel cell polyomavirus-specific CD^{8+} and CD^{4+} T-cell responses identified in Merkel cell carcinomas and blood. *Clin Cancer Res*. 2011;17(21):6671—6680.

140. Paulson KG, Carter JJ, Johnson LG, et al. Antibodies to merkel cell polyomavirus T antigen oncoproteins reflect tumor burden in merkel cell carcinoma patients. *Cancer Res*. 2010;70(21):8388—8397.

141. Paulson KG, Lewis CW, Redman MW, et al. Viral oncoprotein antibodies as a marker for recurrence of Merkel cell carcinoma: a prospective validation study. *Cancer*. 2017;123(8):1464—1474.

142. Chapuis AG, Afanasiev OK, Iyer JG, et al. Regression of metastatic Merkel cell carcinoma following transfer of polyomavirus-specific T cells and therapies capable of re-inducing HLA class-I. *Cancer Immunol Res*. 2014; 2(1):27—36.

143. Paulson KG, Perdicchio M, Kulikauskas R, et al. Augmentation of adoptive T-cell therapy for Merkel cell carcinoma with avelumab. *J Clin Oncol*. 2017:35.

144. Paulson KG, Tegeder A, Willmes C, et al. Downregulation of MHC-I expression is prevalent but reversible in Merkel cell carcinoma. *Cancer Immunol Res*. 2014;2(11): 1071—1079.

145. Ritter C, Fan K, Paulson KG, Nghiem P, Schrama D, Becker JC. Reversal of epigenetic silencing of MHC class I chain-related protein A and B improves immune recognition of Merkel cell carcinoma. *Sci Rep*. 2016;6:21678.

146. Afanasiev OK, Nagase K, Simonson W, et al. Vascular E-selectin expression correlates with CD8 lymphocyte infiltration and improved outcome in Merkel cell carcinoma. *J Invest Dermatol*. 2013;133(8):2065—2073.

147. Bhatia S, Iyer J, Ibrani D, et al. Intratumoral delivery of Interleukin-12 DNA via in vivo electroporation leads to regression of injected and non-injected tumors in Merkel cell carcinoma: final Results of a phase 2 study. *Eur J Cancer*. 2015;51:S104.

148. Bhatia S, Miller N, Lu HL, et al. fPilot trial of intratumoral (IT) G100, a toll-like receptor-4 (TLR4) agonist, in patients (pts) with Merkel cell carcinoma (MCC): final clinical results and immunologic effects on the tumor microenvironment (TME). *J Clin Oncol*. 2016;34(15).

149. Lipson EJ, Vincent JG, Loyo M, et al. PD-L1 expression in the Merkel cell carcinoma microenvironment: association with inflammation, Merkel cell polyomavirus and overall survival. *Cancer Immunol Res*. 2013;1(1):54—63.

150. Nghiem PT, Bhatia S, Lipson EJ, et al. PD-1 blockade with pembrolizumab in advanced Merkel-cell carcinoma. *N Engl J Med*. 2016;374(26):2542—2552.

151. Kaufman HL, Russell J, Hamid O, et al. Avelumab in patients with chemotherapy-refractory metastatic Merkel cell carcinoma: a multicentre, single-group, open-label, phase 2 trial. *Lancet Oncol*. 2016;17(10):1374—1385.

152. D'Angelo SP, Russell J, Hassel JC, et al. First-line (1L) avelumab treatment in patients (pts) with metastatic Merkel cell carcinoma (mMCC): preliminary data from an ongoing study. *J Clin Oncol*. 2017:35.

153. Topalian SL, Bhatia S, Hollebecque A, et al. Abstract CT074: non-comparative, open-label, multiple cohort, phase 1/2 study to evaluate nivolumab (NIVO) in patients with virus-associated tumors (CheckMate 358): efficacy and safety in Merkel cell carcinoma (MCC). In: *Paper Presented at: AACR Annual Meeting; Washington, DC. 2017*.

154. Surdu S. Non-melanoma skin cancer: occupational risk from UV light and arsenic exposure. *Rev Environ Health*. 2014;29(3):255—264.

155. Rogers HW, Weinstock MA, Feldman SR, Coldiron BM. Incidence estimate of nonmelanoma skin cancer (keratinocyte carcinomas) in the U.S. population, 2012. *JAMA Dermatol*. 2015;151(10):1081—1086.

156. Katalinic A, Kunze U, Schafer T. Epidemiology of cutaneous melanoma and non-melanoma skin cancer in Schleswig-Holstein, Germany: incidence, clinical subtypes, tumour stages and localization (epidemiology of skin cancer). *Br J Dermatol*. 2003;149(6): 1200—1206.

157. Lomas A, Leonardi-Bee J, Bath-Hextall F. A systematic review of worldwide incidence of nonmelanoma skin cancer. *Br J Dermatol*. 2012;166(5):1069—1080.

158. Lipson EJ, Lilo MT, Ogurtsova A, et al. Basal cell carcinoma: PD-L1/PD-1 checkpoint expression and tumor regression after PD-1 blockade. *J Immunother Cancer*. 2017;5:23.

159. Borradori L, Sutton B, Shayesteh P, Daniels GA. Rescue therapy with anti-programmed cell death protein 1 inhibitors of advanced cutaneous squamous cell carcinoma and basosquamous carcinoma: preliminary experience in five cases. *Br J Dermatol*. 2016;175(6):1382–1386.

160. Papadopoulos K, Owonikoko T, Johnson M, et al. REGN2810: a fully human anti-PD-1 monoclonal antibody, for patients with unresectable locally advanced or metastatic cutaneous squamous cell carcinoma (CSCC)— initial safety and efficacy from expansion cohorts (ECs) of phase I study. *J Clin Oncol*. 2017; 35(suppl); abstr 9503.

161. Falchook GS, Leidner R, Stankevich E, et al. Responses of metastatic basal cell and cutaneous squamous cell carcinomas to anti-PD1 monoclonal antibody REGN2810. *J Immunother Cancer*. 2016;4:70.

CHAPTER 3

The Current Status of Immunotherapy in Thoracic Malignancies

SUNYOUNG S. LEE, MD, PHD • GRACE K. DY, MD

INTRODUCTION

Lung cancer is the leading cause of cancer-related death in the United States and worldwide. The American Cancer Society estimates that there will be approximately 222,500 new cases and 155,870 deaths from lung cancer in 2017.[1] Non-small-cell lung cancer (NSCLC) and small-cell lung cancer (SCLC) comprise approximately 95% of lung cancer cases (80% NSCLC and 15% SCLC). Mesothelioma and thymic tumors are less common thoracic malignancies, but often present at an advanced stage with conventional systemic agents demonstrating modest efficacy. The management of advanced thoracic malignancies is multidisciplinary in nature, involving expertise in surgery, radiation oncology, medical oncology, and pathology. Beyond platinum-based cytotoxic chemotherapy which remains a core treatment option for all thoracic malignancies, paradigmatic changes in the systemic treatment approach since the new millennium have evolved mainly in NSCLC, with the development of algorithms defining optimal choice of systemic agents in terms of efficacy and/or safety profile as influenced by the histologic subtype (examples include pemetrexed,[2] bevacizumab,[3] and necitumumab[4]). In addition, variations in the prevalence of actionable oncogenic driver genetic alterations, such as mutations arising from nucleotide alterations in epidermal growth factor receptor (EGFR)[5] and B-Raf proto-oncogene, serine/threonine kinase (BRAF)[6] or fusion kinases such as with anaplastic lymphoma kinase (ALK)[7] and c-ros oncogene 1 (ROS1),[8] susceptible to targeted agents have led to routine tumor genomic sequencing, which is of significance for patients with NSCLC, particularly nonsquamous type, wherein prevalence of these actionable mutations is higher particularly in patients who are nonsmokers. We endeavor to provide an overview of the development of immunotherapies that have galvanized the field of cancer therapeutics. Detailed discussion on toxicities and their management is provided in Chapter 11. Antibody-drug conjugates represent a novel mechanism of using passive immunotherapy to deliver cytotoxic chemotherapy in a targeted manner. They are beyond the scope of this discussion and not covered in this chapter.

IMMUNE CHECKPOINT INHIBITION

Major histocompatibility complex (MHC) molecules present tumor-associated antigens (TAAs), and this process can trigger an antitumor immune response as one of the steps in the cancer immunity cycle and cancer-immune set point of each individual as described in Chapter 1. Multiple TAAs have been recognized, including cancer/testis antigens and aberrantly glycosylated surface proteins such as gangliosides.[9–11] These generally represent germline, differentiation or overexpressed self-antigens found on cancer cells. In comparison, tumor-specific neoantigens originating from somatic gene mutations are thought to be most immunogenic as central tolerance mechanisms have not been developed. Effector T-cells (Teff) and regulatory T-cells (Treg) are essential to the activation, maintenance, and inhibition of the immune system. Teffs and Tregs are regulated by cytokines that can both potentiate or inhibit the immune response. Teffs are primed and activated via the specific interaction of T-cell receptors (TCRs) and TAAs expressed on MHC molecules. This pathway requires co-stimulation via ligand-receptor interactions between T cells (CD80, CD86, CD137L, and CD27) and antigen-presenting cells (CD28, CD137, and CD70). Overactivation of the immune system is regulated or prevented by immune checkpoint inhibition. Prolonged activation of the immune pathway by chronic infection or malignancy can result in signal inhibition of immune system activation.[12] Malignant cells can further modulate the immune checkpoint pathway and evade surveillance of the native immune system. Key molecules of immune checkpoints have been identified, and these include programmed death-ligand 1 (PD-1, CD279), programmed death-ligand 1 (PD-L1, CD274 or B7-H1), cytotoxic T-lymphocyte–associated antigen 4 (CTLA-4), lymphocyte-activation gene 3 (LAG-3), T-cell membrane protein 3 (TIM-3), V-domain Ig suppressor of T-cell activation (VISTA), B- and T-cell lymphocyte attenuator, and killer-cell immunoglobulin-like receptors.[13–16]

Immune checkpoint inhibition has now been incorporated as a standard approach in the therapy for various malignancies. Among the potential immune checkpoints mentioned above, PD-1/PD-L1 and CTLA-4 are two targets that have been extensively studied. PD-1 is expressed on immune cells including T and B cells. Various tissues including cancer cells express PD-1 ligands (PD-L1 and PD-L2). The complementary binding of PD-1 and PD-L1/PD-L2 results in immune system exhaustion and Treg upregulation, which handicaps the immune system surveillance system to eliminate malignant cells.[17] CTLA-4 molecules are also responsible for muting the immune response. CTLA-4 is regulated by negative feedback, whereby increasing activation of TCRs results in increased CTLA-4 expression. Upregulated CTLA-4 molecules inhibit the co-stimulatory pathway needed for T-cell activation via direct competition with CD28 ligands. The expression of PD-1/PD-L1 and CTLA-4 increases with increasing proinflammatory cytokine concentrations released during chronic infections or malignancies.[18,19] Immune checkpoint inhibitors antagonizing PD-1/PD-L1 and CTLA-4 have been shown to restore patient's own antitumor activities in many solid and hematologic malignancies.

Several immune checkpoint inhibitors have been extensively investigated. Nivolumab is a fully human IgG4 monoclonal antibody that binds to PD-1 and inhibits PD-1 and PD-L1/PD-L2 interaction.[20] It has been approved for renal cell carcinoma, urothelial carcinoma, head and neck squamous cell carcinoma, Hodgkin lymphoma, melanoma, microsatellite instability-high colorectal cancer, and NSCLC. Pembrolizumab is a humanized IgG4 monoclonal antibody against PD-1,[21] and it has been approved for melanoma, head and neck squamous cell carcinoma, Hodgkin lymphoma, urothelial carcinoma, microsatellite instability-high cancer, and NSCLC.

Atezolizumab and durvalumab are humanized IgG1 monoclonal antibodies, and avelumab is a fully human IgG1 monoclonal antibody. These antibodies selectively bind to PD-L1, inhibiting the interaction between PD-L1 and PD-1 or CD80. Their specificity allows for preservation of interactions between PD-1 and PD-L2.[22]

Atezolizumab, durvalumab, and avelumab are engineered to prevent antibody-dependent cell-mediated cytotoxicity of T cells that also express PD-L1. Atezolizumab has been approved for metastatic NSCLC and advanced urothelial carcinoma. Durvalumab received an FDA-accelerated approval for advanced bladder cancer.[23] Avelumab is approved for the treatment of metastatic Merkel cell carcinoma.[24] Ipilimumab is a recombinant human IgG1 monoclonal antibody that binds to CTLA-4. Ipilimumab was first approved by the FDA for the treatment of unresectable or metastatic melanoma in 2011.[25] Since then, ipilimumab has been extensively studied in many clinical studies including lung cancer. Tremelimumab is a fully human monoclonal IgG2 antibody against CTLA-4 and has been actively tested for many solid cancers including malignant mesothelioma.[26]

NON-SMALL-CELL LUNG CANCER

As mentioned earlier, the management of NSCLC is multidisciplinary in approach, with surgical resection often favored as a curative modality for early-stage diseases, whereas systemic and radiation therapies are integrated into the treatment plan when disease is metastatic either locoregionally or distantly. To this date, platinum-based cytotoxic chemotherapy forms the backbone of the systemic treatment plan for many patients in various settings: perioperatively as neoadjuvant or adjuvant therapy, concurrently with radiation as curative bimodality approach in the management of patients with locoregionally advanced disease, and palliatively as first-line treatment in patients with distant metastases. We hereby, in this section, provide an overview of how immunotherapy has changed and is changing the therapeutic landscape in the management of NSCLC. Multiple clinical trials of immune checkpoint inhibitors either alone or in combination with other treatment modalities including chemotherapy, radiation therapy, or targeted therapy in adjuvant or neoadjuvant settings are underway listed in Table 3.1. Table 3.2. summarizes the key clinical features of pivotal trials of immune checkpoint inhibitors in NSCLC.

NSCLC is genetically heterogeneous with a wide spectrum in terms of tumor mutational burden.[27] Prevalence of PD-L1 expression also varies, with a range of expression between 21% and 95%.[28] The aggregate of studies to date suggest that there is some correlation between the degree of PD-L1 expression with a better response to anti-PD-1/PD-L1 antibodies,[29] although clinical responses can be seen in approximately 10%–15% of

TABLE 3.1
NSCLC Phase 3 Trials

Agent	Trial	Histology	Treatment	Line of Therapy
Nivolumab	ANVIL, NCT02595944	All	Nivolumab versus Best Supportive Care	Adjuvant therapy
Nivolumab	CheckMate 026, NCT02041533	All	Nivolumab versus Chemo	First line therapy for Stage IV or recurrent PD-L1 positive disease
Nivolumab	CheckMate 027, NCT02477826	All	Nivolumab, or Nivolumab + Ipilimumab, or Nivolumab + Chemo versus Chemo	First line therapy for Stage IV or recurrent disease
Nivolumab	CheckMate 816, NCT02998528	All	Nivolumab + Ipilimumab versus Chemo	First line therapy
Nivolumab	CheckMate 057, NCT01673867	Non-squamous	Nivolumab versus Docetaxel	Second line therapy post platinum chemo
Nivolumab	CheckMate 017, NCT01642004	Squamous	Nivolumab versus Docetaxel	Second line therapy post platinum chemo
Nivolumab	NCT02768558	All	RT + Chemo + Nivolumab or Placebo	First line therapy
ONO-4538 (Nivolumab)	NCT03117049	Non-squamous	Carboplatin, paclitaxel + bevacizumab + ONO-4538 or placebo	First line therapy or second line in patients unsuitable for RT
Nivolumab/ Ipilimumab	CheckMate 722, NCT02864251	All	Nivolumab + Chemo or Nivolumab + Ipilimumab + Chemo versus Chemo	First line therapy in Stage IV or recurrent disease
Nivolumab	CheckMate 384, NCT02713867			
Nivolumab/ Ipilimumab	NCT02869789	All	Nivolumab + Ipilimumab	First line therapy in Stage IV or recurrent disease
Pembrolizumab	Keynote 091, NCT02504372	All	Pembrolizumab versus Placebo	Second line therapy, post resection
Pembrolizumab	Keynote 024, NCT02142738	All	Pembrolizumab versus Chemo	First line therapy in Stage IV disease
Pembrolizumab	Keynote 407, NCT02775435	Squamous	Chemo + Pembrolizumab versus Chemo	First line therapy in metastatic squamous
Pembrolizumab	Keynote 010, NCT01905657	All, PD-L1 positive	Pembrolizumab versus Docetaxel	Second line therapy
Pembrolizumab	Keynote 189, NCT02578680	Non-squamous	Chemo versus Chemo + Pembrolizumab	First line therapy in metastatic non-squamous
Pembrolizumab	NCT02864394	All, PD-L1 positive	Pembrolizumab versus Docetaxel	Second line therapy
Atezolizumab	Oak, NCT02008227	All	Atezolizumab versus Docetaxel	Second line therapy
Atezolizumab	IM Power 210, NCT02813785	All	Atezolizumab versus Docetaxel	Second line therapy
Atezolizumab	IM Power 132, NCT02657434	Non-squamous	Chemo + Atezolizumab versus Chemo	First line therapy for Stage IV disease

Continued

TABLE 3.1
NSCLC Phase 3 Trials—cont'd

Agent	Trial	Histology	Treatment	Line of Therapy
Atezolizumab	IM Power 130, NCT02367781	Non-squamous	Chemo + Atezolizumab versus Chemo	First line therapy for Stage IV disease
Atezolizumab	IM Power 150, NCT02366143	Non-squamous	Chemo + Atezolizumab + Bevacizumab versus Chemo + Bevacizumab	First line therapy for Stage IV disease
Atezolizumab	IM Power 010, NCT02486718	All	Atezolizumab versus Best Supportive Care	Adjuvant therapy
Atezolizumab	IM Power 110, NCT02409342	Non-squamous	Atezolizumab versus Chemo	First line therapy in Stage IV disease
Atezolizumab	IM Power 131, NCT02367794	Squamous	Chemo + Atezolizumab versus Chemo	First line therapy in Stage IV disease
Avelumab	Javelin Lung 200, NCT02395172	All	Avelumab versus Docetaxel	Second line therapy
Durvalumab/ Tremelimumab	NEPTUNE, NCT02542293	All	Durvalumab + Tremelimumab versus Chemo	First line therapy
Durvalumab	Pacific, NCT02125461	All	Duvalumab versus Best Supportive Care	Adjuvant therapy
AZD9291/ Durvalumab	Caural, NCT02454933	All, T790 positive	AZD9291 + Durvalumab versus Durvalumab	Adjuvant therapy
Durvalumab	Arctic, NCT02352948	All	Durvalumab versus Durvalumab + Tremelimumab	Adjuvant therapy
Durvalumab	NCT03003962	All	Durvalumab versus Chemo	First line therapy
Durvalumab/ Tremelimumab	POSEIDON, NCT03164616	All	Durvalumab + Chemo versus Durvalumab + Tremelimumab + Chemo	First line therapy
Durvalumab	Mystic, NCT02453282	All	Durvalumab + Tremelimumab versus Durvalumab versus Chemo	First line therapy
Durvalumab	NCT02273375	All	Durvalumab versus Best Supportive Care	Adjuvant therapy

PD-L1 negative tumors.[30,31] Other independent factors, such as mutational burden and presence of tumor-infiltrating lymphocytes, also need to be considered.[27] Table 3.1 summarizes phase 3 trials in NSCLC of major anti-PD-1/PD-L1 inhibitors that are ongoing or underway as of the last quarter of 2017. Table 3.2 provides an outline of the key results from the pivotal randomized trials of these agents in NSCLC.

Treatment of Metastatic Non-Small-Cell Lung Cancer
PD-1 inhibitors
Nivolumab is the first immune checkpoint inhibitor approved for NSCLC. In March 2015, it was FDA approved for metastatic squamous cell carcinoma that progressed during or after first-line chemotherapy. Approval was based on results from CHECKMATE-017: a

TABLE 3.2
Key Clinical Features of Pivotal Trials of Immune Checkpoint Inhibitors in NSCLC

Trial	Phase	Histology	Biomarker Selection	Treatment	N	RR 95% CI	PFS 95% CI	OS 95% CI	Reference
SECOND-LINE, METASTATIC STAGE IV									
CheckMate 017	3	Squamous	None	Nivolumab	135	20% (14–28)	3.5 mo (2.1–4.9)	9.2 mo (7.3–13.3)	Brahmer NEJM
				Docetaxel	137	9% (5–15)	2.8 mo (2.1–3.5)	6.0 mo (5.1–7.3)	
CheckMate 057	3	Nonsquamous	None	Nivolumab	292	19% (15–24)	2.3 mo (2.2–3.3)	12.2 mo (9.7–15.0)	Borghaei NEJM
				Docetaxel	290	12% (9–17)	4.2 mo (3.5–4.9)	9.4 mo (8.1–10.7)	
Keynote 010	3	NSCLC	PD-L1 > 1%	Pembrolizumab 2 mg/kg	345	18.0% (14.1–22.5)	5.0 mo (4.0–6.5)	14.9 mo (10.4–NR)	Herbst Lancet
				Pembrolizumab 10 mg/kg	346	18.5% (14.5–23.0)	5.2 mo (4.1–8.1)	17.3 mo (11.8–NR)	
				Docetaxel	343	9.3% (6.5–12.9)	4.1 mo (3.6–4.3)	8.2 mo (6.4–10.7)	
OAK	3	NSCLC	None	Atezolizumab	425	14% (NA)	2.8 mo (2.6–3.0)	13.8 mo (11.8–15.7)	Rittmeyer Lancet
				Docetaxel	425	13% (NA)	4.0 mo (3.3–4.2)	9.6 mo (8.6–11.2)	
FIRST-LINE, METASTATIC STAGE IV									
Keynote 024	3	NSCLC	PD-L1 > 50%	Pembrolizumab	154	44.8% (36.8–53.0)	10.3 mo (6.7–NR)	NR	Reck NEJM
				Platinum-based chemotherapy	151	27.8% (20.8–35.7)	6.0 mo (4.2–6.2)	NR	
CheckMate 026	3	NSCLC	PD-L1 > 1%	Nivolumab	271	34% (24–45)	4.2 mo (3.0–5.6)	14.4 mo (11.7–17.4)	Carbone NEJM
				Platinum-based chemotherapy	270	39% (30–48%)	5.9 mo (5.4–6.9)	13.2 mo (10.7–17.1)	
Keynote 021	2	Nonsquamous	None	Pembrolizumab + Carboplatin + Pemetrexed	60	54.5% (NA)	13.0 mo (8.3–NR)	NA	Langer Lancet Oncology
				Carboplatin + Pemetrexed	63	32.0 (NA)	8.9 mo (4.4–10.3)	NA	

Continued

TABLE 3.2
Key Clinical Features of Pivotal Trials of Immune Checkpoint Inhibitors in NSCLC—cont'd

Trial	Phase	Histology	Biomarker Selection	Treatment	N	RR 95% CI	PFS 95% CI	OS 95% CI	Reference
Keynote 189	3	Nonsquamous	None	Pembrolizumab + Cisplatin or Carboplatin+ Pemetrexed	410	47.6% (42.6–52.5)	8.8 mo (7.6–9.2)	NR	Gandhi NEJM
				Cisplatin or Carboplatin + Pemetrexed	206	18.9% (13.8–25)	4.9 mo (4.7–5.5)	11.3 (8.7–15.1)	
MYSTIC*	3	NSCLC	PD-L1 25%	Durvalumab+ Tremeliumumab Platinum-based chemotherapy					

CONSOLIDATION AFTER CONCURRENT CHEMORADIATION, STAGE III

Trial	Phase	Histology	Biomarker Selection	Treatment	N	RR 95% CI	PFS 95% CI	OS 95% CI	Reference
PACIFIC	2	NSCLC	None	Durvalumab	473	28.4% (24.3–32.9)	16.8 mo (13.0–18.1)	NA	Antonia NEJM
				Placebo	236	16.0% (11.3–21.6)	5.6 mo (4.6–7.8)	NA	

NA: not available; NR, not reached
*Data not yet publicly released

randomized, open-label, phase 3 study,[32] which evaluated nivolumab at 3 mg/kg administered every 2 weeks compared with docetaxel at 75 mg/m^2 every 3 weeks as second-line therapy for 272 patients with stage IIIB or IV squamous cell carcinoma. The primary endpoint of overall survival (OS) was met. The median OS and OS rate at 1 year was 9.2 months and 42% with nivolumab, while in the docetaxel cohort, these were 6.0 months and 20%, respectively. There was 41% lower risk of death with nivolumab than docetaxel (hazard ratio [HR], 0.59; 95% confidence interval [CI] 0.44−0.79). This survival benefit was observed regardless of the expression of the PD-L1. The counterpart study in 582 patients with stage IIIB or IV nonsquamous histology was CHECKMATE-057. Patients with EGFR mutations or ALK translocations comprised 14% and 4% of the study population, respectively. Similar to CHECKMATE-017, the primary endpoint was met in this study, with median OS of 12.2 months and an OS rate at 1 year of 51% in patients who received nivolumab,[33] while the median OS was 9.4 months and the OS rate at 1 year was 39% in the docetaxel treatment arm. The objective response rate (ORR) was 19% versus 12% in each cohort, respectively. In contrast to the findings in CHECKMATE-017, there appeared to be a strong predictive association between PD-L1 expression and efficacy outcomes of response rate and survival (OS and progression-free survival [PFS]), regardless of the expression levels chosen for analysis (1%, 5%, and 10%). A relevant observation was that although the presence of PD-L1 expression was associated with higher ORR of 31%−37% in the cohorts with PD-L1 above the 1%−10% cutoff relative to the cohorts with lower expression levels, there was an approximately 10% ORR in patients with low PD-L1 expression, with median duration of response similar to that observed in the higher PD-L1 expression group. Moreover, survival in PD-L1 low-expression groups with nivolumab was at least similar to docetaxel.

These two studies thus provide the rationale for the use of nivolumab in the second-line setting without prerequisite ascertainment of PD-L1 status for treatment selection. This has prompted several economic analyses which have demonstrated improved quality-adjusted life year (QALY) with nivolumab but with associated increased cost of therapy of an estimated additional $155,000 and $187,000 per QALY gained compared with docetaxel in squamous and nonsquamous NSCLC, respectively.[34−36] This may potentially be mitigated by PD-L1 testing which can improve the incremental cost-effectiveness ratio by up to 65%.[36] Nonetheless, the experience gained from nivolumab

monotherapy in the second-line setting indicates that patient selection will be crucial to demonstrate superiority to first-line chemotherapy particularly in the nonsquamous cohort, as there is a higher bar for efficacy to be surpassed for the first 6 months of treatment with first-line chemotherapy.

Pembrolizumab, on the other hand, was brought into the clinic later compared with nivolumab. Nonetheless, its eventual successful clinical development in NSCLC ensued from data generated from the cohort of patients enrolled in the phase 1 KEYNOTE-001 study.[37] Four hundred ninety-five patients with advanced NSCLC were enrolled, of which 80% of patients received prior systemic therapy, receiving pembrolizumab either 2 mg/kg or 10 mg/kg every 3 weeks or 10 mg/kg every 2 weeks. Patients with EGFR mutations or ALK translocations represented approximately 15.5% and 2% of the study population, respectively. With emerging data supporting a potential relationship between PD-L1 expression and the efficacy of pembrolizumab, the trial was amended to add a co-primary endpoint to evaluate the efficacy in NSCLC patients with a high level of PD-L1 expression, in addition to enriching for enrollment of patients with tumor PD-L1 expression of at least 1%.[38] In the total population, the ORR was 19.4%, and the median duration of response was 12.5 months. The median PFS was 3.7 months with the median OS of 12.0 months. In patients with tumor PD-L1 expression $\geq$50%, the ORR was 45%, while PD-L1 expression between 1% and 49% had an ORR of 16.5%, and in patients with negative PD-L1 expression, the ORR was 10.7%. These data led to FDA approval of pembrolizumab in October 2015 to treat patients with disease progression after platinum-based chemotherapy in metastatic NSCLC with PD-L1 $\geq$1%, which comprised nearly 80% of all treated patients (or approximately 60% of patients screened). Confirmatory findings were demonstrated in KEYNOTE-010 trial,[39] wherein patients with previously treated NSCLC with PD-L1 expression $\geq$1% were randomized to pembrolizumab 2 mg/kg (345 patients), pembrolizumab 10 mg/kg (346 patients), or docetaxel 75 mg/m^2 (343 patients) every 3 weeks. Primary endpoints were OS and PFS both in the entire treatment population and in the cohort of patients with PD-L1 $\geq$50%, which represented approximately 28% of all patients (or 23% of all screened patients). The median OS for the entire population was 10.4 months, 12.7 months, and 8.5 months, respectively. The median PFS showed no significant difference in the entire population. In comparison, patients with PD-L1 $\geq$50% showed significantly longer

OS of 14.9, 17.3, and 8.2 months as well as a PFS of 5.0, 5.2, and 4.1 months, respectively.

The use of pembrolizumab was further expanded in October 2016 to first-line therapy for patients with metastatic NSCLC whose tumors express PD-L1 ≥50%. This FDA approval was based on results from an open-label, phase 3 trial enrolling 305 patients, who met its primary endpoint of PFS benefit (KEYNOTE-024).[40] In the nearly 1,700 specimens submitted where PD-L1 expression can be ascertained, approximately 30% met the threshold of ≥50%. Patients with EGFR mutations or ALK translocations were not eligible for this trial. The OS at 6 months was 80.2%, and the PFS was 10.3 months in the pembrolizumab cohort; the OS at 6 months was 72.4%, and the PFS was 6.0 months in the chemotherapy cohort. In contrast against expectations, nivolumab as a single agent did not meet its primary endpoint of superior PFS in stage IV NSCLC with PD-L1 expression ≥5% compared with platinum-based chemotherapy (CHECKMATE-026).[41] The OS was also not significantly different, in contrast to the KEYNOTE-024 study. One of the reasons proposed to explain the difference in outcome between these two agents that have similar clinical activity in the second-line setting and across different malignancies was the selection of PD-L1 cutoff in patient inclusion. However, in the exploratory subgroup analysis of patients in CHECKMATE-026 with PD-L1 ≥50%, no difference was observed in ORR: 34% in the nivolumab group and 39% in the chemotherapy group. The HR for disease progression or death was 1.07 (95% CI, 0.77–1.49). Hence, even the potentially "best" cohort did not experience superior results compared to chemotherapy. Because the antibodies used in determining PD-L1 expression are different for the CHECKMATE and KEYNOTE studies, the ideal cutoff to be used for nivolumab is in question, though clearly not the main reason for the trial outcomes since a prior study comparing various PD-L1 immunohistochemical assays demonstrated that the DAKO 22C3 antibody (used for pembrolizumab studies) and DAKO 28-8 (used for nivolumab studies) demonstrated similar analytical performance of PD-L1 expression in NSCLC.[42] Thus, an additional reason proposed that may account for the negative results in CHECKMATE-026 was noted imbalance in clinical characteristics between the treatment groups, with prognostically worse features in the nivolumab group, such as male gender (68% in nivolumab group vs. 55% in chemotherapy group) and the presence of hepatic metastases (20% vs. 13%, respectively). Although CHECKMATE-026 included patients with prior radiation (approximately 40%), whereas this was more limited in enrollment to KEYNOTE-024, retrospective analyses associated prior exposure to radiation therapy with better outcomes to pembrolizumab treatment, and thus unlikely to account for the difference in outcomes between the two studies.[43] Another potential factor that may influence the observed difference in outcomes may relate to subsequent therapy received in the control group. While 60% of patients in the control arm of CHECKMATE-026 received subsequent treatment with nivolumab, only 43.7% of patients in the control arm of KEYNOTE-024 received pembrolizumab.

On May 10, 2017, the US FDA granted accelerated approval for combination of pembrolizumab with pemetrexed and carboplatin as first-line therapy for metastatic nonsquamous NSCLC.[44] This was based on a randomized, phase 2, multicohort KEYNOTE-021 study, where previously untreated patients with stage IIIB or IV nonsquamous NSCLC were randomly assigned to pembrolizumab plus chemotherapy or chemotherapy alone. Chemotherapy consisted of four cycles of carboplatin with pemetrexed, followed by optional maintenance pemetrexed indefinitely. Pembrolizumab was administered along with chemotherapy for up to 24 months. Patients in the chemotherapy alone arm were allowed to crossover to receive pembrolizumab monotherapy upon disease progression. Primary endpoint was ORR. Patients with EGFR or ALK gene alterations were excluded. In the nonsquamous cohort where carboplatin and pemetrexed regimen was assigned, the distribution of patients with PD-L1 expression <1% was relatively similar between the two treatment arms. There was slightly greater proportion of patients with PD-L1 ≥50% in the pembrolizumab combination group (33%) compared with the chemotherapy only control group (27%). There was also slightly higher proportion of women enrolled in the pembrolizumab combination group. The ORR in the pembrolizumab plus chemotherapy cohort was 55%, and that in the chemotherapy alone cohort was 29%. This absolute 26% difference was statistically significant (95% CI, 9%–42%; $P = .0016$). The ORR in patients treated in the pembrolizumab combination group was similar between those with <1% (57%; 95% CI, 34%–79%) and ≥1% (54%; 95% CI 37%–70%) PD-L1 expression. In comparison, for the chemotherapy-alone group, the ORR in PD-L1 <1% was 13% (95% CI, 3%–34%), PD-L1 ≥1%–49% was 39% (95% CI, 20%–51%), and PD-L1 ≥50% was 35% (95% CI, 14%–62%). The median PFS was 13 months for the pembrolizumab combination group versus 8.9 months for the chemotherapy-alone group. However, grade 3 or higher adverse events attributed to treatment occurred more frequently in patients receiving the pembrolizumab plus chemotherapy combination (39%) versus chemotherapy alone (26%). Approximately 32% of patients (20 patients) in the control group crossed-over to receive pembrolizumab within the study. There was no difference in OS noted (HR 0.9; 95% CI, 0.42−1.91; $P = .39$). The accelerated approval for this combination with chemotherapy is contingent on the results from the international, randomized, double-blind, confirmatory phase 3 trial KEYNOTE-189 evaluating the combination of either cisplatin or carboplatin plus pemetrexed in combination with either pembrolizumab or placebo. Co-primary endpoints in this study are PFS and OS. This study showed improvement in OS seen across all PD-L1 categories. The estimated 12-month OS was 69.2% (95% CI, 64.1%−73.8%) in the pembrolizumab plus chemotherapy group versus 49.4% (95% CI, 42.1−56.2) in the placebo group (HR for death 0.49; 95% CI, 0.38−0.64; $P < .001$). Notable as well is that all subgroups appeared to benefit from the pembrolizumab plus chemotherapy combination, including patients who were never-smokers (HR, 0.23; 95% CI, 0.1−0.54). This is an important and relevant distinction from KEYNOTE-024, which showed an HR for death of 0.9 for pembrolizumab monotherapy as first-line treatment in PD-L1-high NSCLC, with 95% CI estimate crossing 1.0 (95% CI, 0.11−7.59). Another key information that may influence the OS outcomes in KEYNOTE-189 is that in the placebo-combination group, only 41.3% received immunotherapy after disease progression (either crossover in the trial to receive pembrolizumab or receiving immunotherapy outside the trial).

PD-L1 inhibitors

Atezolizumab has been evaluated in multiple clinical trials for solid malignancies including NSCLC. Data from the phase 3 OAK trial meanwhile showed slightly different results for the biomarker analyses.[45] In 425 NSCLC patients who received atezolizumab at 1,200 mg every 3 weeks as a second line therapy, the OS was statistically superior at 13.8 months, whereas those who received docetaxel had an OS of 9.6 months. However, in contrast to the phase 2 study, this phase 3 study showed improved survival regardless of the PD-L1 expression level in both squamous and nonsquamous histology. The results from these studies led to FDA approval for the use of atezolizumab in the treatment of metastatic NSCLC with any PD-L1 expression level as a second line therapy. More recently, results from the three-arm phase III IMpower150 study

evaluating the combination of atezolizumab with (arm B) or without bevacizumab (arm A) in combination with carboplatin and paclitaxel in patients with NSCLC were reported.[46] The control group (arm C) was carboplatin and paclitaxel plus bevacizumab, Co-primary endpoints in this study were PFS and OS, and PFS benefit was seen regardless of PD-L1 status. The OS benefit was also demonstrated in arm B compared to arm C, with details to be reported in another major meeting in 2018. Landmark analysis of the intention-to-treat population showed 6-month and 12-month OS of 56% and 18% in the control carboplatin/paclitaxel/bevacizumab group versus 67% and 37% in the atezolizumab combination with carboplatin/paclitaxel/bevacizumab group. Moreover, this study permitted patients with EGFR mutation or ALK translocation to be enrolled after disease progression to one or more approved targeted therapies. While anti-PD-1/anti-PD-L1 therapy as monotherapy has not demonstrated significant benefit in NSCLC with alterations in EGFR/ALK, this study demonstrated that in this molecular subgroup, chemotherapy plus bevacizumab and atezolizumab conferred improved median PFS of 9.7 months versus 6.1 months with chemotherapy plus bevacizumab only, with an HR of 0.59 (95% CI, 0.37−0.94). Clinical benefit was even better defined for patients with EGFR exon 19 deletion or L858R mutation, with an HR of 0.41 (95% CI, 0.22−0.78) and a median PFS of 10.2 months.

An open-label, phase 1/2 study evaluated the clinical activity of durvalumab in multiple solid tumors including NSCLC. Two hundred patients with advanced NSCLC refractory to all standard therapies were followed. The ORR was 16% overall and 27% in patients with PD-L1 ≥25%. The ORR was higher in squamous (21%) than nonsquamous patients (13%).[47] In the single-arm, phase 2 ATLANTIC study of durvalumab administered at 10 mg/kg every 2 weeks for up to 12 months as third (or higher) line of therapy in patients with locally advanced or metastatic NSCLC, patient cohorts were defined by the presence of activating mutations in EGFR or ALK translocation and tumor PD-L1 expression, with ORR as the primary endpoint. In cohort 1 (EGFR mutation/ALK positive patients), patients with PD-L1 ≥25% of tumor cells with membrane staining had an ORR of 12%, with a median PFS and an OS of 1.9 and 13.3 months. Patients with PD-L1 <25% or negative status had an ORR of 3.6%, with a median PFS and an OS of 1.9 and 9.9 months.[48] In the EGFR/ALK wild-type cohort[49] where tumor PD-L1 <25%, the ORR was 7.5%, whereas the ORR was 16.4% in PD-L1 ≥25%. Cohort 3 consisted of patients with PD-L1 ≥90% of tumor cells. In this group, the ORR was 30.9%, with median PFS of 2.4 months. One-year OS was 34.5%, 47.7%, and 50.8% from the lowest to the highest PD-L1 cutoffs, respectively.

Another PD-L1 inhibitor, avelumab, showed an acceptable safety profile and antitumor activity in patients with progressive or treatment-resistant NSCLC in an open-label, phase 1b clinical trial.[50] The trial enrolled 184 previously treated patients with metastatic or recurrent NSCLC with a median follow-up duration of 8.8 months. Twenty-two patients (12%) achieved a confirmed objective response including 1 complete response and 21 partial responses. Seventy patients (38%) had stable disease. Overall, 92 (50%) of 184 patients achieved disease control.

Cytotoxic T-lymphocyte–associated antigen 4 inhibitors in combination trials

The activity of ipilimumab in advanced NSCLC was first investigated in a randomized, phase 2 study,[51] wherein 204 patients were assigned 1:1:1 to receive paclitaxel and carboplatin with either placebo or ipilimumab in one of the following two regimens: concurrent ipilimumab (four doses of ipilimumab plus paclitaxel and carboplatin followed by two doses of placebo plus paclitaxel and carboplatin) or phased ipilimumab (two doses of placebo plus paclitaxel and carboplatin followed by four doses of ipilimumab plus paclitaxel and carboplatin). A subset analysis of this study showed that phased ipilimumab combined with paclitaxel and carboplatin met the primary endpoint of improved immune-related PFS. However, due to toxicities and limited benefit, this was not further evaluated. However, on the heels of the clinical successes seen in melanoma with the combination of PD-1/PD-L1 and CTLA-4 inhibitors, the development of ipilimumab in NSCLC is resurrected, with over 1,000 trials ongoing in NSCLC evaluating different combinations with anti-PD-1/PD-L1 agents, including combinations with anti-CTLA-4 agents.

An open-label, phase 1 clinical trial studying the combination of nivolumab and ipilimumab for patients with recurrent stage IIIB/IV chemotherapy-naive NSCLC was shown to have clinical activity.[52] Patients were assigned 1:1:1 to nivolumab 1 mg/kg every 2 weeks plus ipilimumab 1 mg/kg every 6 weeks, nivolumab 3 mg/kg every 2 weeks plus ipilimumab 1 mg/kg every 12 weeks, or nivolumab 3 mg/kg every 2 weeks plus ipilimumab 1 mg/kg every 6 weeks. Objective responses were 47% and 38% in the ipilimumab every 12-weeks cohort and ipilimumab every 6-weeks cohort, respectively. Median duration of response was not

reached in either cohort with median follow-up times of 12.8 and 11.8 months, respectively. Objective responses in patients with PD-L1 ≥1% were achieved in 57% of each cohort. The combination regimen was well tolerated, and there was no treatment-related death. This study revealed encouraging clinical activity with a high response rate and durable response, as well as a tolerable safety profile.

Several ongoing randomized trials are aimed at assessing the combination of PD-1/PD-L1 and CTLA-4 inhibitors. These are listed in Table 3.1. Tremelimumab is another fully human anti-CTLA4 which had been in clinical development for more than a decade. The initial results from the ongoing randomized, phase 3 MYSTIC study comparing the combination of durvalumab plus tremelimumab with durvalumab or standard platinum-based chemotherapy as a first-line treatment for patients with locally advanced or metastatic NSCLC were first announced in a press release on July 27, 2017. The primary endpoint of PFS superiority compared to chemotherapy alone in patients with PD-L1 expression of ≥25% (as determined by the VENTANA Sp263 assay) was not met. The final OS result, a co-primary endpoint, is still pending and is expected to be announced by the second half of 2018. Details of the results have not yet been released. Biomarker development is thus one of the "hot" areas of research as there is a keen need to optimize selection of patients who require combination therapy for optimal tumor control and to spare patients who benefit from anti-PD-1/PD-L1 therapy alone to avoid the toxicities of combination treatment.

Treatment in the Neoadjuvant, Adjuvant, and Postchemoradiation Setting

A number of neoadjuvant and adjuvant trials are currently ongoing in NSCLC, with patient inclusion not necessarily restricted according to PD-L1 expression. Nivolumab was tested in the neoadjuvant setting, and the results were presented at the 2017 ASCO Annual Meeting.[53] Twenty-two patients with stage IB–IIIA NSCLC received two doses of nivolumab 3 mg/kg over 4 weeks before surgery. Neoadjuvant nivolumab in resectable NSCLC did not delay surgery. 43% of patients had a major pathologic response (<10% viable tumor cells in resection specimen), in contrast to the radiographic response rate of 10%. Pretreatment tumor PD-L1 staining did not correlate with the major pathologic response rate. Of interest is that T cells specific for the dominant tumor-specific mutation-associated neoantigen expanded in the peripheral blood following neoadjuvant treatment with nivolumab. 86% of patients remained alive and recurrence free with a median post-op follow-up of 9 months.

PACIFIC study is a randomized, double-blinded, placebo-controlled, phase 3 trial designed to assess the efficacy of durvalumab for patients with locally advanced, unresectable stage III NSCLC, whose disease did not progress after standard concurrent chemoradiation therapy.[54] Patients were randomized in a 2:1 ratio to durvalumab 10 mg/kg every 2 weeks or placebo for up to 12 months, with treatment starting within 1−42 days after completing chemoradiation. The ORR was higher in the durvalumab group than the placebo group (28.4% vs. 16%; $P < .001$). The median PFS with durvalumab was 16.8 months (95% CI, 13.0−18.1 months) with durvalumab versus 5.6 months with placebo (95% CI, 4.6−7.8 months). The 12-month PFS rate was 55.9% in patients randomized to receive durvalumab versus 35.3% in the placebo group. The median time to death or distant metastasis was 23.2 months with durvalumab versus 14.6 months with placebo treatment (HR, 0.52; 95% CI 0.39−0.69). Notably, pneumonitis or radiation pneumonitis of any grade occurred in 33.9% of patients who received durvalumab versus 24.8% in the placebo group, while Common Terminology Criteria (CTC) grade 3 or 4 pneumonitis or radiation pneumonitis rates were 3.4% and 2.6%, respectively. The OS is not mature yet at the time of publication of the results.

Small-Cell Lung Cancer

Despite its chemosensitivity and radiosensitivity, more than 80% of patients with limited stage (LS)-SCLC and nearly all patients with extensive stage (ES)-SCLC eventually succumb to this disease.[55–57] Aside from oral topotecan that received approval in 2007 for SCLC (the intravenous formulation had been in use for SCLC since the late 90s), there has been no new effective therapeutic agent identified in nearly 20 years for SCLC, despite numerous clinical trials evaluating multiple new cytotoxic and targeted therapies over the years.

Ipilimumab was the first immune checkpoint inhibitor to be investigated in SCLC.[58] In a randomized, double-blind, phase 2 trial, 130 chemotherapy-naïve patients with ES-SCLC were randomized (1:1:1) to receive ipilimumab concurrently with chemotherapy (using carboplatin and paclitaxel) or phased with chemotherapy initially followed by chemotherapy plus ipilimumab or to standard chemotherapy without ipilimumab. Phased ipilimumab improved immune-related PFS (HR 0.64; $P = .03$), but there was no statistically significant improvement in PFS (HR 0.93; $P = .37$) or OS (HR 0.75; $P = .13$). In a follow-up phase 3 study,[59] 954 patients with newly diagnosed ES-SCLC were randomized 1:1 to receive etoposide and platinum

(cisplatin or carboplatin) plus ipilimumab 10 mg/kg or etoposide and platinum plus placebo, followed by ipilimumab or placebo maintenance. Median PFS was 4.6 months in the first group; 4.4 months in the latter group. There was no prolongation of OS with the addition of ipilimumab to chemotherapy (11.0 vs. 10.9 months, respectively).

In contrast, the combination of ipilimumab with nivolumab demonstrated signs of clinical activity in early phase trials of ES-SCLC to date. In the SCLC cohort of CHECKMATE-032, a phase 1/2 study of nivolumab alone versus nivolumab in combination with ipilimumab in patients with advanced or metastatic solid tumors, 216 patients with relapsed SCLC with disease progression after at least one previous platinum-containing regimen were enrolled into three cohorts, regardless of PD-L1 expression. 98 patients received nivolumab alone at 3 mg/kg (N3), 3 patients received nivolumab 1 mg/kg plus ipilimumab 1 mg/kg (N1-I1), 61 patients received nivolumab 1 mg/kg plus ipilimumab 3 mg/kg (N1-I3), and 54 patients received nivolumab 3 mg/kg plus ipilimumab 1 mg/kg (N3I-1). Tumor responses were seen regardless of PD-L1 expression. As expected, CTC grade 3 or 4 treatment-related adverse events were the highest in the N1-I3 cohort (30%). Primary endpoint of ORR was 10%, 23%, and 19% in the N3, N1-I3, and N3-I1 cohorts, respectively, with corresponding median OS of 4.4, 7.7, and 6.0 months. The corresponding 1-year OS rates were 33%, 43%, and 35%, respectively.[60,61] Among patients with tumor response, duration of response was not yet reached at the time of publication for the N3 cohort (95% CI, 4.4 months−not reached), 7.7 months for the N1-I3 cohort (95% CI 4.0 months−not reached), and 4.4 months for the N3-I1 cohort (95% CI, 3.7 months−not reached). The dose-schedule of N1-I3 as induction for four cycles followed by nivolumab alone at 240 mg flat dose every 2 weeks for a maximum of 12 months from the start of consolidation/maintenance therapy is currently being investigated in the randomized phase 2 study STIMULI, evaluating the effect of this regimen versus observation with the primary endpoint of OS and PFS in LS-SCLC after standard of care chemoradiotherapy.

Although it may be hypothesized that selection of SCLC patients based on PD-L1 expression may enrich for potential responders to anti-PD-1/PD-L1 therapies similar to the experience seen in NSCLC, a number of studies, including CHECKMATE-032 have demonstrated that this biomarker is not predictive of response in this patient population. In the cohort of patients with relapsed SCLC demonstrating PD-L1 expression of ≥1% (either on tumor cells, inflammatory cells, or stroma[62]) in KEYNOTE-028, pembrolizumab administered at 10 mg/kg every 2 weeks showed a response rate of 33%, with median duration of response of 19.4 months (range 3.6 to ≥20 months). The median PFS was 1.9 months, with a 1-year OS rate of 37.7%, similar to the nivolumab-only cohort in CHECKMATE-032. In another phase 2 study, the role of maintenance pembrolizumab in patients with ES-SCLC who had a response or achieved stable disease after four to six cycles of platinum/etoposide was evaluated.[63] Tumor PD-L1 ≥1% expression was a prerequisite for study enrollment. The median PFS observed in this single-arm study was 1.4 months (90% CI 1.3−4.0 months) with a median OS of 9.2 months, clearly highlighting the need for better biomarkers to identify patients who benefit from anti-PD-1 monotherapy.

Due to the high association of carcinogenesis of SCLC with smoking, it is not surprising that there is high mutational burden associated with this malignancy.[64,65] Despite these features, the outcome of treatment with immune checkpoint inhibitors in SCLC is far less impressive as illustrated above, especially when compared to NSCLC. The mechanism behind this is unclear. While the prevalence of PD-L1 expression is relatively lower compared to NSCLC (only 31.7% of SCLC had PD-L1 expression ≥1% in KEYNOTE-028 vs. 60.9% of NSCLC with PD-L1 ≥1% in KEYNOTE-001), the lack of association between response to treatment and PD-L1 expression alludes to other immune evasion mechanism, such as immunosuppressive local environment and/or lack of tumor-infiltrating lymphocytes. Several ongoing randomized phase 3 clinical trials of immune checkpoint inhibitors are highlighted in Table 3.3.

Mesothelioma

Malignant pleural mesothelioma (MPM) is a rare malignancy with a poor prognosis. Untreated patients have a median OS of 9.3 months; patients treated with a platinum-based agent and pemetrexed have a median OS of 12.1 months,[66] which can be further improved with the addition of bevacizumab (median OS of 18.8 months compared to cisplatin and pemetrexed alone of 16.1 months).[67] However, the addition of bevacizumab may not be consistently demonstrated, as the combination with gemcitabine and cisplatin did not show an improvement in PFS or OS.[68] To date, no molecular targeted therapy specific to a driver oncogene in MPM has been identified.

Immune checkpoint inhibitors have shown potential, albeit limited benefit in MPM. Perhaps, this may be attributable to its relatively lower mutational burden.[69] In addition, the pathobiology of MPM is mainly driven by atypical inflammation with a low lymphocyte-to-monocyte ratio and a large number of tumor-associated macrophages (TAMs) in the tumor microenvironment (TME).[70,71] This unique immune environment results in a complex immunosuppressive network. The prevalence of PD-L1 expression is 20.7%,[72] also relatively low compared with other solid malignancies such as NSCLC, renal cell carcinoma, and melanoma. The level of PD-L1 expression in MPM has not yet been robustly associated with clinical response to treatment. Clinical trials of immune checkpoint inhibitors for the treatment of MPM are summarized in Table 3.4.

An open-label, single-arm, phase 2 trial tested tremelimumab in 29 patients with chemotherapy-resistant advanced malignant mesothelioma.[26] The ORR was 6.9%, and the duration of response was 12.4 months. When including stable disease, the disease control rate (DCR) was 31%. The median PFS was 6.2 months, and the median OS was 10.7 months. Although it did not statistically meet its endpoint, tremelimumab seemed to have an encouraging clinical activity. However, when it was further investigated in a randomized, phase 2 clinical trial as second- or third-line treatment, tremelimumab monotherapy failed to improve OS, compared with placebo for patients with unresectable malignant mesothelioma.[73]

NivoMes (nivolumab in MPM) is a phase 2 study which tested nivolumab 3 mg/kg every 2 weeks in 38 patients with MPM.[74] The DCR was 50% at 12 weeks. Five patients (13%) showed a partial response, and 12 patients (32%) showed stable disease. A nonrandomized, open-label, phase 1b trial (KEYNOTE-028) also showed that pembrolizumab may have antitumor activity in patients with PD-L1 positive MPM.[75] Twenty-five patients (88% were previously treated) were treated with pembrolizumab: 5 patients had a partial response and 13 of 25 had stable disease. The median response duration was 12.0 months. More convincingly, a randomized, phase 2 trial randomizing 108 MPM patients who progressed from first or second line chemotherapy 1:1 to receive nivolumab 3 mg/kg every 2 weeks or nivolumab 3 mg/kg every 2 weeks plus ipilimumab 1 mg/kg every 6 weeks suggests that immune checkpoint inhibitors may provide new options for relapsed MPM.[76] The DCR at 12 weeks was a primary endpoint. The DCR in the nivolumab cohort was 42.6% and 51.9% in the nivolumab plus ipilimumab cohort. The ORR was 16.7% and 25.9%, respectively. Given the clinical activity seen with immune checkpoint inhibition in MPM, similar to NSCLC and SCLC, these agents are being tested for

TABLE 3.3
SCLC Clinical Trials

		SCLC PHASE 3 CLINICAL TRIALS		
Agent	**Trial**	**Stage**	**Treatment**	**Line of Therapy**
Nivolumab	CheckMate 451, NCT02538666	ES-SCLC	Nivolumab versus Nivolumab + Ipilimumab	Maintenance therapy
Nivolumab	CheckMate 331, NCT02481830	ES-SCLC	Nivolumab versus Chemo	Second line therapy
Pembrolizumab	Keynote-604, NCT03066778	ES-SCLC	Pembrolizumab + Chemo versus Chemo	First line therapy
Atezolizumab	IM Power 133, NCT02763579	ES-SCLC	Atezolizumab + Chemo versus Chemo	First line therapy
Durvalumab/ Tremelimumab	Caspian, NCT03043872	ES-SCLC	Durvalumab + Chemo versus Durvalumab + Tremelimumab + Chemo	First line therapy

		SCLC PHASE 1 AND 2 CLINICAL TRIALS			
Agent	**Trial**	**Phase**	**Stage**	**Treatment**	**Line of Therapy**
Durvalumab/ Tremelimumab/ SGI-110	NCT03085849	Phase 1	ES-SCLC	SGI-110 + Durvalumab + Tremelimumab	Second line therapy
Durvalumab/ Tremelimumab	NCT02701400	Phase 2	Relapsed SCLC	Durvalumab + Tremelimumab + XRT versus Durvalumab + Tremelimumab	Second line therapy
Durvalumab/ Tremelimumab	NCT02937818	Phase 2	ES-SCLC	Durvalumab + Tremelimumab versus Chemo	Second line therapy
Durvalumab/ Tremelimumab	NCT02658214	Phase 1b	Locally advanced or metastatic	Chemo + Durvalumab + Tremelimumab versus Durvalumab + Tremelimumab	First line therapy
Durvalumab	MEDIOLA, NCT02734004	Phase 1/2	Relapsed SCLC	Durvalumab + Olaparib versus Durvalumab	Second line therapy
Trilaciclib/ Atezolizumab	NCT03041311	Phase 2	ES-SCLC	Trilaciclib + Atezolizumab + Chemo versus Trilaciclib + Atezolizumab	First line therapy
Atezolizumab	NCT02748889	Phase 1	ES-SCLC	Chemo versus Chemo + Atezolizumab	First line therapy
Atezolizumab	NCT03059667	Phase 2	ES-SCLC	Atezolizumab versus Chemo	Second line therapy
Nivolumab/ Ipilimumab	NCT03126110	Phase 1/2	ES-SCLC	INCAGN001876 + Nivolumab + Ipilimumab versus Nivolumab + Ipilimumab	First line therapy
Nivolumab/ Ipilimumab	NCT01928394	Phase 1/2	ES-SCLC	Nivolumab + Ipilimumab versus Nivolumab	First line therapy

Continued

TABLE 3.3
SCLC Clinical Trials—cont'd

			SCLC PHASE 1 AND 2 CLINICAL TRIALS		
Agent	**Trial**	**Phase**	**Stage**	**Treatment**	**Line of Therapy**
Pembrolizumab	Keynote 011, NCT01840579	Phase 1	Advanced NSCLC and ES-SCLC	Pembrolizumab versus Pembrolizumab + Ipilimumab versus Pembrolizumab + Chemo	First line therapy
Nivolumab/Ipilimumab	Stimuli, NCT02046733	Phase 2	LS-SCLC	Nivolumab + Ipilimumab	Adjuvant therapy
Nivolumab/Ipilimumab	NCT03043599	Phase 1/2	ES-SCLC	Nivolumab + Ipilimumab + XRT	Adjuvant therapy
Rovalpituzumab/Nivolumab/Ipilimumab	NCT03026166	Phase 1/2	ES-SCLC	Rovalpituzumab + Nivolumab + Ipilimumab versus Rovalpituzumab + Nivolumab	Second line therapy
Nivolumab	NCT02247349	Phase 1/2	Relapsed or Refractory SCLC	Nivolumab + BMS-986012	Second line therapy
Nivolumab	NCT03071757	Phase 1	ES-SCLC and advanced NSCLC	Nivolumab + ABBV-368	Second line therapy
Pembrolizumab	NCT02963090	Phase 2	ES-SCLC	Pembrolizumab versus Topotecan	Second line therapy
Pembrolizumab	NCT02934503	Phase 2	ES-SCLC	Pembrolizumab + Chemo + XRT versus Pembrolizumab + Chemo	First line therapy
Pembrolizumab	NCT02580994	Phase 2	ES-SCLC	Pembrolizumab + chemo versus pembrolizumab	First line therapy
Pembrolizumab	NCT02402920	Phase 1	ES-SCLC	Pembrolizumab + Chemo + XRT versus Pembrolizumab + Chemo	First line therapy
Pembrolizumab/Itacitinib	NCT02646748	Phase 1b	ES-SCLC	Pembrolizumab + Itacitinib versus Pembrolizumab + INCB050465	Second line therapy
Pembrolizumab	Pembro+, NCT02331251	Phase 1b/2	ES-SCLC	Pembrolizumab + Chemo (multiple regimens)	First line therapy
ID-LV305	NCT02122861	Phase 1	ES-SCLC	ID-LV305 versus Best Supportive Care	Second line therapy
Pembrolizumab	Keynote-158, NCT02628067	Phase 2	ES-SCLC	Pembrolizumab versus Best Supportive Care	Second line therapy

TABLE 3.4
Malignant Pleural Mesothelioma Clinical Trials

Agent	Trial	Phase	Treatment	Line of Therapy
Nivolumab/ Ipilimumab	INITIATE, NCT03048474	Phase 2	Nivolumab + Ipilimumab versus Placebo	Second line therapy
Nivolumab/ Ipilimumab	CheckMate 743, NCT02899299	Phase 3	Nivolumab + Ipilimumab versus Chemo	First line therapy
Pembrolizumab	NCT02707666	Phase 1	Pembrolizumab versus Placebo	Neoadjuvant therapy prior to decortication
Pembrolizumab	NCT02959463	Phase 1	Pembrolizumab verus Placebo	Adjuvant therapy
Pembrolizumab	PROMISE-meso, NCT02991482	Phase 3	Pembrolizumab versus Chemo	First line therapy
Pembrolizumab/ Anetumab	NCT03126630	Phase 1/2	Pembrolizumab versus Pembrolizumab + Anetumab	Second line therapy
Pembrolizumab	NCT02784171	Phase 2	Pembrolizumab versus Chemo versus Pembrolizumab + Chemo	First line therapy
Pembrolizumab	NCT02399371	Phase 2	Pembrolizumab versus Placebo	Second line therapy
Atezolizumab	NCT02458638	Phase 2	Atezolizumab versus Placebo	Second line therapy
Atezolizumab	NCT03074513	Phase 2	Atezolizumab + Bevacizumab versus Placebo	Second line therapy
Durvalumab/ Tremelimumab	NCT03075527	Phase 2	Durvalumab + Tremelimumab versus Placebo	Second line therapy
Durvalumab/ Tremelimumab	NCT02592551	Phase 2	Durvalumab versus Durvalumab + Tremelimumab	Second line therapy
Durvalumab	PRE0505, NCT02899195	Phase 2	Durvalumab + Chemo versus Chemo	First line therapy
Durvalumab/ Tremelimumab	NIBIT-MESO-1, NCT02588131	Phase 2	Durvalumab + Tremelimumab	First line or second line therapy

various clinical indications, such as in the neoadjuvant or in the metastatic first-line setting in combination with chemotherapy. Combination with antiangiogenesis inhibitors such as bevacizumab is also being tested.

Thymoma and Thymic Carcinoma

No well-proven standard treatment exists for patients whose disease progressed on or after platinum-based chemotherapeutic regimens for thymoma and thymic carcinoma. The potential role of immune checkpoint inhibitors in this disease was demonstrated in two separate single-arm, phase 2 trials of pembrolizumab. In a Korean study, 33 patients with thymic epithelial tumors[77] (26 thymic carcinoma, 7 thymoma) received pembrolizumab upon disease progression after platinum-based chemotherapy. The ORR was 24.2% (8 partial responses, 17 with stable disease, and 8

with disease progression). The median PFS was 6.2 months for thymic carcinoma, but the PFS in thymoma was not yet reached at the time of study presentation. In a North American single-institution phase 2 clinical trial of pembrolizumab, 40 patients with thymic carcinoma (of which 14 patients with squamous carcinoma histology)[78] were enrolled. Twenty-nine patients had tumor specimen available for PD-L1 testing, of which eight patients had high PD-L1 expression ($\geq$50%). The ORR in this population was 22.5% (1 complete response, 8 partial responses, 20 patients with stable disease, and 11 patients with disease progression), in which 6 out of the 9 responders had high PD-L1 expression. Of interest is the spectrum of treatment-related, immune-related toxicities reported in both studies. In aggregate, CTC grade 3 or higher myocarditis, hepatitis, and myasthenia gravis appeared

TABLE 3.5 Thymic Cancer Clinical Trials				
Agent	**Trial (NCT)***	**Phase**	**Treatment**	**Line of Therapy**
Nivolumab	NIVOTHYM, NCT03134118	Phase 2	Nivolumab versus placebo	Second line therapy
Pembrolizumab	NCT02607631	Phase 2	Pembrolizumabe versus placebo	Second line therapy

to occur at relatively higher incidences of 7%, 11%, and 4% in comparison to pembrolizumab trials enrolling other malignancies. Clinical trials of immune checkpoint inhibitors for the treatment of thymic cancer are summarized in Table 3.5.

BIOMARKERS OF RESPONSE OR RESISTANCE TO IMMUNE CHECKPOINT INHIBITOR THERAPY

As discussed above, tumor PD-L1 expression is closely associated with tumor response to immune checkpoint inhibitors in NSCLC, particularly pembrolizumab, whereas its correlation in other histologic types is tenuous. Nonetheless, it is to be noted that there is significant intratumoral heterogeneity in PD-L1 expression.[79] Moreover, the presence of PD-L1 expression in the stroma (i.e., tumor-infiltrating immune cells) may also be the phenomenon of why clinical responses are seen even when tumors are considered negative for PD-L1 expression. There can also be significant analytical performance variability across different antibodies used. Four PD-L1 assays are commercially available to quantify PD-L1 expression, including Dako 28-8 pharmDx, Dako 22C3 pharmDx, Ventana SP263, and Ventana SP142. Different clinical trials have used different assays with different cut-points, and the clinical correlation among these assays is not clear. One study showed that the percentage of PD-L1-stained tumor cells was comparable to 28-8, 22C3, and SP263 assays, whereas SP142 exhibited fewer stained tumor cells. This study raised a valid concern about interchanging assays and cutoff values, as it could result in misclassifying patients, improper patient care, and treatment decision-making.[42] Additionally, tumors can be temporally and spatially heterogeneous. A primary tumor and its associated metastatic lesions may have different PD-L1 expression in space and over time, with a discordant rate as high as 25%, depending on the study.[80] PD-L1 expression is dynamic and can also be affected by prior treatments including radiation and chemotherapy.[37,39] The method of scoring expressivity also varied according to the platform used. SP142 used for determining

the PD-L1 status in the atezolizumab studies assessed PD-L1 expression on tumor cells and tumor-infiltrating immune cells. A prospective assessment of pathologist scoring in fact showed that while there is high concordance when scoring tumor cells stained with several anti-PD-L1 antibodies, there is poor concordance in scoring immune cells with any antibodies. This may provide an explanation for the different biomarker correlation seen between the phase 2 POPLAR and phase 3 OAK trials of atezolizumab in NSCLC.[81]

In addition to PD-L1 expression, other biomarkers have been suggested. These include smoking status in NSCLC or exposure to other carcinogens (e.g., ultraviolet light).[42,82] These clinical features are likely correlated due to the fact that carcinogen-associated malignancies have higher mutational burden. In fact, tumor mutational burden quantified by the total number of nonsynonymous somatic mutations detected by whole-exome sequencing is emerging to be another putative replicable predictor of the immunotherapy response rate.[83] In fact, in the CHECKMATE-026 study, a higher response rate (47% vs. 28%) and PFS (9.7 months vs. 5.8 months) were demonstrated with nivolumab compared with chemotherapy, respectively, in patients with high tumor mutational burden (243 or more mutations/megabase [Mb]). Similarly, an exploratory analysis in CHECKMATE-032 revealed that the ORR, 1-year PFS, and 1-year OS rates were the highest for SCLC patients with high tumor mutational burden (defined as >248 mutations/Mb). In the high-tumor burden subgroup, survival outcomes were even higher in the nivolumab-ipilimumab group, compared to nivolumab treatment alone[84] (ORR 46.2% vs. 21.3%, 1-year PFS 30% vs. 21.2%, and 1-year OS 62.4% vs. 35.2%). Indeed, tumors with aberrant DNA repair mechanisms that result in high neoantigen load, such as microsatellite instability or mismatch repair defects, have clearly shown benefit from immune checkpoint inhibitor therapy, and this led to the first tumor-agnostic approval of pembrolizumab using this biomarker approach.[42,82] Based on the understanding of the cancer immunity cycle, the presence of an inflamed TME as manifested by the number of tumor-infiltrating CD8+ lymphocytes in the pretreatment specimen can also be used as biomarker to assess response to immune checkpoint inhibitors.[85,86]

Specific genetic or molecular profiles may also be correlated with treatment outcomes with checkpoint inhibitor therapy. NSCLC with EGFR mutations or ALK translocation, despite frequent upregulation of PD-L1,[87,88] did not experience greater benefit with immune checkpoint inhibitors compared to chemotherapy.[33,89] Patients with ALK translocations are too few to draw any definite conclusions from randomized studies, but the same phenomenon as patients with EGFR mutations is observed, with low responses seen in single-arm studies, due to the association with nonsmoking status and low somatic mutational burden.[48] On the other hand, NSCLC with compound KRAS and STK11 mutations expressed lower levels of PD-L1 (compared to KRAS without STK11 loss), and demonstrated reduced number of tumor-infiltrating lymphocytes and resistance to anti-PD-1 antibody therapy.[90,91] Other potential causes of lack of T-cell infiltration that underlies resistance to immune checkpoint inhibitors may be driven by an activation of the Wnt/B-catenin pathway,[92] phosphatase and tensin homolog (PTEN), NF-KB, STAT3, and GAS6/AXL pathways.[93] From an epigenetic standpoint, a number of clinical metagenomics studies have also revealed the influence of specific gut bacteria in association with response to anti-PD-1/PD-L1 blockade, with evidence supporting the beneficial effect of the relative abundance of certain species such as *Akkermansia* and *Ruminococcaceae* bacteria.[94] More recently, a mathematical model to predict response and resistance to immune checkpoint inhibitors was described. This model utilized information on immunogenicity of tumor neoantigens in terms of neoantigen fitness, as determined by relative MHC binding affinity compared with its wildtype and T-cell recognition, as well as inclusion of gene expression analysis of the TME incorporated as a cytolytic score.[95] This framework can potentially be further extended with additional information, such as host microbiome, to enhance its predictive capability.

Mechanisms of adaptive resistance to immune checkpoint inhibitor therapy are beginning to be characterized. These include upregulation of alternative immune checkpoints such as TIM-3[96] and VISTA[97]; inactivation of antigen processing and presentation such as with acquired mutations in genes encoding JAK1, JAK2, and β-2-microglobulin (B2M[98]); downregulation of tumor histocompatibility leukocyte antigen (HLA)-A expression, as well as changes in TCR clonality and neoantigen loss[99]; or activation of pathways associated with T-cell exclusion such as Wnt/β-catenin.

FUTURE DIRECTIONS
Other Modulators of the Cancer Immunity Cycle

Although inhibitors of PD-1/PD-L1 and CTLA-4 have shown promising results, there are still a large number of patients who fail to respond to these agents even when used in combination. Multiple other key immune checkpoint regulators have been identified, such as LAG-3, TIM-3, B7-H3, OX-40, 4-1BB, TIGIT, etc., for which therapeutic agents have been developed in early clinical investigations and are further discussed in another chapter of this book. As always with combination strategies, investigators should be mindful of potential sequence-dependent interactions that may undermine the antitumor efficacy of each individual agent. Conversely, increased immune-related toxicity is a concern with any combinatorial approach and thus the "winning" combination must demonstrate a delicate balance between enhancing antitumor efficacy while minimizing adverse reactions to therapy in patients.

Various metabolic perturbations in the TME have also been demonstrated to exert immunosuppressive functions. These include changes in oxygen and potassium levels that impact directly not just on T cells but on additional immune cells in the TME.[100] *Indoleamine 2,3 dioxygenase 1(IDO1)* is an enzyme that converts tryptophan into the toxic metabolite kynurenine in a pathway associated with immune cell regulation. Many tumors have increased IDO activity therapy with increased stromal kynurenine levels that lead to immunosuppression.[101] Therefore, IDO1 has been considered a potential target to increase the activity of antitumor immunity. Epacadostat is an orally available selective inhibitor of IDO1, which has demonstrated hints of at least additive efficacy in a phase I/II trial evaluating its combination with pembrolizumab as second-line therapy in NSCLC. Among 40 efficacy-evaluable patients, the ORR was 35% (ORR in PD-L1 ≥50% was 43%, in PD-L1 <50% was 35%).[102] Further development of the combination of epacadostat with anti-PD-1 agents in the first-line setting for NSCLC has been terminated following the failure to meet the primary endpoint of PFS benefit (nor was the secondary endpoint of OS expected to meet statistical significance) from epacadostat in combination with pembrolizumab in the phase III ECHO 201-/KEYNOTE-252 trial in patients with metastatic melanoma. *Adenosine* is produced within the hypoxic cancer microenvironment to limit the inflammatory response and reduce damage of normal tissue by a direct inhibition of T cells via the G-protein—coupled A2A receptor (A2AR or ADORA2A), one of four receptors (A1R, A2AR, A2BR, and A3R) that bind adenosine. In addition, cancer-associated fibroblasts expressing A2AR promote tumor growth, progression, and angiogenesis. Therefore, anti-A2AR therapy has been considered a potential anticancer target. Preclinical murine models demonstrate that A2AR antagonists decreased the tumor burden and induced apoptosis of NSCLC xenografts. Reduction in the proliferation of cancer-associated fibroblasts is also seen.[103] CPI-444, PBF-509, and NIR178 are oral A2AR antagonists in development. 5'-nucleotidase (CD73) on the other hand is the enzyme that catalyzes the conversion of adenosine monophosphate to adenosine. Inhibition of adenosine signaling via A2AR blockade improves lymphocyte trafficking into the tumor but results in upregulation of CD73 which may represent an immune escape mechanism. Indeed, co-inhibition of A2AR and CD73 augmented the antitumor efficacy of each antagonist administered as monotherapy.[104] Anti-CD73 antibodies in development include MEDI9447 and IPH53. The role of protumorigenic activity of TAMs and myeloid-derived suppressor cells (MDSCs) is increasingly recognized. One of the mechanisms by which these cells suppress effector T-cell functions is mediated by depletion of *arginine*, such as with high level expression of arginase I which mediates catabolism of arginine.[105] Arginase inhibitor agents in development include orally administered INCB001158 or parenterally administered pegylated drugs such as AEB1102 and PEG-BCT-100.

Colony-stimulating factor 1 (CSF1) and its receptor CSF1R activate a key pathway in the regulation of TAMs.[106] Poor prognosis is associated with overexpression of CSF1 in patients with epithelial malignancies, including NSCLC.[107–110] In animal models, CSF1R inhibition strongly reduced TAMs.[111] Several agents targeting this pathway are in evaluation, with or without the combination of immune checkpoint blockade in solid tumors including NSCLC. These agents include monoclonal antibodies emactuzumab (RG7155) and cabiralizumab (FP-008) and the selective oral kinase inhibitor ARRY-382. However, results from early clinical studies of CSF1 inhibitors have generally been lackluster, except in patients with tenosynovial giant cell tumor and pigmented villonodular synovitis with the CSF1R translocation (which results in aberrant CSF1 overexpression and pathway activation). A potential explanation for the ineffectiveness of CSF1R blockade may be attributable to the recruitment of MDSCs[112] via increased CXCL1 production by cancer-associated fibroblasts, even while TAMs were being reduced. Indeed, combination of CSF1R inhibitor with blockade of CXCL1/CXCR2 pathway inhibitor and anti-PD-1 antibody demonstrated tumor growth inhibition in a preclinical model. On the other hand, the effect of immune checkpoint blockade in TAMs or MDSCs in the TME is not well understood. *In vivo* imaging studies in mice revealed that anti-PD-1 antibodies are engaged on the surface of T cells at an early stage of antibody administration but are subsequently sequestered by TAMs within minutes of drug administration via Fcγ receptor (FcγR)-mediated antibody transfer, which is dependent on the drug's Fc domain glycan composition and TAM surface FcγR expression.[113] This study showed enhancement of immune checkpoint inhibitor-induced tumor regression when FcγRs on myeloid cells are blocked before anti-PD-1 antibody administration. Conversely, PD-1/PD-L1 blockade appeared to mediate its efficacy in a macrophage-dependent fashion by a different group of investigators. PD-1 expression on TAMs increases over time in mouse models of cancer and with increasing cancer stage in humans. TAM PD-1 expression is negatively associated with phagocyte potency against tumors.[114] These studies suggest that immune checkpoint inhibitors exert their therapeutic effects via a complex interplay of immune cells in the TME.

COMBINATION THERAPY WITH OTHER IMMUNOTHERAPY
Adoptive T-cell transfer therapy
Adoptive T-cell transfer therapy pertains to the passive introduction of tumor-specific T cells. Initial approaches for this involve the isolation and expansion ex vivo of tumor-specific T cells arising either from vaccination or from tumor-infiltrating lymphocytes, and reinfused back into patients. Newer methodologies take this a step further by genetic modification of T cells, either to express a defined antigen-specific TCR or antigen-specific engineered antibody-like receptors called chimeric antigen receptor (CAR)-T cell. In CAR-T cells, each synthetic receptor consists of an extracellular antigen-binding single-chain variable antibody fragment (scFv) domain, a hinge/spacer domain derived from CD8 or IgG4, transmembrane domain, and a cytoplasmic signaling/activation domain that is responsible for T-cell proliferation and persistence.[115] While resembling the TCR, the scFv domain enables HLA-independent binding to a variety of different

antigens to bypass MHC requirements, a distinct advantage to overcome downregulated MHC expression induced by tumor cells. When scFvs are murine in origin, disadvantages include potential for anaphylactic reactions and generation of neutralizing human anti-murine antibody responses. Design of the hinge/spacer region is also critical to the CAR function, for example, to eliminate cognate binding that causes "off-target" activation-induced T-cell death.[116] In addition to the activation signal conferred through CD3 zeta chain that is fused to the scFv in first-generation CARs, newer generation CARs designed to confer better in vivo effect and overcome transience of earlier generation of CAR-T cells generally include one or more co-stimulatory domains (e.g., CD28, 4-1BB, and OX40) to enhance proliferation and persistence of cytotoxicity.[117] Additional gene modification can also be introduced, such as co-engineering the expression of stimulatory cytokines. Expression of CARs can be temporary, such as through RNA electroporation, or be stably integrated through lentiviral or retroviral transduction, or transposon systems.[118] CAR-T cells can be either autologous or allogeneic in origin, with the latter off-the-shelf capability providing advantages of faster availability but potential risk for graft-versus-host disease (GVHD). Newer engineering strategies include bispecific tandem CARs wherein the extracellular domain can bind two distinct antigens,[119] combinatorial antigen-sensing CARs engineered to facilitate the second CAR-T activation upon initial activation by the first CAR,[120] or inclusion of inducible "suicide" genes to abrogate adverse reactions by introducing a means to initiate rapid T-cell destruction.

CAR-T cell therapy has been extensively studied in hematologic malignancies, with the first CAR-T cell Tisagenlecleucel-T (CTL019) approved by the FDA for relapsed, refractory B-cell acute lymphoblastic leukemia in July 2017.[121,122] CAR-T cells have also been tested for solid malignancies,[123–125] although there are several hurdles to the successful implementation of this strategy in solid tumors. Various tumor or host factors, such as spatial and temporal heterogeneity in tumor antigen expression, suppressive TME with hostile metabolic conditions or nonconducive vasculature and extracellular matrix that limits T-cell infiltration can reduce CAR-T efficacy. In addition, issues of specificity/cross-reactivity with nontargeted protein or differential antigen expression in normal tissue underlie toxicity concerns, such as fatal pulmonary toxicity encountered after infusion of a third generation HER2 CAR attributed to low-level expression of HER2 on lung epithelial cells.[126] Efficacy of CAR-T cells in vivo is largely influenced by target antigen density and thus toxicity may potentially be modulated when there is low-target antigen expression in normal cells with the use of affinity-tuned CAR-T cells.[127] Regional delivery of CAR-T cells is also an approach being evaluated to overcome obstacles of T-cell trafficking into the tumor site. Furthermore, another technical factor that influences CAR-T cell efficacy in vivo is the culture condition that optimizes the desired subset of CAR-T cell amplified and transferred, with studies demonstrating better functional properties of expansion, persistence, and antitumor efficacy with the transfer of cells with less differentiated phenotype, such as the central memory T cells.[128]

A limited number of clinical trials are underway to validate the clinical efficacy of CAR-T cells for patients with thoracic malignancies. An EGFR CAR-T trial was recently reported in 11 patients with relapsed or refractory NSCLC with ≥50% EGFR expression.[129] There were three cohorts of treatment: one without conditioning regimen prior to CAR-T cell infusion, the other two cohorts had cyclophosphamide in combination with different cisplatin-based regimen (pemetrexed or docetaxel). This study demonstrated that two patients obtained partial response and five had stable disease for 2–8 months. Further extending the concept of EGFR targeting, CARs targeting the entire ErbB family (EGFR, HER2, HER3, HER4) have been engineered, with proposed intracavitary immunotherapy of this "T4" CAR-T in mesothelioma patients.[130] Various CAR-T cells targeting cell surface glycoproteins, such as aberrantly glycosylated mucin 1 (MUC1) and prostate stem cell antigen overexpressed in many malignancies including NSCLC,[131,132] have shown preclinical proof-of-concept and are underway on clinical testings. Mesothelin is a cell surface protein overexpressed in MPM, ovarian cancer, pancreatic cancer, and NSCLC that also functions as the receptor of CA125 (MUC16)-mediating cell adhesion.[133,134] Multiple clinical trials of mesothelin-targeting CAR-T cells have been performed and are ongoing, including CAR-T cells deployed regionally via intrapleural instillation.[135,136] Fibroblast activation protein is a transmembrane serine protease that is highly expressed in all subtypes of MPM but only detected weakly in few adult tissues (pancreas, placenta, cervix, and uterus).[137,138] It is another target antigen against which CAR-T cell therapies are in clinical evaluation for patients with MPM.

Cancer Vaccines

In contrast to adoptive cell transfer therapy which is passive in nature, the process of active immunotherapy generally invokes antigen-specific stimulation of the immune system through vaccination approaches.[139]

However, a lack of demonstrable benefit from earlier cancer vaccination trials may be attributable to multiple factors: the choice of antigens used in the cancer vaccine, the multiple steps required in the cancer immunity cycle which may be thwarted by various host or tumor-specific factors preventing antigen presentation and trafficking of T cells, and a complex immunosuppressive network with local immunosuppression and evasion of immune system surveillance in the TME.[140] Limitations of older generation vaccine strategies thus include the use of single-antigen/monovalent approach; central and peripheral tolerance mechanisms elicited due to the "shared" nature of epitopes that exist with TAAs, such as mesothelin or MUC1 (differential expression in tumor cells compared to normal tissues), or cancer testis antigens, such as MAGE or NY-ESO-1 (absent from mature adult cells except in certain reproductive tissues); as well as the activation of immunosuppressive pathways, such as induction PD-L1 expression in tumor and PD-1 expression on T effector cells by vaccination.[141,142] Contemporary advancements in next-generation sequencing technologies and bioinformatics as well as novel immunotherapy agents provide new strategies in cancer vaccination approaches, such as the identification and use of individualized tumor neoantigen vaccines and combination strategies with immune checkpoint modulators. Table 3.6 provides a summary of relevant randomized phase 2b/3 cancer vaccine trials completed to date in NSCLC.

NON-SMALL-CELL LUNG CANCER
Tumor Cell-Derived Vaccines

Belagenpumatucel-L (Lucanix) is an allogeneic cancer vaccine derived from four NSCLC cell lines (H460 large cell carcinoma, SK-LU1 adenocarcinoma, H520 squamous cell carcinoma, and RH2 squamous cell carcinoma). Each cell line was nonvirally transfected by electroporation with the TGF-β2 antisense, with the rationale that suppressing TGF-β2 secretion upon antigen processing may improve dendritic cell chemotaxis, activation, and cross-priming. The TGF-β pathway is a complex signal network with both stimulatory and inhibitory effects on tumor proliferation.[139] TGF-β inhibits cancer proliferation at an early stage of cancer, while it promotes angiogenesis and epithelial-to-mesenchymal transition at later stages of cancer.[143–145] It also enhances immune tolerance by stimulating the development of Tregs.[146] Several studies have demonstrated that an elevated level of

TGF-β was associated with a poor prognosis.[147,148] Although there were hints of clinical activity based on a partial response of 15% in a small phase 2 study, the confirmatory phase 3 trial of belagenpumatucel-L as maintenance therapy after platinum-based chemotherapy for patients with NSCLC did not show OS benefit (NCT00676507).[149] This vaccine is no longer in clinical development.

Viagenpumatucel-L (HS-110, Ad100-gp96Ig-HLA A1; Gp96-Ig) is also an allogeneic cancer vaccine using an adenocarcinoma backbone cell line with expression of known shared tumor antigens (such as melanoma-associated antigen 3 (MAGE-A3), NY-ESO-1, or LAGE-1), modified to secrete the heat shock protein gp-96-Ig, which chaperones these cell-derived tumor antigens to the vaccine recipient's antigen-presenting cells.[150] A phase 2 study in combination with nivolumab (DURGA trial) is currently ongoing (NCT02439450).

Tergenpumatucel-L (HyperAcute lung) consists of allogeneic lung cancer cell lines genetically modified to express the carbohydrate xenoantigen α(1,3) Gal epitope, which is thought to provide the basis for hyperacute rejection of foreign tissues (such as porcine bioprosthesis).[151] A single-arm, phase 2 study of this agent to be administered as maintenance therapy in NSCLC, first initiated in 2007 with anticipated enrollment of 82 patients was terminated in 2011 due to poor accrual (6 patients enrolled at the time of study closure). An open-label randomized study (NLG0301) of tergenpumatucel-L as second-line treatment versus docetaxel completed accrual in 2016. A trial in combination with an IDO inhibitor indoximod is ongoing (NCT02460367).

DPV-001 is an allogeneic, autophagosome-enriched vaccine which is composed of defective ribosomal products (DRiPs) and short-lived proteins (SLiPs) from two human cancer cell lines: UbiLT3 and UbiLT6.[152] It is thought that DRiPs and SLiPs are rapidly degraded by the proteasomal system in cancer cells and thus not cross-presented by dendritic cells. A group of investigators demonstrated that upon inhibition of proteasomal and lysosomal degradation of these products, the derived autophagosome-enriched product, also known as DRibbles (DRiPs and SLiPs-containing blebs), may be an innovative way of cross-priming of tumor-specific T cells. Vaccination with DPV-001 induced antibody responses against a variety of antigens overexpressed in NSCLC.[153] Combination with anti-OX40 is being planned based on preclinical studies demonstrating apparent synergy.[154]

TABLE 3.6
Completed Randomized Cancer Vaccine Trials in NSCLC

Clinical Setting	Drug vs Control Target (STUDY NAME)	Total Accrual	Trial Accrual Period	Primary Endpoint in Months (vs Control)	Vaccine Route of Administration/ Schedule
STAGE IB-IIIA					
ADJUVANT	GSK1572932A vs placebo MAGE-A3 (MAGRIT)	Phase 3 N=2272	2007–2012	DFS: 60.5 vs 57.9 (p=0.74)	IM (q3 weeks x 5, q 12 weeks x 8)
UNRESECTABLE STAGE III					
POST-CHEMORT	Tecemotide (L-BLP25) vs placebo MUC1 (START)	Phase 3 N=1239	2007–2011	OS: 25.6 vs 22.3 (p=0.123)	Subcutaneous (Cyclophosphamide -3, then q week x 8, q 6 weeks until progression)
POST-CONCURRENT CHEMORT	Tecemotide (L-BLP25) vs placebo MUC1 (START2)	Phase 3 N=32 (~1000)	April to September 2014	Early termination due to futility	Subcutaneous (Cyclophosphamide -3, then q week x 8, q 6 weeks until progression)
STAGE IV					
FIRST-LINE COMBINATION WITH CHEMO	TG4010 vs placebo MUC1-IL12 (TIME)	Phase 2b N=222	2012–2014	PFS: 5.9 vs 5.1 (1-sided α p=0.019) Exploratory OS: (nonsquamous): 14.6 vs 10.8 (p=0.03) (Low TrPAL): 13 vs 10.4 (p=0.018)	Subcutaneous q week x 6, q 3 weeks until progression
MAINTENANCE AFTER FIRST-LINE CHEMO	Belagenpumatucel vs placebo Shared tumor antigens (STOP)	Phase 3 N=532	2008–2012	OS: 20.3 vs 17.8 (p=0.594)	Intradermal monthly x 18 + two quarterly doses
	CIMAvax-EGF vs best supportive care EGF	Phase 3 N=405	2006–2012	OS (safety population): 10.8 vs 8.9 (p=0.1) OS (per-protocol): 12.4 vs 9.4 (p=0.036)	IM (Cyclophosphamide -3, Q 2 weeks x 4, monthly until progression)
	Racotumomab* vs placebo NeuGcGM3	176 1082	2006–2010 2010–2016	OS: 8.23 vs 6.8 (p=0.004)	Intradermal q 2 weeks x 5, q 4 weeks x 10 doses

Tumor-Associated or Cancer-Testis Antigen-Based Vaccines

Epidermal growth factor

Epidermal growth factor (EGF) is the founding member of the EGF-family of proteins and one of the major signaling growth factors implicated in the activation of the EGF receptor ErbB-1 (also known as EGFR). EGFR is overexpressed in many epithelial-derived malignancies, including NSCLC, and modulation of this pathway has led to the successful approval of multiple drugs in several solid malignancies. CIMAvax-EGF, a therapeutic vaccine targeting EGF, was first developed in Cuba[155] in the 1990s. The vaccine consists of EGF conjugated to a carrier protein P64 from *Neisseria meningitides* and emulsified in montanide-ISA 51.[156] In an open-labeled, multicenter, phase 3 clinical trial conducted in Cuba, 405 patients with advanced NSCLC[157] were randomized 1:1 for treatment with either CIMAvax or best supportive care post chemotherapy as maintenance therapy. In the safety population (patients who received at least one dose of the vaccine), survival benefit, while numerically higher in the vaccinated group, did not reach statistical significance. In the prespecific analysis of OS in the "per-protocol" population based on analysis of patients completing the induction period (four doses of CIMAvax-EGF) and control patients surviving through the same induction period, the OS difference was statistically significant, with HR of 0.77, $P = .036$. The five-year survival rate was 16.6% versus 6.2% in the vaccinated and nonvaccinated group, respectively. Additional observations seen during the earlier phase 2 trial with baseline serum EGF levels as potentially predicting benefit of the vaccine was redemonstrated in this study. Patients with high serum EGF levels who received vaccination had better OS compared to no vaccination (14.66 months vs. 8.63 months, $P = .0001$). As a corollary observation, a significant inverse relationship was observed between anti-EGF antibody titers and serum EGF concentration in vaccination patients. Of further interest is the remarkable safety profile in this anti-EGF vaccination approach. In contrast to currently utilized anti-EGFR antibody or EGFR tyrosine kinase inhibitor therapies which are associated with frequent dermatologic and gastrointestinal side effects, adverse event reported with CIMAvax-EGF was mostly injection-site pain and fever. A global phase 3 trial of first-line chemotherapy in combination with either CIMAvax-EGF or best supportive care only in patients with metastatic NSCLC launched in 2014 is ongoing (NCT02187367). A single-arm phase1/2 study of CIMAvax-EGF in combination with nivolumab is also ongoing (NCT02955290) since early 2017.

Mucin 1

MUC1 is a tumor-associated cell surface antigen overexpressed in many solid malignancies, particularly in nonsquamous histologies. The MUC1 protein expressed in the tumor is abnormally glycosylated, and this aberrant glycosylation is the target of various vaccination studies. TG4010 is a cancer vaccine designed to optimize MUC1-specific T-cell activation. It consists of a suspension of a recombinant modified vaccinia Ankara virus that codes for the MUC1 TAA

and interleukin-2.[158,159] A randomized, double-blinded, placebo-controlled, phase 2b/3 trial was tested in combination with platinum-based combination chemotherapy in the first-line setting for patients with stage IV nonmutated EGFR NSCLC and MUC1 expression in at least 50% of tumor cells.[159] The primary endpoint of median PFS in the overall population was 5.9 months in the TG4010 group and 5.1 months in the placebo group (HR, 0.74; CI, 0.55−0.97; $P = .019$). No grade 3 and 4 adverse events deemed to be related to TG4010 alone were observed. The study was also prespecified to analyze the utility of a companion diagnostic biomarker that was co-developed. This blood-based biomarker analyzes, using flow cytometry, the percentage of activated killer cell phenotype of CD16+/CD56+/CD69+ triple-positive activated lymphocytes (TrPALs) in circulation. The PFS and OS were also significantly improved in patients with nonsquamous histology, with the highest benefit noted in the subgroup of patients with low TrPAL value receiving TG4010 versus placebo (mPFS 6.0 vs. 4.9 months, $P = .0033$; mOS 15.1 vs. 10.3 months, $P = .0072$). Additional exploratory analysis of tumor PD-L1 expression revealed a significant difference in PFS between TGF4010 versus placebo in patients with low PD-L1 expression in the immune infiltrate but not in tumor with intermediate or high level of PD-L1 expression in the immune infiltrate. However, recruitment into the study had been suspended since 2015 and the phase 3 portion of the study was officially terminated as of January 2017, as new developmental strategies evolved with changes in the therapeutic landscape. It is currently being investigated in combination with nivolumab in a single-arm, phase 2 study in patients with nonsquamous NSCLC (NCT02823990). It also received FDA clearance in September 2017 to proceed with a phase 2 trial of TG4010 in combination with nivolumab and chemotherapy as first-line treatment in nonsquamous NSCLC. Additional viral vector-based vaccines in clinical development against MUC1 include Ad-sig-hMUC-1/ecdCD40L (adenovirus vector encoding human MUC1 and CD40 ligand,[160] NCT02140996), ETBX-061 (using adenovirus serotype 5 as gene delivery platform[161]), and the bivalent CV301 containing transgenes for both CEA and MUC-1 (using modified vaccinia Ankara virus as the primer, followed by fowlpox virus-based vaccination as booster) as well as three human costimulatory molecules (B7.1, ICAM-1, and LFA-3, designated as TRICOM), the latter two vaccines being tested in combination with anti-PD-1/PD-L1 monoclonal antibodies (NCT03169738 and NCT02840994). Nucleic-acid-based vaccine approaches have recently been developed, and CV9202/BI 136849 is an mRNA-based polyvalent vaccine which includes MUC1 as one of the six antigens in its platform (NCT03164772).

Tecemotide (L-BLP25, emepepimut, Stimuvax) is a synthetic peptide-based cancer vaccine designed to induce an immune response to MUC1 using a liposomal formulation. A randomized, open-label, phase 2b clinical trial of this vaccine as maintenance therapy versus best supportive care in patients with stage IIIB or IV NSCLC who responded to or were stable after first-line therapy demonstrated a trend toward OS benefit (HR, 0.739; 95% CI, 0.509−1.073; $P = .112$).[162] It was tolerated well without significant toxicities. This provided the basis for the double-blind, randomized, placebo-controlled, phase 3 trial (START) evaluating the role of tecemotide in patients with unresectable stage III NSCLC who had completed chemoradiotherapy (NCT00409188).[163] The median OS was 25.6 months in the tecemotide group and 22.3 months in the placebo group (HR, 0.88; 95% CI, 0.75−1.03; $P = .123$). In particular, exploratory analysis of those who received previous concurrent chemoradiation showed median OS of 30.8 and 20.6 months (HR, 0.78; 95% CI, 0.64−0.95; $P = .016$) in the vaccine and placebo groups, respectively. This served as the rationale for activating START2 in April 2014, a phase 3 study enrolling patients who completed concurrent chemoradiation to receive tecemotide versus placebo. However, this trial was terminated early in September 2014 following the results of a phase 1/2 study in Japanese patients with unresectable stage III NSCLC, majority of whom received concurrent chemoradiation.[164] No apparent trend toward increased OS was observed with tecemotide over placebo (32.4 vs. 32.2 months, HR, 0.95; 95% CI, 0.61−1.48; $P = .83$) in this study, which led to the early study closure. This agent is no longer in clinical development.

Melanoma-associated antigen 3

MAGE-A3 is a cancer testis antigen that is expressed in approximately 30% of NSCLCs, as well as other malignancies, but not expressed in benign human tissues.[165,166] It is thus an attractive target with multiple trials, both completed and ongoing, of vaccination strategies in NSCLC. GSK1572932A is the first recombinant MAGE-A3 protein-based vaccine that had been evaluated as adjuvant therapy in patients with completely resected MAGE-A3-positive NSCLC, with MAGE-A3 positivity determined by quantitative polymerase chain reaction (qPCR) of MAGE-A3 RNA expression on fresh tumor tissue samples. MAGE-A3 positivity was defined as 1% of the positive MAGE-A3 control. Patients with

stage IB or II NSCLC were randomized to MAGE-A3 (n = 122) or placebo (n = 60) in the initial randomized, phase 2 study.[167] Although there was no statistically significant improvement in disease-free interval (DFI; HR, 0.75; 95% CI, 0.46−1.23; $P = .254$), disease-free survival (DFS) (HR, 0.7; 95% CI, 0.48−1.23; $P = .248$), or OS (HR, 0.81; 95% CI, 0.47−1.40; $P = .454$), the numerical trend toward improvement in DFI, DFS, and OS provided the basis for the conduct of the confirmatory double-blind, placebo-controlled, randomized phase 3 MAGRIT study which enrolled patients with completely resected stages IB, II, and IIIA MAGE-A3-positive NSCLC (using qPCR analysis on formalin-fixed paraffin-embedded surgical specimens), with stratification for adjuvant chemotherapy. A total of 13,849 patients had tumor tissue screened, with approximately 33% of patients identified to have a MAGE-A3-positive tumor. The final total treated population in the study was 2,272: MAGE-A3 group of 1,515 patients and placebo group of 757 patients. There were no unusual safety signals, with new onset of autoimmune diseases occurring equally in 2% of either vaccine or placebo group. Unfortunately, adjuvant treatment with MAGE-A3 vaccine did not increase DFS despite a demonstrable immunological response as measured by the anti-MAGE-A3 IgG antibody seropositivity rate from 9% at baseline to 100% after four treatment doses, compared with placebo in these patients (9% baseline and with placebo treatment). Based on this result, further development of GSK1572932A for use in NSCLC was stopped.[166] Nonetheless, there is continued interest in developing alternative vaccine strategies targeting MAGE-A3 and/or other cancer testis antigens such as NY-ESO-1. Viral-vector transgenic expression of MAGE-A3, such as MG1-MAGEA3 and Ad-MAGEA3 vaccines, are currently being tested in combination with pembrolizumab (NCT02879760). Polyvalent vaccine approaches, either peptide-based (e.g., OSE2101, previously known as IDM-2101, which incorporates synthetic epitopes encompassing TAAs, CEA, p53, HER2, MAGE-2, and MAGE-3 for HLA-A2-positive NSCLC) or nucleic acid-based (e.g., CV9202/BI 1361849 targeting NY-ESO-1, MAGE C1, MAGE C2, 5T4, survivin, and MUC1) platforms, are also currently in clinical evaluation in NSCLC.

Neu-glycolyl (NeuGc)-containing gangliosides are not present in normal human tissues but are expressed on cancer cells including melanoma, breast, or NSCLC.[168,169] In particular, NeuGc ganglioside GM3 (NeuGcGM3) is known to be a potent immunosuppressive molecule and TAA.[170] Racotumomab-alum is an anti-idiotype antibody that acts as a vaccine targeting

NeuGcGM3. Several early phase clinical trials were conducted in patients with melanoma, breast, and lung cancer.[171] A randomized, double-blind, placebo-controlled, phase 2 clinical trial of the vaccine as maintenance therapy was performed in Cuban patients with stage IIIB and stage IV NSCLC who had at least stable disease after first-line chemotherapy.[172] The median OS was 8.23 and 6.80 months in the racotumomab-alum group and the placebo group, respectively (HR, 0.63; 95% CI, 0.46−0.87; $P = .004$). The PFS was 5.33 versus 3.90 months (HR, 0.73; 95% CI, 0.53−0.99; $P = .039$). Furthermore, among vaccinated patients, serum IgM binding to and cytotoxicity against NGcGM3-expressing L1210 cells appear to be associated with survival. Treatment-related adverse events were similar between the vaccine and control groups. Results from the confirmatory phase 3 trial which completed accrual in mid-2016 are awaited.

INDIVIDUALIZED TUMOR NEOANTIGEN-BASED VACCINES

Tumor-specific mutations generate cancer neoantigens that represent the epitome of foreignness. Neoantigens if presented are highly immunogenic and have been considered the ideal targets by cancer vaccines as they represent the highest degree of potential immunogenicity and lowest concern for autoimmunity.[173] However, the identification and quantification of tumor-specific mutations and their associated neoantigens have not been technically feasible until recently. With advancements in machine-learning and sequencing technologies as well as algorithms to predict neoepitope affinity to MHC proteins, individualized cancer vaccination approaches have become feasible and demonstrated proof-of-concept in early trials in melanoma patients.[174,175] A number of both peptide- and mRNA-based individualized neoantigen vaccine trials in combination with anti-PD-1/PD-L1 inhibitors are currently ongoing in a variety of malignancies including NSCLC, and results are eagerly awaited.

Malignant pleural mesothelioma

A number of tumor cell-based vaccines have been conducted to evaluate their feasibility in mesothelioma as well. Various strategies have been adopted, using either autologous or allogeneic tumor cells directly or dendritic cells pulsed with tumor cell lysates. Whereas a tumor-specific immune response can be elicited in a fraction of patients, objective tumor responses are not generally seen, similar to the experience with other cancer vaccine

approaches in other malignancy types. These vaccines have not moved further beyond early phase testing.

In comparison, vaccines against the TAAs Wilm's tumor protein (WT-1) and mesothelin have been developed further in the clinic. The results from a double-blind, randomized, phase II trial of the WT-1 peptide vaccine galinpepimut-S (with GM-CSF and montanide as adjuvants) administered as adjuvant therapy after multimodality therapy with surgery were recently published.[176] Although 78 patients were planned for enrollment, prespecified futility analysis resulted in the early closure of the control arm, and the treatment arm was also subsequently closed due to the unblinding, with a total of 41 patients accrued for randomization. An improvement in 1-year PFS from 50% to 70% was the primary endpoint. The PFS rate in the galinpepimut arm was 45%. The 1-year PFS-rate in the control arm was 33%. Although not meeting the primary endpoint, due to the numerically better PFS outcomes in the experimental group, a larger randomized trial is being planned to further evaluate the role of galinpepimut-S in the treatment of MPM.

CRS-207 is a live-attenuated *Listeria monocytogenes* (*Lm*) bacterial vector transgenically modified to express mesothelin. Selection of *Lm* as the vaccine vector is based on this intracellular pathogen's ability to target dendritic cells in vivo. A phase I study of CRS-207 administered as intravenous infusion showed that multiple doses can be administered safely, along with demonstration of mesothelin-specific T-cell responses.[177] A phase Ib study of CRS-207 in combination with cisplatin and pemetrexed in MPM demonstrated an ORR of 59% with median PFS of 8.5 months.[178] A phase II, single-arm study of pembrolizumab in combination with CRS-207 for patients with MPM after platinum-failure started enrollment in June 2017. Primary endpoint of this study is ORR. However, due to the failure of this vaccine in other trials, along with analysis of data collectively in mesothelioma and ovarian studies, the company made a decision in December 2017 to terminate development of CRS-207, including halting further recruitment into any of the ongoing studies such as the combination study with pembrolizumab.

CONCLUSION

Cytotoxic chemotherapy has been the core backbone of systemic treatment approach for advanced or recurrent thoracic malignancies up until recently. Targeted therapies introduced at the turn of the 21st century have extended the treatment options for patients with actionable mutations. Improvements in technology and the understanding of the immunological basis of cancer have recently provided new avenues of immunotherapy that are poised to revolutionize how cancer will be treated in the years to come. In this decade alone, the standard of care has markedly changed within a few years for a large majority of patients, including patients with lung cancer and MPM. The role of immunotherapy in cancer treatment paradigm is in its "infancy" stages. Despite the breath-taking successes seen to date, we take heed of the lessons past in recognition of the swift evolution of cancer cells that gives rise to treatment resistance. Moreover, we are in the midst of an immunotherapy "bubble" as the pharmaceutical industry has rushed in headlong with a singular focus of finding the next big winner. As of the last quarter of 2017, there are over 3,000 active clinical trials of immune oncology agents with a target enrollment of over 577,000 patients.[179] With the increasing complexity of clinical trials and stringency in eligibility criteria, we now face a crisis that critically requires partnerships across all stakeholders to facilitate smooth and rapid development of drug combinations. Beyond this, the rising cost of care mandates the necessity of translational biomarkers to identify and select patients who stand to benefit the most from such expensive treatments in addition to a rationale-driven approach for allocating studies efficiently.

ACKNOWLEDGMENTS

We are very grateful to Dr. Matthew Loecher from Department of Urology, Temple University Hospital, for organizing the tables and other editorial assistance with this book chapter.

REFERENCES

1. National Cancer Institute. *Surveillance, Epidemiology, and End Results (SEER) 18 Registries.* 2016.
2. Senan S, Brade A, Wang LH, et al. PROCLAIM: randomized phase III trial of pemetrexed-cisplatin or etoposide-cisplatin plus thoracic radiation therapy followed by consolidation chemotherapy in locally advanced non-squamous non-small-cell lung cancer. *J Clin Oncol.* 2016;34(9):953−962.
3. Wakelee HA, Dahlberg SE, Keller SM, et al. Adjuvant chemotherapy with or without bevacizumab in patients with resected non-small-cell lung cancer (E1505): an open-label, multicentre, randomised, phase 3 trial. *Lancet Oncol.* 2017;18(12):1610−1623.
4. Thatcher N, Hirsch FR, Luft AV, et al. Necitumumab plus gemcitabine and cisplatin versus gemcitabine and cisplatin alone as first-line therapy in patients with stage IV squamous non-small-cell lung cancer (SQUIRE): an open-label, randomised, controlled phase 3 trial. *Lancet Oncol.* 2015;16(7):763−774.
5. He M, Capelletti M, Nafa K, et al. EGFR exon 19 insertions: a new family of sensitizing EGFR mutations in lung adenocarcinoma. *Clin Cancer Res.* 2012;18(6):1790−1797.
6. Brustugun OT, Khattak AM, Tromborg AK, et al. BRAF-mutations in non-small cell lung cancer. *Lung Cancer.* 2014;84(1):36−38.
7. Kwak EL, Bang YJ, Camidge DR, et al. Anaplastic lymphoma kinase inhibition in non-small-cell lung cancer. *N Engl J Med.* 2010;363(18):1693−1703.
8. Shaw AT, Ou SH, Bang YJ, et al. Crizotinib in ROS1-rearranged non-small-cell lung cancer. *N Engl J Med.* 2014;371(21):1963−1971.
9. Gure AO, Chua R, Williamson B, et al. Cancer-testis genes are coordinately expressed and are markers of poor outcome in non-small cell lung cancer. *Clin Cancer Res.* 2005;11(22):8055−8062.
10. Dai L, Tsay JC, Li J, et al. Autoantibodies against tumor-associated antigens in the early detection of lung cancer. *Lung Cancer.* 2016;99:172−179.
11. Taneja TK, Sharma SK. Markers of small cell lung cancer. *World J Surg Oncol.* 2004;2:10.
12. Freeman GJ, Long AJ, Iwai Y, et al. Engagement of the PD-1 immunoinhibitory receptor by a novel B7 family member leads to negative regulation of lymphocyte activation. *J Exp Med.* 2000;192(7):1027−1034.
13. Woo SR, Turnis ME, Goldberg MV, et al. Immune inhibitory molecules LAG-3 and PD-1 synergistically regulate T-cell function to promote tumoral immune escape. *Cancer Res.* 2012;72(4):917−927.
14. Ngiow SF, von Scheidt B, Akiba H, Yagita H, Teng MW, Smyth MJ. Anti-TIM3 antibody promotes T cell IFN-gamma-mediated antitumor immunity and suppresses established tumors. *Cancer Res.* 2011;71(10):3540−3551.
15. Le Mercier I, Chen W, Lines JL, et al. VISTA regulates the development of protective antitumor immunity. *Cancer Res.* 2014;74(7):1933−1944.
16. Fourcade J, Sun Z, Pagliano O, et al. CD8(+) T cells specific for tumor antigens can be rendered dysfunctional by the tumor microenvironment through upregulation of the inhibitory receptors BTLA and PD-1. *Cancer Res.* 2012;72(4):887−896.
17. Spranger S, Spaapen RM, Zha Y, et al. Up-regulation of PD-L1, IDO, and T(regs) in the melanoma tumor microenvironment is driven by CD8(+) T cells. *Sci Transl Med.* 2013;5(200):200ra116.
18. Pardoll DM. Immunology beats cancer: a blueprint for successful translation. *Nat Immunol.* 2012;13(12):1129−1132.
19. Kinter AL, Godbout EJ, McNally JP, et al. The common gamma-chain cytokines IL-2, IL-7, IL-15, and IL-21 induce the expression of programmed death-1 and its ligands. *J Immunol.* 2008;181(10):6738−6746.

20. Robert C, Long GV, Brady B, et al. Nivolumab in previously untreated melanoma without BRAF mutation. *N Engl J Med.* 2015;372(4):320−330.

21. Robert C, Ribas A, Wolchok JD, et al. Anti-programmed-death-receptor-1 treatment with pembrolizumab in ipilimumab-refractory advanced melanoma: a randomised dose-comparison cohort of a phase 1 trial. *Lancet.* 2014;384(9948):1109−1117.

22. Rosenberg JE, Hoffman-Censits J, Powles T, et al. Atezolizumab in patients with locally advanced and metastatic urothelial carcinoma who have progressed following treatment with platinum-based chemotherapy: a single-arm, multicentre, phase 2 trial. *Lancet.* 2016; 387(10031):1909−1920.

23. Massard C, Gordon MS, Sharma S, et al. Safety and efficacy of durvalumab (MEDI4736), an anti-programmed cell death ligand-1 immune checkpoint inhibitor, in patients with advanced urothelial bladder cancer. *J Clin Oncol.* 2016;34(26):3119−3125.

24. Kaufman HL, Russell J, Hamid O, et al. Avelumab in patients with chemotherapy-refractory metastatic merkel cell carcinoma: a multicentre, single-group, open-label, phase 2 trial. *Lancet Oncol.* 2016;17(10):1374−1385.

25. Wolchok JD, Neyns B, Linette G, et al. Ipilimumab monotherapy in patients with pretreated advanced melanoma: a randomised, double-blind, multicentre, phase 2, dose-ranging study. *Lancet Oncol.* 2010;11(2):155−164.

26. Calabro L, Morra A, Fonsatti E, et al. Tremelimumab for patients with chemotherapy-resistant advanced malignant mesothelioma: an open-label, single-arm, phase 2 trial. *Lancet Oncol.* 2013;14(11):1104−1111.

27. Rizvi NA, Hellmann MD, Snyder A, et al. Cancer immunology. mutational landscape determines sensitivity to PD-1 blockade in non-small cell lung cancer. *Science.* 2015;348(6230):124−128.

28. Patel SP, Kurzrock R. PD-L1 expression as a predictive biomarker in cancer immunotherapy. *Mol Cancer Ther.* 2015;14(4):847−856.

29. Topalian SL, Hodi FS, Brahmer JR, et al. Safety, activity, and immune correlates of anti-PD-1 antibody in cancer. *N Engl J Med.* 2012;366(26):2443−2454.

30. Taube JM, Klein A, Brahmer JR, et al. Association of PD-1, PD-1 ligands, and other features of the tumor immune microenvironment with response to anti-PD-1 therapy. *Clin Cancer Res.* 2014;20(19):5064−5074.

31. Garon EB, Gandhi L, Rizvi N, et al. Antitumor activity of pembrolizumab (pembro; mk-3475) and correlation with programmed death ligand 1 (pd-l1) expression in a pooled analysis of patients (pts) with advanced non−small cell lung carcinoma (NSCLC). *Ann Oncol.* 2014; 25(5):1−41.

32. Brahmer J, Reckamp KL, Baas P, et al. Nivolumab versus docetaxel in advanced squamous-cell non-small-cell lung cancer. *N Engl J Med.* 2015;373(2):123−135.

33. Borghaei H, Paz-Ares L, Horn L, et al. Nivolumab versus docetaxel in advanced non-squamous non-small-cell lung cancer. *N Engl J Med.* 2015;373(17):1627−1639.

34. Goeree R, Villeneuve J, Goeree J, Penrod JR, Orsini L, Tahami Monfared AA. Economic evaluation of nivolumab for the treatment of second-line advanced squamous NSCLC in Canada: a comparison of modeling approaches to estimate and extrapolate survival outcomes. *J Med Econ.* 2016;19(6):630−644.

35. Matter-Walstra K, Schwenkglenks M, Aebi S, et al. A cost-effectiveness analysis of nivolumab versus docetaxel for advanced non-squamous NSCLC including PD-L1 testing. *J Thorac Oncol.* 2016;11(11):1846−1855.

36. Aguiar PN, Perry LA, Penny-Dimri J, et al. The effect of PD-L1 testing on the cost-effectiveness and economic impact of immune checkpoint inhibitors for the second-line treatment of NSCLC. *Ann Oncol.* 2017;28(9):2256−2263.

37. Garon EB, Rizvi NA, Hui R, et al. Pembrolizumab for the treatment of non-small-cell lung cancer. *N Engl J Med.* 2015;372(21):2018−2028.

38. Gandhi L, Balmanoukian A, Hui R, et al. MK-3475 (anti-PD-1 monoclonal antibody) for non-small cell lung cancer (NSCLC): antitumor activity and association with tumor PD-L1 expression. *Cancer Res.* 2014;74(suppl 19):nr CT105.

39. Herbst RS, Baas P, Kim DW, et al. Pembrolizumab versus docetaxel for previously treated, PD-L1-positive, advanced non-small-cell lung cancer (KEYNOTE-010): a randomised controlled trial. *Lancet.* 2016;387(10027): 1540−1550.

40. Reck M, Rodriguez-Abreu D, Robinson AG, et al. Pembrolizumab versus chemotherapy for PD-L1-positive non-small-cell lung cancer. *N Engl J Med.* 2016;375(19): 1823−1833.

41. Carbone DP, Reck M, Paz-Ares L, et al. First-line nivolumab in stage IV or recurrent non-small-cell lung cancer. *N Engl J Med.* 2017;376(25):2415−2426.

42. Hirsch FR, McElhinny A, Stanforth D, et al. PD-L1 immunohistochemistry assays for lung cancer: results from phase 1 of the blueprint PD-L1 IHC assay comparison project. *J Thorac Oncol.* 2017;12(2):208−222.

43. Shaverdian N, Lisberg AE, Bornazyan K, et al. Previous radiotherapy and the clinical activity and toxicity of pembrolizumab in the treatment of non-small-cell lung cancer: a secondary analysis of the KEYNOTE-001 phase 1 trial. *Lancet Oncol.* 2017;18(7):895−903.

44. Langer CJ, Gadgeel SM, Borghaei H, et al. Carboplatin and pemetrexed with or without pembrolizumab for advanced, non-squamous non-small-cell lung cancer: a randomised, phase 2 cohort of the open-label KEYNOTE-021 study. *Lancet Oncol.* 2016;17(11):1497−1508.

45. Rittmeyer A, Barlesi F, Waterkamp D, et al. Atezolizumab versus docetaxel in patients with previously treated non-small-cell lung cancer (OAK): a phase 3, open-label, multicentre randomised controlled trial. *Lancet.* 2017;389(10066):255−265.

46. Kowanetz M, Socinski MA, Zou W, et al. IMpower150: efficacy of atezolizumab plus bevacizumab and chemotherapy in 1L metastatic nonsquamous NSCLC across key subgroups. Abstract CT076. In: *Presented at American*

Association for Cancer Research Annual Meeting; April 14–18, 2018; Chicago. 2018.

47. Antonia S, Rizvi S, Brahmer J, et al. Safety and clinical activity of durvalumab (MEDI4736), an anti-programmed cell death ligand-1 (PD-L1) antibody, in patients with non-small cell lung cancer (NSCLC). *Cancer Immunol Res.* 2016;4(suppl 1):nr A047.

48. Garassino M, Cho BC, Gray JE, et al. Durvalumab in ≥ 3rd-line EGFR mutant/ALK+, locally advanced or metastatic NSCLC: results from the phase 2 ATLANTIC study. *Ann Oncol.* 2017;28:ii51.

49. Garassino M, Vansteenkiste J, Kim JH, et al. Durvalumab in ≥3rd-line locally advanced or metastatic, EGFR/ALK wild-type NSCLC: results from the phase 2 ATLANTIC study. *J Thorac Oncol.* 2017;12:S10–S11.

50. Gulley JL, Rajan A, Spigel DR, et al. Avelumab for patients with previously treated metastatic or recurrent non-small-cell lung cancer (JAVELIN solid tumor): dose-expansion cohort of a multicentre, open-label, phase 1b trial. *Lancet Oncol.* 2017;18(5):599–610.

51. Lynch TJ, Bondarenko I, Luft A, et al. Ipilimumab in combination with paclitaxel and carboplatin as first-line treatment in stage IIIB/IV non-small-cell lung cancer: results from a randomized, double-blind, multicenter phase II study. *J Clin Oncol.* 2012;30(17):2046–2054.

52. Hellmann MD, Rizvi NA, Goldman JW, et al. Nivolumab plus ipilimumab as first-line treatment for advanced non-small-cell lung cancer (CheckMate 012): results of an open-label, phase 1, multicohort study. *Lancet Oncol.* 2017;18(1):31–41.

53. Chaft JE, Forde PM, Smith KN, et al. Neoadjuvant nivolumab in early-stage, resectable non-small cell lung cancers. *J Clin Oncol.* 2017;35(suppl 15):8508.

54. Antonia SJ, Villegas A, Daniel D, et al. Durvalumab after chemoradiotherapy in stage III non–small-cell lung cancer. *N Engl J Med.* 2017;377:1919–1929.

55. Puglisi M, Dolly S, Faria A, Myerson JS, Popat S, O'Brien ME. Treatment options for small cell lung cancer - do we have more choice? *Br J Cancer.* 2010;102(4):629–638.

56. Byers LA, Rudin CM. Small cell lung cancer: where do we go from here? *Cancer.* 2015;121(5):664–672.

57. Chute JP, Chen T, Feigal E, et al. Twenty years of phase III trials for patients with extensive-stage small-cell lung cancer: perceptible progress. *J Clin Oncol.* 1999;17(6):1794–1801.

58. Reck M, Bondarenko I, Luft A, et al. Ipilimumab in combination with paclitaxel and carboplatin as first-line therapy in extensive-disease-small-cell lung cancer: results from a randomized, double-blind, multicenter phase 2 trial. *Ann Oncol.* 2013;24(1):75–83.

59. Reck M, Luft A, Szczesna A, et al. Phase III randomized trial of ipilimumab plus etoposide and platinum versus placebo plus etoposide and platinum in extensive-stage small-cell lung cancer. *J Clin Oncol.* 2016;34(31):3740–3748.

60. Sabari JK, Lok BH, Laird JH, et al. Unravelling the biology of SCLC: implications for therapy. *Nat Rev Clin Oncol.* 2017;14(9):549–561.

61. Antonia SJ, Lopez-Martin JA, Bendell J, et al. Nivolumab alone and nivolumab plus ipilimumab in recurrent small-cell lung cancer (CheckMate 032): a multicentre, open-label, phase 1/2 trial. *Lancet Oncol.* 2016;17(7):883–895.

62. Ott PA, Elez E, Hiret S, et al. Pembrolizumab in patients with extensive-stage small-cell lung cancer: results from the phase ib KEYNOTE-028 study. *J Clin Oncol.* 2017;35(34):3823–3829.

63. Gadgeel SM, Ventimiglia J, Kalemkerian GP, et al. Phase II study of maintenance pembrolizumab (pembro) in extensive stage small cell lung cancer (ES-SCLC) patients (pts). *J Clin Oncol.* 2017;35(suppl 15):8504.

64. Khalil DN, Smith EL, Brentjens RJ, Wolchok JD. The future of cancer treatment: immunomodulation, CARs and combination immunotherapy. *Nat Rev Clin Oncol.* 2016;13(5):273–290.

65. Alexandrov LB, Nik-Zainal S, Wedge DC, et al. Signatures of mutational processes in human cancer. *Nature.* 2013;500(7463):415–421.

66. Vogelzang NJ, Rusthoven JJ, Symanowski J, et al. Phase III study of pemetrexed in combination with cisplatin versus cisplatin alone in patients with malignant pleural mesothelioma. *J Clin Oncol.* 2003;21(14):2636–2644.

67. Zalcman G, Mazieres J, Margery J, et al. Bevacizumab for newly diagnosed pleural mesothelioma in the mesothelioma avastin cisplatin pemetrexed study (MAPS): a randomised, controlled, open-label, phase 3 trial. *Lancet.* 2016;387(10026):1405–1414.

68. Kindler HL, Karrison TG, Gandara DR, et al. Multicenter, double-blind, placebo-controlled, randomized phase II trial of gemcitabine/cisplatin plus bevacizumab or placebo in patients with malignant mesothelioma. *J Clin Oncol.* 2012;30(20):2509–2515.

69. Bueno R, Stawiski EW, Goldstein LD, et al. Comprehensive genomic analysis of malignant pleural mesothelioma identifies recurrent mutations, gene fusions and splicing alterations. *Nat Genet.* 2016;48(4):407–416.

70. Yamagishi T, Fujimoto N, Nishi H, et al. Prognostic significance of the lymphocyte-to-monocyte ratio in patients with malignant pleural mesothelioma. *Lung Cancer.* 2015;90(1):111–117.

71. Ceresoli GL, Mantovani A. Immune checkpoint inhibitors in malignant pleural mesothelioma. *Lancet Oncol.* 2017;18(5):559–561.

72. Cedres S, Ponce-Aix S, Zugazagoitia J, et al. Analysis of expression of programmed cell death 1 ligand 1 (PD-L1) in malignant pleural mesothelioma (MPM). *PLoS One.* 2015;10(3):e0121071.

73. Calabro L, Morra A, Fonsatti E, et al. Efficacy and safety of an intensified schedule of tremelimumab for chemotherapy-resistant malignant mesothelioma: an open-label, single-arm, phase 2 study. *Lancet Respir Med.* 2015;3(4):301–309.

74. Quispel-Janssen J, Zago G, Schouten R, et al. OA13.01 A phase II study of nivolumab in malignant pleural mesothelioma (NivoMes): with translational research (TR) biopies. *J Thorac Oncol.* 2017;12(1):S292−S293.

75. Alley EW, Lopez J, Santoro A, et al. Clinical safety and activity of pembrolizumab in patients with malignant pleural mesothelioma (KEYNOTE-028): preliminary results from a non-randomised, open-label, phase 1b trial. *Lancet Oncol.* 2017;18(5):623−630.

76. Scherpereel A, Mazieres J, Greillier L, et al. Second- or third-line nivolumab (nivo) versus nivo plus ipilimumab (ipi) in malignant pleural mesothelioma (MPM) patients: results of the IFCT-1501 MAPS2 randomized phase II trial. *J Clin Oncol.* 2017;35(suppl 18):LBA8507.

77. Cho J, Ahn M-J, Yoo KH, et al. A phase II study of pembrolizumab for patients with previously treated advanced thymic epithelial tumor. *J Clin Oncol.* 2017;35(suppl 15): 8521.

78. Giaccone G, Thompson J, McGuire C, et al. Pembrolizumab in patients with recurrent thymic carcinoma: results of a phase II study. *J Clin Oncol.* 2017;35(suppl 15):8573.

79. McLaughlin J, Han G, Schalper KA, et al. Quantitative assessment of the heterogeneity of PD-L1 expression in non-small-cell lung cancer. *JAMA Oncol.* 2016;2(1): 46−54.

80. Kim S, Koh J, Kwon D, et al. Comparative analysis of PD-L1 expression between primary and metastatic pulmonary adenocarcinomas. *Eur J Cancer.* 2017;75: 141−149.

81. Rimm DL, Han G, Taube JM, et al. A prospective, multi-institutional, pathologist-based assessment of 4 immunohistochemistry assays for PD-L1 expression in non-small cell lung cancer. *JAMA Oncol.* 2017;3(8): 1051−1058.

82. Grigg C, Rizvi NA. PD-L1 biomarker testing for non-small cell lung cancer: truth or fiction? *J Immunother Cancer.* 2016;4:48.

83. Kowanetz M, Koeppen H, Boe M, et al. Spatiotemporal effects on programmed death ligand 1 (PD-L1) expression and immunophenotype of non-small cell lung cancer (NSCLC). *J Thorac Oncol.* 2015;9(suppl 2):S199.

84. Rizvi N, Antonia S, Callahan MK, et al. Impact of tumor mutation burden on the efficacy of nivolumab or nivolumab plus ipilimumab in small cell lung cancer: an exploratory analysis of CheckMate 032. In: *World Conference on Lung Cancer.* 2017.

85. Mitchell P, Murone C, Asadi K, et al. Programmed death ligand-1 (PD-L1) expression in non-small cell lung cancer (NSCLC): analysis of a large early stage cohort; and concordance of expression in paired primary-nodal and primary-metastasis tumour samples (ID 3226). In: *World Conference on Lung Cancer.* 2015.

86. Twyman-Saint Victor C, Rech AJ, Maity A, et al. Radiation and dual checkpoint blockade activate non-redundant immune mechanisms in cancer. *Nature.* 2015; 520(7547):373−377.

87. Azuma K, Ota K, Kawahara A, et al. Association of PD-L1 overexpression with activating EGFR mutations in surgically resected nonsmall-cell lung cancer. *Ann Oncol.* 2014;25(10):1935−1940.

88. Ota K, Azuma K, Kawahara A, et al. Induction of PD-L1 expression by the EML4-ALK oncoprotein and downstream signaling pathways in non-small cell lung cancer. *Clin Cancer Res.* 2015;21(17):4014−4021.

89. Lee CK, Man J, Lord S, et al. Checkpoint inhibitors in metastatic EGFR-mutated non-small cell lung cancer-A meta-analysis. *J Thorac Oncol.* 2017;12(2):403−407.

90. Skoulidis F, Byers LA, Diao L, et al. Co-occurring genomic alterations define major subsets of KRAS-mutant lung adenocarcinoma with distinct biology, immune profiles, and therapeutic vulnerabilities. *Cancer Discov.* 2015;5(8): 860−877.

91. Koyama S, Akbay EA, Li YY, et al. STK11/LKB1 deficiency promotes neutrophil recruitment and proinflammatory cytokine production to suppress T-cell activity in the lung tumor microenvironment. *Cancer Res.* 2016;76(5): 999−1008.

92. Spranger S, Bao R, Gajewski TF. Melanoma-intrinsic beta-catenin signalling prevents anti-tumour immunity. *Nature.* 2015;523(7559):231−235.

93. Aguilera TA, Giaccia AJ. Molecular pathways: oncologic pathways and their role in T-cell exclusion and immune evasion-A new role for the AXL receptor tyrosine kinase. *Clin Cancer Res.* 2017;23(12):2928−2933.

94. Gopalakrishnan V, Spencer CN, Nezi L, et al. Gut microbiome modulates response to anti-PD-1 immunotherapy in melanoma patients. *Science.* 2018;359(6371):97−103.

95. Łuksza M, Riaz N, Makarov V, et al. A neoantigen fitness model predicts tumour response to checkpoint blockade immunotherapy. *Nature.* 2017;551(7681):517−520.

96. Koyama S, Akbay EA, Li YY, et al. Adaptive resistance to therapeutic PD-1 blockade is associated with upregulation of alternative immune checkpoints. *Nat Commun.* 2016;7:10501.

97. Kakavand H, Jackett LA, Menzies AM, et al. Negative immune checkpoint regulation by VISTA: a mechanism of acquired resistance to anti-PD-1 therapy in metastatic melanoma patients. *Mod Pathol.* 2017;30(12):1666−1676.

98. Zaretsky JM, Garcia-Diaz A, Shin DS, et al. Mutations associated with acquired resistance to PD-1 blockade in melanoma. *N Engl J Med.* 2016;375(9):819−829.

99. Anagnostou V, Smith KN, Forde PM, et al. Evolution of neoantigen landscape during immune checkpoint blockade in non-small cell lung cancer. *Cancer Discov.* 2017;7(3):264−276.

100. Gurusamy E, Clever D, Eil R, et al. Novel "Elements" of immune suppression within the tumor microenvironment. *Cancer Immunol Res.* 2017;5(6):426−433.

101. Hwu P, Du MX, Lapointe R, et al. Indoleamine 2,3-dioxygenase production by human dendritic cells results in the inhibition of T cell proliferation. *J Immunol.* 2009; 164(7):3596−3599.

102. Gangadhar TC, Schneider BJ, Bauer TM, et al. Efficacy and safety of epacadostat plus pembrolizumab treatment of NSCLC: preliminary phase I/II results of ECHO-202/KEYNOTE-037. *J Clin Oncol.* 2017;35(suppl 15):9014.
103. Mediavilla-Varela M, Luddy K, Noyes D, et al. Antagonism of adenosine A2A receptor expressed by lung adenocarcinoma tumor cells and cancer associated fibroblasts inhibits their growth. *Cancer Biol Ther.* 2013;14(9):860–868.
104. Young A, Ngiow SF, Barkauskas DS, et al. Co-inhibition of CD73 and A2AR adenosine signaling improves anti-tumor immune responses. *Cancer Cell.* 2016;30:391–403.
105. Rodriguez PC, Quiceno DG, Zabaleta J, et al. Arginase I production in the tumor microenvironment by mature myeloid cells inhibits T-cell receptor expression and antigen-specific T-cell responses. *Cancer Res.* 2004;64(16):5839–5849.
106. Strachan DC, Ruffell B, Oei Y, et al. CSF1R inhibition delays cervical and mammary tumor growth in murine models by attenuating the turnover of tumor-associated macrophages and enhancing infiltration by CD8+ T cells. *Oncoimmunology.* 2013;2(12):e26968.
107. Pei BX, Sun BS, Zhang ZF, Wang AL, Ren P. Interstitial tumor-associated macrophages combined with tumor-derived colony-stimulating factor-1 and interleukin-6, a novel prognostic biomarker in non-small cell lung cancer. *J Thorac Cardiovasc Surg.* 2014;148(4):1216. e2.
108. Sharma M, Beck AH, Webster JA, et al. Analysis of stromal signatures in the tumor microenvironment of ductal carcinoma in situ. *Breast Cancer Res Treat.* 2010;123(2):397–404.
109. Lin EY, Gouon-Evans V, Nguyen AV, Pollard JW. The macrophage growth factor CSF-1 in mammary gland development and tumor progression. *J Mammary Gland Biol Neoplasia.* 2002;7(2):147–162.
110. Mantovani A, Sica A. Macrophages, innate immunity and cancer: balance, tolerance, and diversity. *Curr Opin Immunol.* 2010;22(2):231–237.
111. Ries CH, Cannarile MA, Hoves S, et al. Targeting tumor-associated macrophages with anti-CSF-1R antibody reveals a strategy for cancer therapy. *Cancer Cell.* 2014;25(6):846–859.
112. Kumar V, Donthireddy L, Marvel D, et al. Cancer-associated fibroblasts neutralize the anti-tumor effect of CSF1 receptor blockade by inducing PMN-MDSC infiltration of tumors. *Cancer Cell.* 2017;32(5):668. e5.
113. Arlauckas SP, Garris CS, Kohler RH, et al. In vivo imaging reveals a tumor-associated macrophage-mediated resistance pathway in anti-PD-1 therapy. *Sci Transl Med.* 2017;9(389). pii: eaal3604.
114. Gordon SR, Maute RL, Dulken BW, et al. PD-1 expression by tumour-associated macrophages inhibits phagocytosis and tumour immunity. *Nature.* 2017;545(7655):495–499.
115. Jin C, Fotaki G, Ramachandran M, Nilsson B, Essand M, Yu D. Safe engineering of CAR T cells for adoptive cell therapy of cancer using long-term episomal gene transfer. *EMBO Mol Med.* 2016;8(7):702–711.
116. Hombach A, Hombach AA, Abken H. Adoptive immunotherapy with genetically engineered T cells: modification of the IgG1 fc 'spacer' domain in the extracellular moiety of chimeric antigen receptors avoids 'off-target' activation and unintended initiation of an innate immune response. *Gene Ther.* 2010;17(10):1206–1213.
117. Finney HM, Akbar AN, Lawson AD. Activation of resting human primary T cells with chimeric receptors: costimulation from CD28, inducible costimulator, CD134, and CD137 in series with signals from the TCR zeta chain. *J Immunol.* 2004;172(1):104–113.
118. Singh H, Huls H, Kebriaei P, Cooper LJ. A new approach to gene therapy using sleeping beauty to genetically modify clinical-grade T cells to target CD19. *Immunol Rev.* 2014;257(1):181–190.
119. Grada Z, Hegde M, Byrd T, et al. TanCAR: a novel bispecific chimeric antigen receptor for cancer immunotherapy. *Mol Ther Nucleic Acids.* 2013;2:e105.
120. Roybal KT, Rupp LJ, Morsut L, et al. Precision tumor recognition by T cells with combinatorial antigen-sensing circuits. *Cell.* 2016;164(4):770–779.
121. Fan F, Zhao W, Liu J, et al. Durable remissions with BCMA-specific chimeric antigen receptor (CAR)-modified T cells in patients with refractory/relapsed multiple myeloma. *J Clin Oncol.* 2017;35(suppl 18):LBA3001.
122. Lee DW, Kochenderfer JN, Stetler-Stevenson M, et al. T cells expressing CD19 chimeric antigen receptors for acute lymphoblastic leukaemia in children and young adults: a phase 1 dose-escalation trial. *Lancet.* 2015;385(9967):517–528.
123. Lamers CH, Klaver Y, Gratama JW, Sleijfer S, Debets R. Treatment of metastatic renal cell carcinoma (mRCC) with CAIX CAR-engineered T-cells-a completed study overview. *Biochem Soc Trans.* 2016;44(3):951–959.
124. Song DG, Ye Q, Poussin M, Chacon JA, Figini M, Powell DJ. Effective adoptive immunotherapy of triple-negative breast cancer by folate receptor-alpha redirected CAR T cells is influenced by surface antigen expression level. *J Hematol Oncol.* 2016;9(1):56.
125. Kershaw MH, Westwood JA, Parker LL, et al. A phase I study on adoptive immunotherapy using gene-modified T cells for ovarian cancer. *Clin Cancer Res.* 2006;12(20 Pt 1):6106–6115.
126. Morgan RA, Yang JC, Kitano M, et al. Case report of a serious adverse event following the administration of T cells transduced with a chimeric antigen receptor recognizing ERBB2. *Mol Ther.* 2010;18(4):843–851.
127. Caruso HG, Hurton LV, Najjar A, et al. Tuning sensitivity of CAR to EGFR density limits recognition of normal tissue while maintaining potent antitumor activity. *Cancer Res.* 2015;75(17):3505–3518.
128. Klebanoff CA, Gattinoni L, Restifo NP. Sorting through subsets: which T-cell populations mediate highly effective adoptive immunotherapy? *J Immunother.* 2012;35(9):651–660.
129. Feng K, Guo Y, Dai H, et al. Chimeric antigen receptor-modified T cells for the immunotherapy of patients

with EGFR-expressing advanced relapsed/refractory non-small cell lung cancer. *Sci China Life Sci.* 2016;59(5): 468−479.

130. Klampatsa A, Achkova DY, Davies DM, et al. Intracavitary 'T4 immunotherapy' of malignant mesothelioma using pan-ErbB re-targeted CAR T-cells. *Cancer Lett.* 2017;393: 52−59.

131. Wei X, Lai Y, Li J, et al. PSCA and MUC1 in non-small-cell lung cancer as targets of chimeric antigen receptor T cells. *Oncoimmunology.* 2017;6(3):e1284722.

132. Posey AD, Schwab RD, Boesteanu AC, et al. Engineered CAR T cells targeting the cancer-associated tn-glycoform of the membrane mucin MUC1 control adenocarcinoma. *Immunity.* 2016;44(6):1444−1454.

133. Chang K, Pastan I. Molecular cloning of mesothelin, a differentiation antigen present on mesothelium, mesotheliomas, and ovarian cancers. *Proc Natl Acad Sci U S A.* 1996;93(1):136−140.

134. Rump A, Morikawa Y, Tanaka M, et al. Binding of ovarian cancer antigen CA125/MUC16 to mesothelin mediates cell adhesion. *J Biol Chem.* 2004;279(10):9190−9198.

135. Beatty GL, Haas AR, Maus MV, et al. Mesothelin-specific chimeric antigen receptor mRNA-engineered T cells induce anti-tumor activity in solid malignancies. *Cancer Immunol Res.* 2014;2(2):112−120.

136. Adusumilli PS, Cherkassky L, Villena-Vargas J, et al. Regional delivery of mesothelin-targeted CAR T cell therapy generates potent and long-lasting CD4-dependent tumor immunity. *Sci Transl Med.* 2014;6(261):261ra151.

137. Schuberth PC, Hagedorn C, Jensen SM, et al. Treatment of malignant pleural mesothelioma by fibroblast activation protein-specific re-directed T cells. *J Transl Med.* 2013;11:187.

138. Petrausch U, Schuberth PC, Hagedorn C, et al. Re-directed T cells for the treatment of fibroblast activation protein (FAP)-positive malignant pleural mesothelioma (FAPME-1). *BMC Cancer.* 2012;12:615.

139. Rijavec E, Biello F, Genova C, et al. Belagenpumatucel-L for the treatment of non-small cell lung cancer. *Expert Opin Biol Ther.* 2015;15(9):1371−1379.

140. Butts CA, Sangha R. TIME for a successful cancer vaccine in NSCLC? *Lancet Oncol.* 2016;17(2):131−132.

141. Soares KC, Rucki AA, Wu AA, et al. PD-1/PD-L1 blockade together with vaccine therapy facilitates effector T-cell infiltration into pancreatic tumors. *J Immunother.* 2015; 38(1):1−11.

142. Remy-Ziller C, Thioudellet C, Hortelano J, et al. Sequential administration of MVA-based vaccines and PD-1/PD-L1-blocking antibodies confers measurable benefits on tumor growth and survival: preclinical studies with MVA-betaGal and MVA-MUC1 (TG4010) in a murine tumor model. *Hum Vaccin Immunother.* 2018;14(1): 140−145.

143. Zhang H, Yang P, Zhou H, et al. Involvement of Foxp3-expressing CD4+ CD25+ regulatory T cells in the development of tolerance induced by transforming growth factor-beta2-treated antigen-presenting cells. *Immunology.* 2008;124(3):304−314.

144. Valcourt U, Kowanetz M, Niimi H, Heldin CH, Moustakas A. TGF-beta and the smad signaling pathway support transcriptomic reprogramming during epithelial-mesenchymal cell transition. *Mol Biol Cell.* 2005;16(4): 1987−2002.

145. Siegel PM, Massague J. Cytostatic and apoptotic actions of TGF-beta in homeostasis and cancer. *Nat Rev Cancer.* 2003;3(11):807−821.

146. Thomas DA, Massague J. TGF-beta directly targets cytotoxic T cell functions during tumor evasion of immune surveillance. *Cancer Cell.* 2005;8(5):369−380.

147. Huang AL, Liu SG, Qi WJ, et al. TGF-beta1 protein expression in non-small cell lung cancers is correlated with prognosis. *Asian Pac J Cancer Prev.* 2014;15(19): 8143−8147.

148. Papadopoulou E, Anagnostopoulos K, Tripsianis G, et al. Evaluation of predictive and prognostic significance of serum TGF-beta1 levels in breast cancer according to HER-2 codon 655 polymorphism. *Neoplasma.* 2008; 55(3):229−238.

149. Giaccone G, Bazhenova LA, Nemunaitis J, et al. A phase III study of belagenpumatucel-L, an allogeneic tumour cell vaccine, as maintenance therapy for non-small cell lung cancer. *Eur J Cancer.* 2015;51(16): 2321−2329.

150. Cohen RB, Nemunaitis J, Gabrail N, et al. A phase II study of viagenpumatucel-l (HS-110) in combination with low-dose cyclophosphamide versus physician's choice in patients with advanced non-small cell lung cancer. *J Immunother Cancer.* 2014;2(suppl 3):P82.

151. Sandrin MS, McKenzie IF. Gal alpha (1,3)gal, the major xenoantigen(s) recognised in pigs by human natural antibodies. *Immunol Rev.* 1994;141:169−190.

152. Page DB, Hulett TW, Hilton TL, Hu H, Urba WJ, Fox BA. Glimpse into the future: harnessing autophagy to promote anti-tumor immunity with the DRibbles vaccine. *J Immunother Cancer.* 2016;4:25.

153. Fox BA, Boulmay BC, Li R, et al. T cell population expansion in response to allogeneic cancer vaccine alone (DPV-001) or with granulocyte-macrophage colony-stimulating factor (GM-CSF) or imiquimod (I) for definitively-treated stage III NSCLC patients (pts). *J Clin Oncol.* 2017;35(suppl 15):E14639.

154. Hilton T, Paustian C, Koguchi Y, et al. A strategy to assess contributions of individual agents in combination immunotherapy trials. *J Immunother Cancer.* 2017; 5(suppl 2):P38.

155. Rodriguez PC, Rodriguez G, Gonzalez G, Lage A. Clinical development and perspectives of CIMAvax EGF, cuban vaccine for non-small-cell lung cancer therapy. *MEDICC Rev.* 2010;12(1):17−23.

156. Neninger E, Diaz RM, de la Torre A, et al. Active immunotherapy with 1E10 anti-idiotype vaccine in patients with small cell lung cancer: report of a phase I trial. *Cancer Biol Ther.* 2007;6(2):145−150.

157. Saavedra D, Crombet T. CIMAvax-EGF: a new therapeutic vaccine for advanced non-small cell lung cancer patients. *Front Immunol.* 2017;8:269.

158. Limacher JM, Quoix E. TG4010: a therapeutic vaccine against MUC1 expressing tumors. *Oncoimmunology.* 2012;1(5):791–792.
159. Quoix E, Lena H, Losonczy G, et al. TG4010 immunotherapy and first-line chemotherapy for advanced non-small-cell lung cancer (TIME): results from the phase 2b part of a randomised, double-blind, placebo-controlled, phase 2b/3 trial. *Lancet Oncol.* 2016;17(2):212–223.
160. Akbulut H, Tang Y, Akbulut KG, et al. Addition of adenoviral vector targeting of chemotherapy to the MUC-1/ecdCD40L VPPP vector prime protein boost vaccine prolongs survival of mice carrying growing subcutaneous deposits of lewis lung cancer cells. *Gene Ther.* 2010;17(11):1333–1340.
161. Tsang KY, Gabitzsch ES, Palena C, et al. The generation and analysis of a novel combination of recombinant adenovirus vaccines targeting three tumor antigens as an immunotherapeutic. *J Immunother Cancer.* 2015;3(suppl 2):P452.
162. Butts C, Murray N, Maksymiuk A, et al. Randomized phase IIB trial of BLP25 liposome vaccine in stage IIIB and IV non-small-cell lung cancer. *J Clin Oncol.* 2005;23(27):6674–6681.
163. Butts C, Socinski MA, Mitchell PL, et al. Tecemotide (L-BLP25) versus placebo after chemoradiotherapy for stage III non-small-cell lung cancer (START): a randomised, double-blind, phase 3 trial. *Lancet Oncol.* 2014;15(1):59–68.
164. Katakami N, Hida T, Nokihara H, et al. Phase I/II study of tecemotide as immunotherapy in Japanese patients with unresectable stage III non-small cell lung cancer. *Lung Cancer.* 2017;105:23–30.
165. Declerck S, Vansteenkiste J. Immunotherapy for lung cancer: ongoing clinical trials. *Future Oncol.* 2014;10(1):91–105.
166. Vansteenkiste JF, Cho BC, Vanakesa T, et al. Efficacy of the MAGE-A3 cancer immunotherapeutic as adjuvant therapy in patients with resected MAGE-A3-positive non-small-cell lung cancer (MAGRIT): a randomised, double-blind, placebo-controlled, phase 3 trial. *Lancet Oncol.* 2016;17(6):822–835.
167. Vansteenkiste J, Zielinski M, Linder A, et al. Adjuvant MAGE-A3 immunotherapy in resected non-small-cell lung cancer: phase II randomized study results. *J Clin Oncol.* 2013;31(19):2396–2403.
168. van Cruijsen H, Ruiz MG, van der Valk P, et al. Tissue micro array analysis of ganglioside N-glycolyl GM3 expression and signal transducer and activator of transcription (STAT)-3 activation in relation to dendritic cell infiltration and microvessel density in non-small cell lung cancer. *BMC Cancer.* 2009;9:180.
169. Alfonso M, Diaz A, Hernandez AM, et al. An anti-idiotype vaccine elicits a specific response to N-glycolyl sialic acid residues of glycoconjugates in melanoma patients. *J Immunol.* 2002;168(5):2523–2529.
170. de Leon J, Fernandez A, Mesa C, et al. Role of tumour-associated N-glycolylated variant of GM3 ganglioside in cancer progression: effect over CD4 expression on T cells. *Cancer Immunol Immunother.* 2006;55(4):443–450.
171. Hernandez AM, Toledo D, Martinez D, et al. Characterization of the antibody response against NeuGcGM3 ganglioside elicited in non-small cell lung cancer patients immunized with an anti-idiotype antibody. *J Immunol.* 2008;181(9):6625–6634.
172. Alfonso S, Valdes-Zayas A, Santiesteban ER, et al. A randomized, multicenter, placebo-controlled clinical trial of racotumomab-alum vaccine as switch maintenance therapy in advanced non-small cell lung cancer patients. *Clin Cancer Res.* 2014;20(14):3660–3671.
173. Schumacher TN, Schreiber RD. Neoantigens in cancer immunotherapy. *Science.* 2015;348(6230):69–74.
174. Ott PA, Hu Z, Keskin DB, et al. An immunogenic personal neoantigen vaccine for patients with melanoma. *Nature.* 2017;547(7662):217–221.
175. Sahin U, Derhovanessian E, Miller M, et al. Personalized RNA mutanome vaccines mobilize poly-specific therapeutic immunity against cancer. *Nature.* 2017;547(7662):222–226.
176. Zauderer MG, Tsao AS, Dao T, et al. A randomized phase II trial of adjuvant galinpepimut-S, WT-1 analogue peptide vaccine, after multimodality therapy for patients with malignant pleural mesothelioma. *Clin Cancer Res.* 2017;23(24):7483–7489.
177. Le DT, Brockstedt DG, Nir-Paz R, et al. A live-attenuated Listeria vaccine (ANZ-100) and a live-attenuated Listeria vaccine expressing mesothelin (CRS-207) for advanced cancers: phase I studies of safety and immune induction. *Clin Cancer Res.* 2012;18(3):858–868.
178. Jahan T, Hassan R, Alley E, et al. 208O_PR: CRS-207 with chemotherapy (chemo) in malignant pleural mesothelioma (MPM): results from a phase 1b trial. *J Thorac Oncol.* 2016;11(suppl 4):S156.
179. Tang J, Shalabi A, Hubbard-Lucey VM. Comprehensive analysis of the clinical immuno-oncology landscape. *Ann Oncol.* 2018;29(1):84–91.

FURTHER READING

1. Gandhi L, Rodriguez-Abreu D, Gadgeel S, et al. Pembrolizumab plus chemotherapy in metastatic non-small cell lung cancer. *N Engl J Med*; 2018 [Epub ahead of print]. https://doi.org/10.1056/NJMoa1801005).

CHAPTER 4

Immune Checkpoint Inhibitors in Gastrointestinal Malignancies

CHRISTOS FOUNTZILAS, MD • SUNYOUNG S. LEE, MD, PHD • RENUKA V. IYER, MD • PATRICK M. BOLAND, MD

INTRODUCTION

Cytotoxic T-lymphocyte antigen 4 (CTLA-4) and Programmed Death Protein 1 (PD-1) are among the many inhibitory molecules (immune checkpoints) that can downregulate immune responses.[1] Binding of the HLA (human leukocyte antigen)/epitope complex to the T-cell receptor is not by itself sufficient to lead to T-cell activation. Antigen-presenting cell (APC) surface molecules B7.1 and 2 bind to the costimulatory CD28 in the surface of T-cell and provide the necessary second signal. CTLA-4 is expressed on T-cells on activation. Preferential binding of CTLA-4 to B7.1 and 2 leads to downregulation of the immune response.[2] PD-1 is another T-cell stimulation inhibitor.[3] Its ligand, PD-L1, can be expressed in both tumor and immune cells within the tumor microenvironment (TME). Cancer immunotherapy refers to the use of systemically or locally administered agents with a goal to stimulate the immune system against cancer. Immune checkpoint inhibitor therapy—the most frequently used clinical form of immunotherapy—can activate the immune system against cancer cells by removing coinhibitory signals. In recent years, immune checkpoint inhibition through CTLA-4 and/or PD-1/PD-L1 blockade has significantly improved outcomes in multiple malignancies.[4–6] Clear benefits have been demonstrated with PD-1 inhibition in non–small cell lung cancer (NSCLC), head and neck squamous cell cancers, urothelial cancer, and renal cell carcinoma, among others.[6–11]

Inflammation is considered to be an enabling characteristic of cancer, and it is closely related to evasion from immune surveillance; malignant tumors arising in the gastrointestinal tract, liver, pancreas, and bile ducts are considered highly inflammatory.[12,13] The success of immunotherapy with checkpoint inhibitors in the treatment of gastrointestinal malignancies has been variable, reflecting the multiple disease types with different pathogeneses, natural histories, and prognoses. Recently, we have seen progress with the approvals of nivolumab for hepatocellular cancer, pembrolizumab for PD-L1+ gastroesophageal cancers (GEC), and both agents for microsatellite instability–high (MSI-H) colorectal cancers. Furthermore, pembrolizumab has been approved for MSI-H cancers of any origin. In this chapter, we discuss the current value and future of immunotherapy with immune checkpoint inhibitors in patients with gastrointestinal malignancies.

GASTROESOPHAGEAL CANCER

GEC is a major cause of cancer-related death worldwide.[14] Most patients are diagnosed at an advanced stage[15] and fluoropyrimidine/platinum-based therapy only provides a modest short-term benefit, improving median overall survival (OS) to approximately 9–11 months.[16,17]

GEC is an attractive disease for the development of immunotherapeutic agents. Gastric cancer can be molecularly classified into four subclasses, (1) the Epstein–Barr virus (EBV) infection–associated, (2) the MSI-associated, (3) the chromosomal instability (CIN)–related, and (4) the genomically stable tumors.[18] EBV-associated gastric cancers exhibit recurrent 9p24.1 amplifications, which contain the *PD-L1/PD-L2* genes; these cancers are characterized by PD-L1 overexpression and presence of tumor-infiltrating lymphocytes (TIL).[19] The MSI-H subtype is estimated to comprise 22% of gastric cancers across all stages.[20] This proportion seems to be less in advanced disease, with 4% of metastatic gastroesophageal patients in KEYNOTE-059 testing MSI-H, and just 6.6% of evaluable tumors in the MAGIC trial, where > two-thirds of patients with available tissue were pathologic stage III.[21] In MSI-H tumors, mismatch repair (MMR) deficiency leads to accumulation of mutations resulting in increased neoantigen burden that correlates with response to immunotherapy.[22–24] *Helicobacter pylori*–induced damage is found to cause genomic alterations in many cases of CIN tumors [25] and can lead to PD-L1 upregulation in preclinical studies.[26] Furthermore, almost half of squamous carcinomas of the esophagus exhibit PD-L1 or PD-L2 expression, which correlates with poor prognosis.[27]

Clinical Trials of Immune Checkpoint Inhibitors in Gastroesophageal Cancer

Immune checkpoint inhibitors as single agent therapy

Tremelimumab, a fully humanized, anti-CTLA4 IgG2 monoclonal antibody, was evaluated in a phase II trial that enrolled patients ($N = 18$) with previously treated, advanced GEC.[28] The overall response rate (ORR) was 5%, and the median OS was 4.8 months. The one patient who responded was continued on treatment for 32.7 months. Furthermore, patients whose lymphocytes had a proliferative response to carcinoembryonic antigen (CEA) in vitro had improved survival compared with nonresponders (17.1 vs. 4.7 months, respectively; $P = .004$). Separately, the anti-CTLA4, fully humanized monoclonal IgG1 antibody, ipilimumab, was tested as sequential or maintenance treatment after first-line chemotherapy in advanced GEC.[29] Patients were randomized 1:1 to ipilimumab versus best supportive care. Although one partial response was observed (1.8%), stable disease was only achieved in a minority (31.6%); neither immune-related progression-free survival (irPFS) nor OS were improved over best supportive care. In fact, irPFS was superior in the BSC arm, particularly owing to events within the first 6 weeks, after which time progression rates appeared similar.

Pembrolizumab and nivolumab are IgG4 monoclonal antibodies, humanized and fully human, respectively, targeting PD-1. KEYNOTE-012 was a multicohort phase I study of pembrolizumab in patients with advanced tumors with at least 1% PD-L1 expression in tumor and contiguous mononuclear inflammatory cells by immunohistochemistry (IHC) using the 22C3 antibody (PD-L1+).[30] The ORR was 22% in patients with advanced gastric or gastroesophageal junction (GEJ) adenocarcinoma. Responses occurred fairly rapidly, at a median of 8 weeks, and they were long lasting, with the median duration of response being 40 weeks. Pembrolizumab therapy was generally well tolerated; five patients experienced grade 3 or 4 adverse events

(AE) with one patient having grade 4 pneumonitis. No patient discontinued therapy secondary to toxicity. The multicohort, phase I KEYNOTE-028 trial enrolled 23 patients with previously treated, PD-L1+, esophageal/GEJ carcinoma and treated them with single-agent pembrolizumab at a dose of 10 mg/kg every 2 weeks. Of the treated patients, 78% had squamous histology and 87% had received at least two prior lines of therapy for advanced disease.[31] Of the enrolled patients, 30% attained a response and almost half of the patients had a decrease in tumor burden; responses were observed regardless of histology and were long-lasting (median 15 months). No new safety signals were observed.

These studies led to KEYNOTE-059, a three cohort phase II trial of pembrolizumab in patients with advanced gastric or GEJ cancer. Cohort 1 enrolled patients who had received two or more lines of prior therapy irrespective of PD-L1 expression ($N = 259$).[32,33] Patients in cohort 1 received pembrolizumab monotherapy. The ORR in cohort 1 was 12%; 17% of the patients achieved stable disease. The ORR was higher in patients receiving pembrolizumab as third-line therapy as compared with fourth-line (14.9% vs. 7.2%) and in patients with PD-L1+ as compared with PD-L1− tumors (15.5% vs. 5.5%), defined as positive staining by IHC in more than 1% of tumor or stromal cells. Furthermore, in MSI-H tumors, ORR was significantly improved at 57%, compared with 9% in the remaining majority. Cohort 3 enrolled treatment-naïve patients with PD-L1+ tumors; ORR was 26% in this patient population. While the median OS was 6 months in cohort 1, it was not reached in cohort 3. Ultimately, these data sets led to the approval of pembrolizumab in the United States in 2017 for PD-L1+ gastric/GEJ cancer after two or more lines of therapy.

CheckMate-032 evaluated nivolumab in patients with pretreated, advanced gastric cancer unselected for PD-L1 tumor status.[34,35] The ORR rate was 12% in patients receiving nivolumab monotherapy, and the 24-month OS rate was 22%; PD-L1+ tumors (>1% PD-L1 expression in tumor cells by IHC using the 28-8 pharmDx assay) appeared to respond more favorably to treatment (19% vs. 12%), but there was no major difference in 12-month OS (39% vs. 34%). Sixty-five patients with treatment-refractory carcinoma of the esophagus were treated in another single-arm, phase II trial with nivolumab monotherapy; 11 patients had an objective response.[36] The toxicity profile of nivolumab was similar as that seen in other cancers.

ONO-4538-12 (ATTRACTION-2) was a randomized (2:1), phase III study of nivolumab compared with placebo in patients with advanced, pretreated gastric or GEJ cancer.[37] More than 80% of patients in this study had gastric cancer, with less than 10% having GEJ tumors; the vast majority had previously received more than three lines of therapy. The ORR rate was 11.2% with nivolumab versus 0% in placebo arm. A significant improvement in the median OS was observed with nivolumab as compared with placebo: 5.32 versus 4.14 months (HR = 0.63; $P < .0001$). Importantly, although median differences were small, there appeared to be a subset of patients with durable benefit. For nivolumab versus placebo, 6 month PFS stood at 7.6% versus 1.5%, respectively. OS at both 12 and 18 months also appeared improve at 26.2% versus 10.9% and 16.2% versus 5%, respectively. The treatment discontinuation rate due to AEs was quite low in both arms (2.7% for nivolumab and 2.5% in the placebo arm); grade 3 or 4 AEs were seen in 11.5% of patients treated with nivolumab versus 5.5% of the placebo-treated patients.

In the JAVELIN trial, avelumab, a fully humanized IgG1 anti-PD-L1 monoclonal antibody, was evaluated as maintenance treatment after first-line ($N = 89$) or as second-line therapy ($N = 62$) in patients with advanced GEC.[38] The median PFS was 12 weeks in the maintenance and 6 weeks in the second-line setting. The ORR as maintenance therapy was 10% in PD-L1 positive and 3% in PD-L1 negative patients; the ORR as second-line therapy was 18.2% in PD-L1 positive and 9.1% in PD-L1 negative patients. AE of any grade occurred in 59% patients, 10% of who had grade 3 or greater toxicity. One treatment-related death occurred due to hepatic failure. There are ongoing phase III trials with avelumab in gastric cancer (NCT02625610, NCT02625623). In a phase I trial, durvalumab, a fully humanized, anti-PD-L1 IgG1 monoclonal antibody showed modest activity in gastric cancer.[39]

Immune checkpoint inhibitor combination strategies

Within KEYNOTE-059, Cohort 2 ($N = 25$) enrolled treatment-naïve patients with metastatic GEC; patients were treated with cisplatin plus fluoropyrimidine in combination with pembrolizumab.[33,40] The ORR was 60%, with 32% of the patients achieving stable disease as best response; the median OS was 14 months. As in other scenarios, the ORR was higher in patients with PD-L1+ tumors (73% vs. 38% in PD-L1- tumors). KEYNOTE-590 is currently evaluating this combination (cisplatin plus 5-fluorouracil) with pembrolizumab or placebo for treatment-naïve patients with esophageal

cancer (NCT03189719). Nivolumab in combination with platinum-fluoropyrimidine chemotherapy is under evaluation in the randomized ATTRACTION-04/ONO-4538-37 study for treatment-naïve patients with advanced gastric or GEJ cancer (NCT02746796) and as adjuvant therapy after curative resection in the ATTRACTION-05/ONO-4538-38 trial (NCT03006705).

In addition to nivolumab monotherapy, CheckMate-032 evaluated nivolumab and ipilimumab at two different dose levels in 101 patients (nivolumab 1 mg/kg plus ipilimumab 3 mg/kg every 3 weeks for four cycles or nivolumab 3 mg/kg plus ipilimumab 1 mg/kg every 3 weeks for four cycles); nivolumab monotherapy followed four cycles of the combination.[34,35] Although preliminary, responses appeared greater for the 3 mg/kg ipilimumab group (24% vs. 8%); this is compared with 12% in the nivolumab monotherapy group. As seen in other diseases, rates of grade 3 or greater toxicities were significantly higher with CTLA-4 and PD-1 combination therapy as compared with PD-1 monotherapy.

To validate this promising data and delineate the most active strategy, the phase III, randomized CheckMate-649 trial will evaluate a nivolumab/ipilimumab combination strategy as compared with nivolumab plus chemotherapy or chemotherapy alone (NCT02872116). Durvalumab is currently being investigated in combination with other classes of immune checkpoint inhibitors in phase I/II clinical trials (NCT02340975, NCT02318277).

Angiogenesis is a relevant treatment target in GEC. Ramucirumab is an IgG1, fully human monoclonal antibody against the vascular endothelial growth factor (VEGF) receptor-2 and has been approved for advanced, platinum/fluoropyrimidine refractory GEC as monotherapy as well as in combination with a taxane.[41,42] Treatment with antiangiogenesis agents can increase effector T-cell infiltration within the tumor and improve its functionality.[43] There is evidence for synergy between anti-VEGF and anti-PD-1 therapy in preclinical colon cancer models.[44] Ramucirumab is combined with pembrolizumab in an ongoing phase I trial enrolling patients with treatment-naïve or pretreated gastric or GEJ cancer (NCT02443324). In the treatment naïve cohort ($N = 28$), the preliminary ORR was 25% and disease controlled was achieved in 68% of enrolled patients; the median PFS and duration of response was 5.3 and 10 months, respectively.[45] Sixty-one percent of patients experienced a grade 3 treatment-related AE, mostly diarrhea and hypertension, and there were no grade 4 or 5 AEs. In the pretreated cohort ($N = 41$, 59% with two prior lines of therapy), the ORR was 7%, 64% of patients achieved disease control with study treatment, and the PFS at 6 months was 22%.[46] Approximately 25% of the patients experienced a grade 3 or 4 AE, mostly colitis or hypertension. In another ongoing phase I study of ramucirumab in combination with durvalumab in pretreated patients (NCT02572687), the preliminary confirmed ORR was 17% (5 out of 29 enrolled patients) and the median PFS was 2.6 months.[47] The ORR in tumors with PD-L1 expression higher than 25% was 36%. Thirty-five percent of patients had a grade 3 treatment-related AE, the most frequent ones being hypertension, fatigue, and diarrhea. There were no grade 4 or 5 AEs. A study evaluating the combination of ramucirumab with nivolumab is also in progress (NCT02999295).

Trastuzumab, a humanized IgG1 monoclonal antibody targeting the extracellular domain of human epidermal receptor 2 (HER2), has been established as standard of care in combination with first-line chemotherapy in patients with HER2-amplified, advanced GEC cancer based on the results of the ToGA study.[48] Immune checkpoint inhibitors are currently in development with anti-HER2 agents in GEC cancer (NCT02689284, NCT02318901). The preliminary results of a phase I/II trial of pembrolizumab in combination with margetuximab, a novel HER2 targeting monoclonal antibody with an optimized Fc domain to increase affinity for activating CD16A Fc-receptors on natural killer (NK) cells, were encouraging with an ORR of 18.4%; stable disease was achieved in 28.9% of patients.[49] The study treatment was well tolerated with only one serious treatment-related AE being observed in the 57 patients enrolled in the dose-escalation and dose-expansion cohorts to date.

Future Directions

T-cell immunoglobulin domain and mucin domain-3 (TIM3) and carcinoembryonic antigen cell adhesion molecule 1 (CEACAM1) are two inhibitory immune checkpoints that form a heterodimer on effector T-cells; CEACAM1 is essential for the surface expression and inhibitory activity of TIM3.[50] CEACAM1 is overexpressed in malignant gastric tissue while not in neighboring benign tissue[51] and can be an important contributor to immune evasion in GEC. A phase I clinical trial evaluation of the combination of pembrolizumab and CM24, a CEACAM1 targeting monoclonal antibody, in multiple tumor types including GEC is underway (NCT02346955). The expression pattern of CEACAM1 is different in intestinal versus diffuse type gastric carcinoma (membranous vs. cytoplasmic respectively),[51] and this can potentially affect the activity of CM24. Hyaluronan is an extracellular glycosaminoglycan in many solid tumors types; ectopic expression is frequent in gastric carcinoma and is associated with the presence of poor clinicopathologic prognostic factors.[52] PEGPH20 can increase the efficacy of immune checkpoint inhibitors in preclinical cancer models[53]; PEGH20 is actively evaluated in combination with immune checkpoint inhibitors in clinical trials in multiple disease types including GEC (NCT02563548).

Claudin-18 isoform 2 (CLDN18.2) is a tight junction protein and a target of interest in gastric and GEJ adenocarcinoma.[54,55] IMAB362 is a CLDN18.2-targeting, chimeric, IgG1 monoclonal antibody that can potentially improve clinical outcomes for patients with advanced disease in combination with chemotherapy.[56] In an open label, phase I study, patients with advanced, pretreated gastric cancer were treated with IMAB362 with or without an immunomodulatory regimen comprising of interleukin-2 and/or zoledronic acid.[57] Increased effector T-cell and NK cell activation as well as antigen-dependent cell cytotoxicity was observed. Based on the observed effects in innate antitumor immunity, it may be an appropriate agent for development in combination with immune checkpoint inhibitors.

Radiotherapy is a standard part of therapy for early stage disease and often used as a means of symptom management in advanced disease. Preclinical models have demonstrated increased T-cell infiltration at sites of radiation, particularly with fractionated therapy, as well as abscopal responses, which appear to be restrained by multiple immune checkpoints.[58,59] Given its potential to enhance immunogenicity of the TME, through multiple mechanisms, there is good rationale for the use of radiotherapy, before or in combination with checkpoint inhibition. Multiple studies are underway looking at PD-1 or PD-L1 inhibition combined with preoperative chemoradiotherapy in the locally advanced setting (NCT02730546, NCT0296063, NCT03087864, NCT02844075). As combinations are within reach, one ongoing phase I study is evaluating PD-1 or dual PD-1/CTLA-4 inhibition before a combination of nivolumab and chemoradiotherapy for resectable gastroesophageal cancer (NCT03044613). The strategy of PD-1 combined with palliative radiation is also being evaluated in the metastatic setting (NCT02830594). These studies should serve to broaden the understanding of optimal incorporation of radiotherapy with checkpoint inhibition in this disease.

HEPATOCELLULAR CARCINOMA

Hepatocellular carcinoma (HCC) is an important global healthcare problem. The incidence varies globally and in certain regions, where hepatitis B and C are endemic and rates are significantly elevated; although hepatitis C remains prominent in the United States, many additional cases can be attributed in part to alcohol-induced cirrhosis, diabetes mellitus, obesity, and nonalcoholic steatohepatitis.[60,61] With an incidence that has almost tripled since the early 1980s, it is currently the fastest rising cause of cancer-related death in the United States.[62,63] Systemic therapy options are limited for patients with advanced disease; sorafenib and regorafenib are the only approved agents in first- and second-line setting, respectively, but their effectiveness is suboptimal.[64,65]

Essential for its function as the main organ that processes molecules absorbed from the gastrointestinal tract, the liver can minimize immune response to intestinal bacteria–derived molecules.[66,67] Hepatocytes and supportive cells within the liver can induce an anergic CD8+ T-cell phenotype[68–70]; liver dendritic cells (DCs) are less immunogenic than those in other organs.[71] In addition, upregulation of immune checkpoints and immunosuppressive cytokines is observed in the setting of chronic viral inflammation leading to immune exhaustion.[72–78] Furthermore, tumor cells interact with supportive cells within the TME through the secretion of immunosuppressive cytokines,[79] which can suppress cytotoxic T- and NK-cells and activate M2 (protumor) TAMs.[80–83]

Clinical Trials of Immune Checkpoint Inhibitors in Hepatocellular Carcinoma

Immune checkpoint inhibitors as single agents
CTLA-4 targeting monotherapy has been investigated in HCC. Tremelimumab resulted in an ORR of 17.6% and a disease control rate of 76.4% in patients with advanced HCC in a phase I trial.[84] A significant decrease in hepatitis C viral load in a subgroup of patients with chronic hepatitis C infection was also noted. CheckMate-040 is a phase I/II trial of nivolumab in patients with sorafenib-naïve or pretreated, advanced HCC.[85] The ORR ranged between 14% and 20% in a mixed population both with and without prior exposure and trial phase (dose-escalation or expansion); the 12-month OS ranged between 58% and 70% (depending on prior therapy and dose cohort). PD-L1 expression did not correlate with the response nor did viral status.[86] Treatment was well

tolerated. Outcomes with nivolumab were considerably improved compared with historical experience with sorafenib. This led to a randomized, controlled phase III trial comparing nivolumab with sorafenib as a primary treatment in patients with advanced HCC; this trial is currently in progress (CheckMate-459, NCT02576509). Pembrolizumab monotherapy as second-line therapy is also under evaluation in advanced HCC. In the phase II KEYNOTE-224 study (NCT02702414), 104 sorafenib pretreated patients have been enrolled to date. Most patients had disease progression on sorafenib, and 63% had extrahepatic disease.[87] The ORR was 16.3%, and 61.5% of patients had stable disease as best response; as in CheckMate-040, responses were unrelated to the underlying etiology of liver disease. The median PFS was tabulated at 4.8 months. Twenty-five percent of patients had a grade 3 or higher treatment-related AE; there was one death on study (ulcerative esophagitis). Importantly, no viral hepatitis flare was observed. KEYNOTE-240 (NCT02702401) is evaluating pembrolizumab compared with placebo in patients with advanced, pretreated HCC; results are expected in 2019. Durvalumab was tested in a phase I trial in patients with advanced HCC; 93% had received prior therapy with sorafenib.[88] Twenty percent of the patients experienced a grade 3 or 4 AE, mainly hepatic enzyme elevation; there were no deaths secondary to study therapy. The ORR was 10.3%. Durvalumab efficacy—contrary to that of nivolumab—appears to be related to viral status, with the highest ORR observed in patients with hepatitis C (25% vs. 0% in patients with hepatitis B vs. 9.5% in patients without hepatitis). Similarly 12-month OS was higher in patients with hepatitis C (83.3% vs. 38.6% vs. 57.1).

Immune checkpoint inhibitor combinations
Dual immune checkpoint inhibition with durvalumab/tremelimumab combination has been tested for patients with advanced HCC in a phase I trial ($N = 40$).[89] One-third of the patients had not received any prior systemic therapy. The combination was safe, with most common serious AE being asymptomatic elevations in transaminases. Three patients had to discontinue treatment for treatment-related AE (grade 3 pneumonitis, grade 3 colitis, and asymptomatic grade 4 transaminase elevation). The ORR was 20%. Contrary to the durvalumab monotherapy study, the combination appears more efficacious in patients without viral hepatitis (39% vs. 9% in patients with hepatitis B vs. 0% in patients with hepatitis C).

Future Directions

Sorafenib can enhance antitumor immunity by improving functionality of effector T-cells, DC, and NK-cells, increasing the effector T-cell/regulatory T-cell (T_{reg}) ratio, enhance cytotoxic T-cells, and suppress immunosuppressive immune cell migration to the liver, as well as decrease the levels of immunosuppressive IL-10 and TGF-β1.[90−94] Thus, sorafenib can be a useful agent to be used in combination with immunotherapeutic agents. Clinical trials evaluating sorafenib in combination with immune checkpoint inhibitors are underway (NCT03211416). Furthermore, TGF-β can act as an immunosuppressive cytokine by enhancing T_{reg} function.[95] Galunisertib, a TGF-β1 inhibitor, in combination with nivolumab is under evaluation in a phase I/II trial, enrolling patients with multiple tumor types including advanced, refractory HCC (NCT02423343).

Ablative therapies are approved treatment options for early or intermediate stage HCC. Tumor destruction by delivering high energy with radiofrequency ablation (RFA) or microwave ablation leads to the release of highly immunogenic intracellular molecules that can be taken up by professional APCs and improve the systemic antitumor cytokine profile.[96−98] RFA can markedly increase cytotoxic T-cells within the tumor and draining lymph nodes as well as delay growth of distant tumors through a T-cell−mediated, antitumor immunity.[99] In addition, as reviewed by Gravante and colleagues, cryoablation causes cellular inflammation through low temperatures and can release intact cellular components that are also immunogenic.[100] Furthermore, transarterial chemoembolization (TACE) has been shown to increase T_{h17} cells, decrease T_{regs}, and alter the systemic cytokine profile and the level of T-cell activation.[101−104] When combined with immune checkpoint inhibitors, these therapies have the potential of having a synergistic antitumor effect. Tremelimumab in combination with subtotal TACE or RFA in patients with advanced HCC was shown to be safe and feasible.[105] Currently, several trials are evaluating the role of liver-directed ablative therapies plus immune checkpoint inhibition in HCC (NCT02821754, NCT01853618, NCT01828762).

Adoptive T-cell therapy is an interesting immunotherapy strategy, where tumor-specific immune cells are modified ex vivo and then infused in human subjects and can be used as an adjunct to immune checkpoint inhibitor therapy. Cytokine-induced killer cells (CIKs) are autologous peripheral mononuclear cells created ex vivo by incubation with cytokines including IFN-γ, IL-1, IL-2, and anti-CD3 antibody.[106] Results from phase III trials of CIKs administration after curative resection or local ablation in patients with early HCC, reveal potentially improved long-term outcomes.[107,108] A clinical trial evaluating CIKs and anti-PD-1 combination therapy is underway (NCT02886897).

CHOLANGIOCARCINOMA

Cholangiocarcinoma (CC) is the second most common hepatic malignancy following HCC. It is categorized into intrahepatic and extrahepatic. Intrahepatic CC originates proximal to the bifurcation of right and left hepatic ducts. Extrahepatic CC is further divided into perihilar CC, originating from the common bile duct distal to the bifurcation of hepatic ducts but proximal to the cystic duct, and distal CC, originating distal to the cystic duct.[109,110] CC is a rare malignancy in the United States, but the incidence of CC has increased gradually over decades worldwide.[111] Patients with early stage disease are usually asymptomatic; most patients with CC have advanced disease at diagnosis.[112,113] Gemcitabine plus cisplatin is the most widely used initial treatment strategy for patients with advanced disease based on the results of the ABC-02 trial, but the overall prognosis is grim with a median OS of less than 1 year.[114]

A characteristic feature of the CC microenvironment is the extensive desmoplasia (accounting for up to 90% of the tumor volume) amidst immunosuppressive inflammatory and stromal cells.[115,116] Desmoplasia can also increase the intratumoral pressure and material density leading to decreased penetration of therapeutic drugs and cytotoxic immune cells.[117] This complex ecosystem has been attributed as the main cause of poor response to immunotherapy. However, PD-L1 expression is present in up to 72% of tumor cells and 63% of immune cells,[112,118,119] and 5%−10% of CC are known to have MMR deficiency.[120] Therefore, immune checkpoint inhibitors could be a promising treatment option, but as the presence of chronic inflammation from underlying infectious or autoimmune diseases (liver fluke infection, hepatitis B and C, bacterial cholangitis, and primary sclerosing cholangitis) is the main predisposing risk factor,[121] patients have the theoretical risk of underlying disease flare when treated with immuno-oncology agents. Clinical trials of immune checkpoint inhibitors are underway as monotherapy or in combination with other treatment modalities for the treatment of CC.

Clinical Trials of Immune Checkpoint Inhibitors in Cholangiocarcinoma

Interim results from the CC cohort of KEYNOTE-028 were presented in 2015.[122] Out of 89 patients with CC, 37 (42%) were positive for PD-L1 expression. Twenty four (24) out of 37 patients were enrolled and were treated with pembrolizumab every 2 weeks for up to 2 years. The ORR was 17% (4 patients), and 4 (17%) patients had stable disease. Median progression-free survival (PFS) was not reached at the time of analysis and presentation. Overall, 15 (63%) patients had treatment-related AEs, mostly pyrexia and nausea. Four (17%) patients experienced grade 3−4 treatment-related AEs including anemia, autoimmune hemolytic anemia, colitis, and dermatitis. Clinical trials of anti-PD-1 (NCT03110328, NCT02628067, and NCT02829918) and anti-CTLA-4 antibodies (NCT01938612) as monotherapy are underway.

Future Directions

In an effort to improve the efficacy of immune checkpoint inhibitors, anti-PD-1 and anti-CTLA-4 antibody combination treatment is currently under evaluation in advanced CC (NCT02834013 and NCT01938612). Furthermore, chemotherapy is known to augment antitumor immunity by inducing immunogenic cell death and disrupting strategies that tumors use to evade immune recognition.[123] Clinical trials of cytotoxic combination chemotherapy plus immune checkpoint inhibition (NCT02268825, NCT03111732, and NCT03046862) and cytotoxic/immune checkpoint inhibitor combination versus dual immune checkpoint inhibitor therapy (NCT03101566) are additionally in progress. As discussed earlier, radiation or ablation leads to the release of intracellular components that can induce immunogenicity, the activation of APCs, and enhancement of local antitumor immunity. An open-label, phase I clinical trial of tremelimumab with chemoembolization or ablation for liver cancer including intrahepatic CC is evaluating the safety of these combined treatment modalities (NCT01853618). Adoptive T-cell strategies can also increase the efficacy of immune checkpoint inhibition. Tran et al. reported that treatment with CD4+ TILs recognizing a specific mutation in HER2 interacting protein (ERBB2IP), led to a partial response in a patient with CC, which was reproduced on retreatment following progression.[124] Based on this promising result, a phase II clinical trial of pembrolizumab with infusion of TILs for patients with metastatic cancer is underway. This study has a subset of CC (NCT01174121).

As previously discussed, CC is characterized by a very complex, immunosuppressive microenvironment with an extensive desmoplastic reaction. Combinations of immune checkpoint inhibitors with immunomodulators such as cytokines (NCT02703714) and peginterferon alfa-2b (NCT02982720) are in progress. A phase I trial of ramucirumab with pembrolizumab with a goal of enhancing T-cell recruitment and normalizing the dysfunctional tumor vasculature is including patients with advanced CC (NCT02443324).[112] The heterogeneity of CC revealed by the whole genome sequencing has opened the possibility of the molecular targeted therapy. Nakamura et al. demonstrated that up to 40% of patients with CC have targetable alterations such as isocitrate dehydrogenase-1/2 (*IDH1/2*), *BRCA1/2* mutations, fibroblast growth factor receptor-2 (*FGFR2*) translocations, MSI, and v-ros UR2 sarcoma virus oncogene homologue 1 (*ROS1*) fusions.[125] Multiple clinical trials are underway to prove the efficacy of targeted agents in CC. A phase I/II trial of INCB054828 (an inhibitor of FGFR1-3) combined with pembrolizumab is to evaluate the safety and efficacy of the combination in advanced malignancies with genetic alterations in FGF or FGFR genes (NCT02393248), including patients with CC.

PANCREATIC ADENOCARCINOMA

Pancreatic ductal adenocarcinoma (PDAC) is the fourth leading cause of cancer-related death in the United States with a 5-year OS of only 5%.[126,127] Almost 80% of the patients present with advanced (locoregional or metastatic) disease for which there is no known cure.[126] The basis of management of advanced PDAC is cytotoxic chemotherapy, gemcitabine- or 5-fluorouracil (5FU)−based.[128−130] Cancer immunotherapy has been proven to be largely ineffective. PDAC is considered an immunologically "quiescent" tumor.[131] As previously discussed, tumor immunogenicity and response to immune checkpoint inhibitors are related to the ability of cancer cells to present neoepitopes and is associated with the mutational burden of the tumor. In general, PDAC is characterized by a low to moderate mutation burden compared with that of other cancers.[132] In fact, the mutational burden of pancreatic cancer is the lowest among gastrointestinal cancers (5 mutations per Mb), with approximately 1% of pancreatic cancers having a high mutation burden (defined as more than 17 mutations per Mb).[133] Furthermore, although MSI correlates with response to immunotherapy, the incidence of MSI-H pancreatic adenocarcinoma is less than 1%.[134,135]

In addition to low mutation and neoepitope burden, PDAC is characterized by a highly immunosuppressive TME.[136,137] Immune cells such as TAMs, T_{regs}, and myeloid derived suppressor cells (MDSCs) are linked to the development of this immune-quiescent microenvironment.[136] T_{regs} and MDSCs are increased in patients with PDAC compared with normal individuals.[138,139] Furthermore, increasing number of MDSCs in peripheral blood has been associated with progressive disease.[140] These immune cells can impair effector T-cell activity through multiple mechanisms such as expression of surface inhibitory proteins, induction of T-cell apoptosis through FAS/FAS-L and TRAIL pathway activation, prevention of T-cell differentiation, secretion of immunosuppressive cytokines and growth factors (e.g., TGF-β, IL-6, IL-10), production of reactive oxygen species, and depletion of amino acids essential for T-cell function and survival such as arginine and tryptophan.[141,142] Furthermore, nonimmune cells within the PDAC microenvironment, such as the fibroblast-activating protein expressing cancer-associated fibroblasts (CAFs), may be associated with impaired effector T-cell accumulation within the tumor through CXCL12 production.[143] Pancreatic stellate cells, a subset of CAFs, secrete IL-6 that can promote differentiation of myeloid cells to functional MDSCs.[144]

Thus, multiple components of the tumor ecosystem should be simultaneously or sequentially modulated to improve the activity of the immune system against tumor cells. Multiple studies incorporating cancer vaccines, immune checkpoint inhibitors, and cytotoxic chemotherapeutics have been launched in a quest for an effective combination. We are discussing the most important clinical efforts in the next section.

Clinical Trials of Immune Checkpoint Inhibitors in Pancreatic Adenocarcinoma
Immune checkpoint inhibitors as single agents
The results of a phase II study of ipilimumab in advanced, pretreated PDAC were in general disappointing with only 1 of the 27 enrolled patients experiencing a delayed response after pseudoprogression.[145] A phase I study of the anti-PD-L1 IgG4 antibody BMS-936559 enrolled 14 patients with PDAC.[131] No clinical responses were noted. Preliminary activity of durvalumab was reported at the 2014 American Society of Clinical Oncology Annual Meeting with some tumor stabilization observed in almost half of the patients with PDAC.[146] These results were not confirmed in a subsequent phase II trial of durvalumab monotherapy or in combination with tremelimumab in patients with previously treated disease (NCT02558894). The study was terminated after enrollment of the first 65 patients for futility, as the disease control rate was 6.1% and 9.4% in the

monotherapy and combination arms, respectively.[147] One patient in the combination arm ($N = 32$) had a durable partial response lasting more than 12 months. There were no new safety signals.

Small molecular inhibitors targeting key enzymes linked to immune tolerance represent a novel class of immunotherapeutic agents. Indoleamine 2, 3-dioxygenase (IDO) is an enzyme that degrades tryptophan through the kynurenine pathway thus leading to decreased T-cell proliferation; most human cancers including PDAC express IDO.[148,149] IDO-expressing tumors in vivo show signs of resistance to peptide vaccine immunotherapy that can be reversed with pharmacologic IDO inhibition.[148] IDO is expressed and can be upregulated with IFN-γ in PDAC.[150] Hydroxyamidine IDO1 inhibitors have in vivo activity against PDAC xenografts in immunocompetent but not immunodeficient mice; activity is not dependent on host IDO expression.[151] Levels of tumor-infiltrating lymphocytes are increased after IDO inhibitor treatment.[151] Indoximod is a competitive IDO inhibitor with a favorable toxicity profile in phase I trials that can be safely combined with cytotoxic chemotherapy.[152,153] There were only three patients with pancreatic cancer in those two studies precluding any meaningful conclusions regarding its activity as single agent.

Immune checkpoint inhibitors in combination with other agents
Immune checkpoint inhibitor and tumor vaccine combinations. The main class of immunotherapeutic agents that have been under investigation in PDAC is therapeutic tumor vaccines. GVAX is an allogeneic, irradiated granulocyte-macrophage colony-stimulating factor (GM-CSF) expressing, whole-cell PDAC vaccine manufactured from the PANC 10.05 and 6.03 cell lines.[154] GVAX has been extensively studied in the adjuvant or advanced disease setting both as a single agent and in combination with chemotherapy or chemoradiotherapy.[155–157] GVAX is very well tolerated, with the most common AE being grade 1 or 2 injection site reactions, but its clinical efficacy appears to be limited. Development of a delayed hypersensitivity reaction (DTH) to the vaccine has been linked to improved long-term outcomes.[155] DTH response to GVAX directly correlates with induction of mesothelin-specific effector T-cell responses.[158] Sustained enhancement of mesothelin peptide–specific effector T-cell responses and expansion in the repertoire of the

targeted mesothelin-derived epitopes appeared to be associated with long (more than 3 years) disease-free survival in patients treated with adjuvant therapy.[156]

There is evidence that GVAX can edit PDAC, converting it to a more "immune active" tumor.[159] Neoadjuvant GVAX can induce formation of organized tertiary intratumoral lymphoid aggregates that contain antigen-experienced T-cells. Presence of these aggregates is a characteristic of more immunogenic tumors such as NSCLC or melanoma.[160,161] T-cells in the aggregates express early activation markers and the activated T-cell, trafficking chemokine receptor CXCR3 but not granzyme B. T_{regs} are present in the aggregates as well as macrophages expressing PD-L1. T_{reg} pathway downregulation and T_{h17} pathway upregulation within the lymphoid aggregates is associated with longer survival. Furthermore, PD-1 upregulation is associated with improved survival, whereas the opposite is true for PD-L1.

A phase Ib study at John Hopkins University evaluated the combination of GVAX with ipilimumab in patients with previously treated advanced PDAC.[162] The study's primary objective was to test the safety of the combination. Individuals were randomized in a 1:1 fashion to ipilimumab alone at the dose of 10 mg/kg or GVAX plus ipilimumab. The occurrence of grade 3 or 4 immune-related AE was 20% for both arms; the rate of events attributed to ipilimumab was consistent to prior knowledge. OS appeared to improve with the combination (5.7 vs. 3.6 months for ipilimumab monotherapy). Increased posttreatment mesothelin-specific T-cell responses (T-cell number and repertoire) were noted in patients surviving more than 4.3 months. Five patients had stable disease as best response in both arms combined, including one case of pseudoprogression in the combination arm.

As discussed earlier, GVAX induces PD-L1 expression in PDAC in vivo; combination of the vaccine plus PD-1–blocking antibody improved survival in a murine PDAC xenograft model compared with either agent as monotherapy.[163] STELLAR is an ongoing randomized phase II study that evaluates GVAX plus CRS-207, a live-attenuated *Listeria monocytogenes* strain genetically modified to express mesothelin,[164] with or without nivolumab (NCT02243371). In a study presented by Nesselhut and colleagues, by the use of an autologous DC vaccine modified in vitro by PDL-1 blockade, secondary disease stabilization (4–8 months) was achieved in 5 out of 10 patients with advanced PDAC, who failed to respond to previous vaccine therapy.[165] In a pilot study from the same group, addition of nivolumab induced partial responses in two out of the seven DC vaccine–treated patients.[166] An ongoing study will evaluate CRS-207, nivolumab, and ipilimumab with or without the GVAX in advanced pancreatic cancer (NCT03190265).

Immune checkpoint inhibitor and oncolytic virus combinations. Oncolytic viruses (either naturally occurring or genetically modified) are characterized by their ability to infect and kill malignant cells while leaving normal neighboring cells unharmed. Treatment with reovirus, a naturally occurring oncolytic virus, can directly and indirectly lead to malignant cell death through dysfunctional RNA-dependent protein kinase signaling in tumors harboring an activated RAS pathway[167] and the induction of tumor-specific adaptive immune responses, respectively.[168] Gemcitabine in combination with reovirus can accelerate antitumor immunity generation most likely by decreasing immunosuppressive cells within the TME.[169]

In a phase II randomized study in patients with treatment-naïve advanced PDAC, addition of oncolytic reovirus to chemotherapy (carboplatin/paclitaxel) did not improve outcomes compared with chemotherapy alone and appeared to increase cells with an immunosuppressive phenotype (T_{regs}, CTLA4+ and TIM3+ T-cells) as detected by flow cytometry.[170] In a single-arm, phase II trial in a similar patient population, the combination of reovirus with gemcitabine prolonged the duration of disease control compared with gemcitabine alone (historical control) with minimal toxicities.[171] Furthermore, when analyzing on-treatment tumor biopsies, apart from viral replication and apoptosis that were observed, upregulation of PD-L1 was demonstrated.[172,173] In the phase I REO 024 trial, reovirus was combined with pembrolizumab and chemotherapy as second-line therapy of patients with advanced disease.[174] Of the 11 patients enrolled, 8 experienced a grade 3 or 4 AE mostly related to chemotherapy or the underlying disease. Of the five patients who were evaluable for efficacy, one had a long-lasting partial response (6 month duration) and two had stable disease (lasting 126 and 221 days). On-treatment biopsies confirmed cancer cell infection with the virus and presence of immune infiltrates.

Immune checkpoint inhibitor and chemotherapy or radiotherapy combinations. T-cells in patients with PDAC treated with gemcitabine exhibit increased IFN-γ and decreased IL-10 production after treatment as well as an increase in T-cells, harboring the early activation marker CD69; overall numbers of T-, B-, and DC precursor cells and activity are not affected.[175] More importantly, cytotoxic agents as well as radiotherapy can prime the immune system against cancer through induction of apoptosis and antigen release.[176,177] Chemotherapeutics such as oxaliplatin can trigger immunologic cell death through release of danger associated molecular patterns such as calreticulin, ATP, and high-mobility group box-1 (HMGB-1) protein. Treatment with platinum agents can also lead to downregulation of PD-L2 through loss of STAT6 phosphorylation.[178] 5FU and gemcitabine can decrease the number of MDSCs in vivo.[179,180] MDSC production of arginase-1, an enzyme associated with induction of T-cell suppression, is not increased when human monocytes are primed with PDAC cell culture supernatant in the presence of gemcitabine.[181] Furthermore, it can decrease T_{regs} and restore the effector T-cell/T_{reg} ratio in patients with PDAC.[182] Thus, studies examining chemoimmunotherapy combinations have been pursued or are underway.

Gemcitabine has been combined with ipilimumab in treatment-naïve patients with advanced PDAC.[183] The maximum tolerated dose was established as 3 mg/kg IV for ipilimumab and 1000 mg/m^2 IV for gemcitabine. The disease control rate in the 16 enrolled patients was 43% with 2 patients having a partial response. Median PFS and OS were 2.5 and 8.5 months, respectively. In a phase I study, nivolumab was combined with nab-paclitaxel (arm A) and nab-paclitaxel/gemcitabine combination (arm B); all medications were given at the Food and Drug Administration (FDA) approved doses.[184] The preliminary results presented at the 2017 ASCO Gastrointestinal Cancers Symposium are promising, with 6 out of 11 patients in arm A and all 6 patients in arm B experiencing disease control (2 and 3 patients had partial response respectively). The combinations were well tolerated with most severe adverse events being myelosuppression secondary to chemotherapy. There were no immune-related AE.

There is in vitro evidence for synergy between IDO downregulation and gemcitabine.[185] In a phase I/II trial, indoximod was combined with nab-paclitaxel/gemcitabine as first-line therapy in patients with advanced PDAC. There was no new safety signals in the phase I part of the study; the recommended phase 2 dose was 1200 mg twice daily orally (the same as the monotherapy dose).[186] Preliminary efficacy results after enrollment of 30 patients are encouraging with an ORR of 37%.[187] There was one case of colitis necessitating withdrawal from the study.

The lymphocyte activation gene-3 (LAG-3 or CD223) is a T-cell surface protein that negatively regulates effector T-cell function; when it binds to major histocompatibility complex (MHC) type II, it promotes the maturation of DCs.[188,189] IMP321 is a chimeric molecule consisting of an extracellular portion of human LAG-3 fused to the F_C fraction of human IgG1 and has been shown to have strong immunostimulatory effects.[190] When combined with gemcitabine in a phase I study in 18 patients with newly diagnosed advanced PDAC, it was proven to be safe and well tolerated; no dose-limiting toxicity related to IMP321 was observed.[191] No immunologic effect was evident with the doses evaluated in this study. IMP321 is not currently in development for pancreatic adenocarcinoma. Other LAG-3 antibodies (BMS-986016) are currently in clinical development for a variety of solid and hematologic tumors.

Stereotactic body radiotherapy (SBRT) was combined with immune checkpoint inhibition for patients with advanced PDAC in a pilot, phase I study.[192] Twenty-four patients with chemotherapy-refractory metastatic disease, with at least one lesion amenable to SBRT, have been enrolled to date. Patients were treated with durvalumab alone or in combination with tremelimumab. The combination was safe, with the most common toxicity being fatigue. Approximately 25% of the patients developed rapid disease progression, and the best response was stable disease in 21% of the patients.

Future Directions

Inhibition of monocyte trafficking to the tumor bed and differentiation to TAMs/M2-polarized monocytes through chemokine axis targeting may be another useful therapeutic strategy to overcome PDAC resistance to immunotherapy.[193] Multiple chemokines orchestrate monocyte migration to tissues in health and disease.[194] Chemokine receptor CXCR2 and its ligands are important for MDSC migration in tumor areas.[195] CXCR2 is overexpressed in tumor-infiltrating neutrophils and associated with poor outcomes. Pharmacologic CXCR2 inhibition in the KPC pancreatic cancer mouse model improved animal survival and prevented metastatic spread; outcomes appeared to improve when CXCR2 inhibitor was administered in combination with gemcitabine or anti-PD1 therapy.[196] In addition, inhibition of the CXCL12 receptor CXCR4 with plerixafor can increase T-cell accumulation within the tumor and lead to growth arrest in the KPC model, effects that are augmented with anti-PD-L1 therapy, while anti-PD-L1 therapy alone is ineffective.[143] Furthermore, targeting myeloid cells within the TME through colony stimulating factor-1 receptor (CSF1R) blockade increases antitumor T-cell responses and can sensitize PDAC to immunotherapy.[197,198] A clinical trial evaluating the anti-CSF1R antibody AMG 820 in combination with pembrolizumab is currently underway (NCT02713529). Acquisition of a tumor-promoting phenotype by TAMs in pancreatic cancer appears to be related to a crosstalk between the TAMs and B-cells, mediated through Bruton tyrosine kinase (BTK) and phosphatidylinositol kinase-3-gamma (PI3Kγ) signaling.[199] Treatment with BTK or PI3Kγ inhibitors appears to reverse immunosuppression and improve the efficacy of gemcitabine in preclinical pancreatic cancer models.[199,200] Preclinical synergy between BTK or PI3Kγ and PD-1/PD-L1 inhibition has been demonstrated in lymphoma and breast cancer, respectively.[201] The potential for synergy with immune checkpoint inhibitors in PDAC remains to be determined.

Focal adhesion kinase (FAK) is a nonreceptor cytoplasmic protein tyrosine kinase that participates in tumor cell–microenvironment crosstalk.[202] FAK is upregulated in PDAC compared with normal pancreatic tissue. High FAK levels in tumor cells correlate with the presence of an immune infiltrate characterized by an abundance of myeloid cells and decreased effector T-cells.[203] FAK inhibition appears to decrease both macrophage and CAF migration in vitro; furthermore, decrease in TAM and CAF was observed in vivo correlating with decrease in tumor cell proliferation and growth.[204] In addition, FAK inhibition has synergistic antitumor activity with immune checkpoint inhibition in vivo. FAK inhibition can also decrease fibrosis within the TME.[203] Prior attempts to target desmoplasia in PDAC with Sonic Hedgehog pathway inhibition have failed with preclinical evidence of acceleration in the disease process and no clinical benefit.[205–207] Depletion of CAF and associated decrease in desmoplasia in PDAC animal models has also lead to more aggressive tumors, inducing epithelial to mesenchymal phenotype and increasing the number of cancer stem cells and T_{regs}; treatment with immune checkpoint inhibitors appears to reverse this process.[208] FAK inhibition appears to decrease desmoplasia without evidence of disease acceleration.[203] Currently, the combination of defactinib, an oral FAK inhibitor, with pembrolizumab is under investigation in clinical trials (NCT02758587, NCT02546531).

CD40 is an APC surface molecule that upon activation by its ligand (CD40L) can lead to increased cytotoxic T-cell priming.[209] The CD40 agonist CP-870,893 was tested in combination with gemcitabine in 21 patients with advanced PDAC as first-line therapy.[210] The most common AE was cytokine release syndrome on the day of CD40 agonist infusion that was transient, mild to moderate in severity, and managed at an outpatient basis. Four patients had a response to therapy, and 11 had stable disease. On-treatment biopsies from two patients who had a response to therapy revealed tumor necrosis and macrophage but no lymphocyte infiltration. Results were similar in the KPC pancreatic cancer model for the combination therapy, whereas monotherapy with gemcitabine resulted in inferior outcomes. CD40 therapy did not lead to T-cell accumulation within the tumor in the KPC model as well. It appears that CD40 agonist therapy promoted migration of macrophages with an M1 antitumor phenotype within the tumor, which are able to degrade the fibrotic tumor stroma. Furthermore, in preclinical models, CD40 agonist therapy with or without cytotoxic chemotherapy in vitro increases the effector T-cell/T_{reg} ratio and sensitizes pancreatic adenocarcinoma to PD-1/CTLA-4 immune checkpoint inhibitors, providing rationale for combination studies in humans.[211,212]

Janus-activated kinases (JAK) phosphorylate and activate STAT proteins.[213] Ruxolitinib is a JAK1/2 inhibitor approved for treatment of essential myelofibrosis. In a phase II, double blind, placebo-controlled trial patients with advanced pretreated PDAC were treated with capecitabine plus ruxolitinib or placebo ($N = 127$).[214] Although combination therapy was not proven superior to capecitabine plus placebo in the intention-to-treat population, in an ad hoc analysis of patients with C-reactive protein (CRP) above the population median, ruxolitinib significantly increased OS (HR 0.47, $P = .011$) but not PFS (HR 0.82, $P = .47$). Improvement in OS was not confirmed in phase III studies preselecting patients with CRP >10 mg/L.[215] Thus, ruxolitinib development was halted for PDAC, but a potential for synergy with immune checkpoint inhibitor therapy exists as ruxolitinib can increase CD8+ T-cell infiltration in vivo.[216]

Furthermore, as summarized by Chiappanelli et al., epigenetic modulation and gene reprogramming with demethylating agents (DAs) and histone deacetylase inhibitors (HDACi) in a variety of human malignancies has the potential for synergy with immunotherapy through upregulation of tumor-associated antigens, activation of INF-related pathways, and decrease in T_{reg} population.[217] Immune-quiescent tumors can be sensitized to immunotherapy with checkpoint inhibitors with DA/HDACi therapy.[218] In preclinical models, PDAC was proven to be amenable to epigenetic modulation with DAs and potentially more responsive to immunotherapy through upregulation of INF-related genes.[219,220] In addition, inhibition of autophagy with hydroxychloroquine in combination with HDACi has been shown to improve the immunologic profile of patients with refractory, metastatic colorectal cancer with decrease in T_{regs} and T-cell exhaustion markers in peripheral blood and can be a useful strategy to be explored in other immune-quiescent tumors such as PDAC.[221] In a phase II trial of preoperative systemic therapy in patients with PDAC amenable to surgical resection, hydroxychloroquine was proven to increase tumor T-cell infiltration and PD-L1 expression when combined with chemotherapy compared with chemotherapy alone.[222]

Germline *BRCA1/2* mutations are present in approximately 5% of unselected patients with pancreatic adenocarcinoma.[223] Twenty-two percent of pancreatic cancer cases tested at a commercial laboratory had *BRCA1/2* mutation (somatic or germline).[224] In addition, almost 15% of pancreatic cancers have evidence of a somatic *BRCA*-like mutational signature.[225] *BRCA2*-positive tumors have a higher rate of PD-1/PD-L1 positivity, *BRCA1*-positive cases have a higher incidence of PD-1+ TILs.[224] Poly-ADP-ribose polymerase (PARP) inhibitors and platinum agents are potential active agents for patients with *BRCA*-deficient pancreatic cancers.[225–227] PARP inhibitor therapy renders *BRCA*-deficient ovarian cancer more susceptible to immune checkpoint inhibition in vivo.[228] Early findings from a phase I trial evaluating PARP and PD-L1 inhibition in a variety of solid tumors are promising, with two patients with PDAC ($N = 3$) treated experiencing prolonged disease stabilization.[229]

COLORECTAL CANCER

Colorectal adenocarcinomas (CRC) represent the most common malignancies originating within the gastrointestinal system. All told, CRC is the second leading cause of cancer-related death in the United States and a major problem globally.[126] Nearly 25% of patients present with metastatic colorectal adenocarcinoma (mCRC) and almost half of all patients will develop recurrent or metastatic disease at some point within their disease course.[230] Although hepatectomy and other local therapies remain options in metastatic disease, chemotherapy remains the mainstay of treatment, with several agents approved over the last 20 years.

Unfortunately, for metastatic disease the 5-year survival still stands at just 14%, leaving great need.[230]

Recently, consensus molecular subtypes were established in colorectal cancer, with the following groups defined: CMS1 (MSI, immune), CMS2 (canonical), CMS3 (metabolic), and CMS 4 (mesenchymal).[231] The CMS1 subtype is characterized by immune infiltration and activation, containing the MSI-H tumors, as well as hypermethylated and hypermutated tumors. The CMS-4 subtype, on the other hand, is characterized by markers of angiogenesis and TGF-β activation. Furthermore, while there is an inflammatory signature, a high density of fibroblasts is present, with abundant expression of monocytic markers, all consistent with a net immunosuppressive environment. Meanwhile, CMS2 and CMS3 subtypes exhibit low immune and inflammatory signatures, most consistent with classic so-called 'cold' tumors.[232] Thus, from the standpoint of CMS-subtyping and successful immunotherapy, immune checkpoint inhibitors might be expected to have efficacy on their own in CMS1 tumors, whereas CMS4 tumors might require additional combinatorial strategies targeting stromal or monocytoid cells. CMS2 and 3 subtypes would seem most likely to require additional proinflammatory stimuli, such as vaccines, Toll-like receptor (TLR) agonists, or radiation, to incite a local immune response.

MSI was first widely recognized in colorectal cancers and deserves some additional attention beyond the prior discussion. MSI is the result of deficient or dysfunctional mismatch repair proteins (dMMR), specifically, inactivation of MLH1, MSH2, MSH6, or PMS2. In colorectal cancer, MSI-H tumors are characterized by markedly elevated mutational rates and dense T-cell infiltrates.[132,233] MSI was historically used to identify patients who might be affected by the hereditary condition, Lynch syndrome, wherein there is a germ-line mutation in the mismatch repair genes. Of note, the PCR-based MSI assay has comparable sensitivity to IHC-based staining as screening for Lynch syndrome.[233] As of 2017, two PD-1 inhibitors, pembrolizumab and nivolumab, are approved in the United States for refractory MSI-H or dMMR colorectal cancers. The studies to date have largely enrolled patients identified through either methodology, IHC (dMMR) or PCR (MSI-H). It is not clear that which methodology should be preferred in the identification of candidates for immune checkpoint inhibitors; however, as stand-alone tests, the IHC-based assay (MMR) remains less expensive and can more readily be performed in most centers as compared with the slightly more complicated PCR-based assay.

Clinical Trials of Immune Checkpoint Inhibitors in Colorectal Cancer

Immune checkpoint inhibitors as single agents

The CTLA-4 inhibitor, tremelimumab, was studied in advanced, refractory CRC as monotherapy. Although there was one clinical response, which was maintained for 6 months, the remaining 46 patients did not demonstrate a clear benefit. Median duration on study was 2.3 months with 6-month PFS standing at 2.1%.[234] Thus, this approach was abandoned. Initial studies of the PD-1–targeting agent, nivolumab, included a cohort of 19 CRC patients. Similar to CTLA-4 monotherapy, there was no generalizable activity, with no responses observed amongst these patients.[235] This lack of activity was later demonstrated with the PD-1 inhibitor, pembrolizumab, which garnered a median PFS of 2.1 months and OS of 5 months, demonstrating that PD-1 monotherapy is of virtually no benefit in unselected CRC patients.[135]

Efficacy in MSI-H/dMMR tumors came to light in a different way. In 2013, a publication drew attention to several patients treated on early nivolumab studies, including one patient with colorectal cancer who achieved a complete response that was ongoing at 3 years. He was 71 years old, his tumor was MSI-H, and the tumor itself was characterized by membranous PD-L1 expression on tumor-infiltrating macrophages and lymphocytes, along with infiltrating CD3+ T-cells.[236] These data and knowledge surrounding the biology of MSI-H tumors prompted dedicated investigation of PD-1 inhibition in MSI-H CRC. In 2015, early data were presented, which demonstrated the compelling efficacy of pembrolizumab in MSI-H/dMMR CRC. A 40% (4/10) response rate was demonstrated with additional durable stable disease—median PFS had not been reached.[135] Additional studies have evaluated pembrolizumab and nivolumab in MSI-H CRC. KEYNOTE-164 evaluated pembrolizumab in mCRC patients who had received at least two prior therapies and demonstrated a response rate of 26.2% with a 50.8% disease control rate. At presentation, with more than 6 months of follow-up for all 61 patients, the median duration of response had not been reached.[237] CheckMate-142 evaluated nivolumab in 74 patients with dMMR/MSI-H mCRC where at least one systemic therapy had been administered. Eighty-four percent of patients had received at least two prior therapies. Here, an investigator-assessed objective response of 31.1% was documented with the achievement of 69% disease control for at least 12 weeks. Responses were again highly durable. The median PFS of the entire population was 14.3 months. Interestingly, this analysis included evaluation of PD-L1 staining intensity and mutational status (BRAF and KRAS). None of these parameters affected the likelihood of response or disease control. Similarly, a clinical history of Lynch syndrome did not affect likelihood of clinical benefit, leaving MSI as the sole indicator of likelihood to respond to therapy.[238]

Immune checkpoint inhibitor combination therapy

CTLA-4 and PD-1 combination therapy has also been tested in advanced CRC. As seen with PD-1 or CTLA-4 monotherapy, combination therapy yields minimal benefit in non-MSI-H (microsatellite-stable, MSS) CRC. KEYNOTE-142 tested two doses of ipilimumab and nivolumab in MSS CRC. Median PFS was 1.4 months, although 1 (5%) patient of 20 did demonstrate a response.[239] On the other hand, in the MSI-H CRC population treated with nivolumab 3 mg/kg plus ipilimumab 1 mg/kg (for four doses), an investigator-assessed objective response rate of 55% was achieved with a 6 month PFS rate of 77%. Here, again, PD-L1 expression and mutational status did not affect clinical benefit.[240] Thus, based on nonrandomized data, there is suggestion that PD-1/CTLA-4 combinatorial therapy may have greater efficacy than PD-1 monotherapy and merits further investigation. Of relevance, the Canadian Cancer Trials Group is conducting a phase III study of CTLA-4 (tremelimumab) and PD-L1 (durvalumab) inhibition versus best supportive care in advanced, refractory CRC, without attention to MSI status (NCT02870920). Given that 97% of mCRC is MSS, this study will be helpful in further defining the activity of this combination in MSS tumors and in delineating whether there are any definable subsets of patients who may benefit.

Immune checkpoint inhibitor and targeted therapy combinations

A novel combinatorial strategy involves dual PD-L1 and MEK inhibition. Mouse models demonstrated that blockade of MEK induces upregulation of MHC class I proteins on tumor cells and increases intratumoral T-cell infiltration. Concurrent inhibition of the PD-1 axis synergizes with MEK inhibition in vivo.[241] Given these findings, MEK and PD-1 inhibition are undergoing testing in multiple settings. Data have been presented surrounding the profile of combined cobimetinib, a MEK-targeting tyrosine kinase inhibitor, and atezolizumab in mCRC. In this phase I study, initial results reported four (17%) patients achieving a partial response with an additional five patients attaining stability. Three of the four responders were established to be non-MSI-H.[242] This exciting preliminary efficacy is being further tested in a randomized phase III trial using atezolizumab and cobimetinib in refractory mCRC (NCT02788279). Results are expected in 2018.

RO6958688 is a carcinoembryonic antigen CD3 T-cell bispecific (CEA CD3 TCB) antibody. In preclinical models, evidence of synergy with anti-PD-L1 antibodies was demonstrated. RO6958688 has been tested as a single agent and in combination with atezolizumab in phase I investigation. Infusion-related reactions and diarrhea were common, although ≥ grade 3 AEs were uncommon. Responses were seen in two (6%) of the patients receiving monotherapy. In combination with atezolizumab, 5 (14%) patients attained a partial response with an additional 17 (47%) attaining stable disease. All but 2 of the 36 patients were established to be MSS.[243] At this point, data are very early, but this combination also appears worthy of further exploration.

Future Directions

At present, we are at a loss as to the optimal means by which to harness the power of the immune system for benefit in MSS CRC. The PD-1 and CTLA-4 combinatorial data from MSI-H colorectal cancer would seem to suggest that the discovery and exploitation of additional immune modulatory factors will ultimately allow us to make significant inroads. Furthermore, the preliminary efficacy of PD-1 and MEK inhibition in MSS tumors has at least given us some initial footholds within which we can begin to climb over these seemingly insurmountable barriers.

The general strategies for MSS CRC are likely to be similar as for other cancers, although aspects of the tumors, such as CMS subtyping may ultimately aid in determination of optimal components of care in specific patients. Multiple studies that combine PD-1/L1 axis blockade with the inhibition of factors, which may preferentially affect myeloid populations, such as CSF-1R, c-fms, CCR5, and CCR2, are underway (NCT02777710, NCT02713529, NCT03274804, NCT03184870). In addition, there are several studies that are evaluating IDO inhibition with PD-1 or combined with additional therapies.

Specific to CRC, antiangiogenic drugs are a mainstay of therapy, with bevacizumab used across multiple lines of therapy and the tyrosine kinase inhibitor, regorafenib, used in the refractory setting. The randomized phase II BACCI trial is evaluating the value of adding

PD-L1 inhibition, via atezolizumab, to a regimen of capecitabine and bevacizumab (NCT02873195). Additional studies are evaluating similar combinations of PD-1 and angiogenic inhibition, via use of bevacizumab, nintedanib, or ziv-aflibercept (NCT03396926, NCT02856425, NCT02298959). Multiple additional studies are evaluating MEK inhibition further, with PD-1 inhibition, dual PD-1/CTLA-4 inhibition, or even in combination with PD-1 inhibition and chemotherapy (NCT03374254, NCT03271047, NCT03-377361, NCT02876224, NCT02060188). Only time will tell the true value of these approaches.

For MSI-H tumors, current efforts are focusing on how and when to best integrate immune checkpoint inhibitors. Based on the success seen thus far, the ATOMIC Study (Alliance A021502) has recently commenced. This study will evaluate the efficacy of adding atezolizumab to 6 months of adjuvant FOLFOX in stage III colon cancer (NCT02912559). In the metastatic setting, two important studies are underway. KEYNOTE-177 is evaluating PD-1 monotherapy with pembrolizumab as compared with standard chemotherapy doublets in treatment-naïve, mCRC patients (NCT02563002). The COMMIT Study (NRG-GI004/S1610) will assess treatment in the same treatment-naïve MSI-H mCRC population, comparing FOLFOX plus bevacizumab with FOLFOX plus bevacizumab and atezolizumab as well as with atezolizumab monotherapy. At the time of this writing, there is not a fully developed study to evaluate the PD-1/CTLA-4 combination more definitively, but the investigation of this regimen in a randomized fashion with well-designed biomarker assays would seem just as important.

ANAL CANCER

Anal squamous cell cancer is a rare disease entity. It is estimated that approximately 8200 new cases with 1100 attendant deaths will be noted in the United States in 2017.[126] Human papilloma virus (HPV) presence has documented association with the vast majority of anal carcinomas (84%) with HPV16 being the dominant subtype.[244] For early stage disease, standard treatment involves definitive chemoradiation, with salvage surgery an option for local failure. Twenty-five percent or more of patients eventually develop distant metastatic disease.[245] In the advanced disease setting, data are limited to guide care, although platinum doublets (cisplatin plus fluoropyrimidine) represent an accepted standard. The HPV E6 and E7 proteins drive oncogenesis, are immunogenic, and are capable of stimulating a host immune response.[246] Given the viral underpinnings of this disease, it seems natural to consider immunotherapy as having promise. To date there has been limited exploration.

Immune checkpoint inhibition using the anti-PD-1 monoclonal antibody, nivolumab, has been tested in metastatic anal squamous cell cancers. NCI9673 was a single-arm phase II study that enrolled patients who had received at least one line of systemic therapy for unresectable or metastatic disease. All patients had distant metastases with a median of 2 (range 1−7) prior therapies. Patients received nivolumab (3 mg/kg) every 3 weeks until progression. Nine (24%) of 37 patients enrolled achieved a partial response, with one of two enrolled HIV-positive patients achieving a response. Seventeen (47%) additional patients achieved disease control. Median PFS was 4.1 months, with 6 month PFS at 38% and median OS of 11.5 months.[247]

Pembrolizumab has also been tested as a therapeutic option in anal carcinomas. As part of the multicohort KEYNOTE-028 study, 43 such patients were evaluated for PD-L1 expression. Of the tumors, 23 (74%) were PD-L1 positive using the 22C3 antibody. Twenty-four patients with squamous histology were ultimately enrolled for treatment, with four (17%) achieving a confirmed partial response. An additional 10 (42%) achieved stable disease. Thus, the majority (58%) of patients achieved disease control.[248] Based on these data sets, PD-1 monotherapy appears to be a promising option in this disease type. Future relevant information on this strategy will be derived from the DART study (SWOG 1609, NCT02834013), which is evaluating dual PD-1 and CTLA-4 inhibition in this rare disease type.

Additional immunotherapy efforts have attempted to target HPV and the E6/E7 proteins. ADXS11-001 is an irreversibly attenuated *L. monocytogenes*−based immunotherapy, which secretes an antigen−adjuvant protein fused to the E7 peptide of HPV 16.[249] Early signs of clinical benefit have been seen in the HPV-related malignancy, cervical cancer. A Phase II study was recently conducted in metastatic or locally recurrent anal squamous cell cancers following failure of at least one line of systemic therapy (NCT02399813). Thirty-one evaluable patients underwent therapy, with one patient (3.5%) achieving a durable partial response and seven (24%) achieving disease. This conferred a 6 month PFS rate of 22%. Grade III toxicities were uncommon but included cytokine-related syndrome ($n = 1$), infusion reactions ($n = 2$), and hypotension ($n = 2$).[250] Thus, there is evident clinical activity−future investigation with immune checkpoint inhibitors or in other disease states would seem warranted.

PATIENT SELECTION FOR IMMUNOTHERAPY AND BIOMARKER DEVELOPMENT

Ideal patient selection remains one of the most important research efforts in cancer medicine. PD-L1 expression has been evaluated as a predictive biomarker of anti-PD-1 therapy in multiple cancers, mostly NSCLC and renal cell cancer.[235,251] In GEC, patients with PD-L1+ tumors appear to derive most of the benefit, but the results of clinical trials up to now cannot provide a definitive answer. The differences in definition of PD-L1 positivity among different studies and agents as well as different antibody clones used to determine positivity preclude meaningful comparisons between studies and pooling of results to increase power. In addition, as with any disease type, PD-L1 expression is subject to temporal and spatial variation. For example, PD-L1 expression can decrease after first-line, platinum-based chemotherapy in patients with metastatic gastric cancer.[252] Furthermore, heterogeneity of biomarker expression in gastric cancer can complicate interpretation of biomarker testing.[253] Specific immune signatures (genes associated with cytotoxic T-cell and APC function and IFN-γ signaling) may be used as predictive biomarkers for response to anti-PD-1 therapies in patients with gastric cancer.[254] In the esophageal/GEJ cohort of KEYNOTE-028, there was a trend for improved PFS and ORR with pembrolizumab therapy in patients with higher composite scores in IFN-γ tumor gene expression signature (*CXCL9/CXCL10/HLA-DRA/IDO1/IFNG/STAT1*).[31] MSI is an approved biomarker for selection of patient with CRC for treatment with immune checkpoint inhibitors.[225] Preliminary data from a phase II trial show evidence of immune checkpoint inhibition efficacy (response in 5 out of 10 evaluable patients) in a variety of dMMR gastrointestinal malignancies beyond CRC, including PDAC and biliary tumors.[255] As mentioned in previous sections in this chapter, increased number of tumor mutations results in increased neoantigen burden that correlates with response to immunotherapy.[22−24] In mCRC, almost 22% of tumors without MSI have a high mutation burden that can expand the patient population who may derive benefit from immune checkpoint inhibitors.[256] Interestingly, PDAC with somatic mutations in MMR genes appears to have a considerably lower mutation burden compared with tumors harboring germline mutations; this may have significant implications for optimal patient selection for immune checkpoint inhibitor therapy.[257] In a comprehensive genomic profiling in 614 consecutive HCC cases, the prevalence of MSI was <1%; point mutations, small indels, copy number changes, and rearrangements in MMR proteins were identified in approximately 2% of cases, and 1% had a mutation burden of >20 mutations/Mb.[258] Given the much higher clinical benefit with immune checkpoint inhibitors in molecularly unselected patients with HCC reported in clinical trials, the MSI/MMR status and high tumor mutation burden may be less relevant biomarkers in this disease.

SUMMARY/CONCLUSION

The history of immune checkpoint inhibitor therapy for gastrointestinal cancers reflects on the differences in pathogenesis and natural history among the many different tumor types. Malignancies associated with direct exposure to strong mutagens, such as tobacco in the case of esophagus cancer and viruses in HCC and anal cancer, appear to benefit the most from therapy in unselected populations, with at least short-term outcomes that parallel to the benefit observed in other disease types. In CRC, a tumor that is generally immune "quiescent," the small subgroup of patients with MSI derives benefit that is equivalent to dual checkpoint inhibitor therapy in melanoma. In fact, pembrolizumab is approved in all MSI gastrointestinal malignancies regardless of histology and or disease site. Despite many efforts, PDAC remains resistant to immune checkpoint inhibitors. This is likely related to an intensively immunosuppressive TME and a low mutation/neoantigen burden. Furthermore, the many times rapid tumor progression and deteriorating health of patients with advanced PDAC may preclude any benefit of immunotherapy from being clinically apparent. Potential strategies for further development in PDAC should include targeting various immunosuppressive components of the TME combined with immunostimulants such as tumor vaccines and oncolytic viruses; chimeric antigen receptor T-cell therapy is a new, promising strategy.[259]

REFERENCES

1. Harris TJ, Drake CG. Primer on tumor immunology and cancer immunotherapy. *J Immunother Cancer.* 2013;1:12.
2. Melero I, Hervas-Stubbs S, Glennie M, Pardoll DM, Chen L. Immunostimulatory monoclonal antibodies for cancer therapy. *Nat Rev Cancer.* 2007;7(2):95–106.
3. Okazaki T, Honjo T. PD-1 and PD-1 ligands: from discovery to clinical application. *Int Immunol.* 2007;19(7): 813–824.
4. Robert C, Thomas L, Bondarenko I, et al. Ipilimumab plus dacarbazine for previously untreated metastatic melanoma. *N Engl J Med.* 2011;364(26):2517–2526.
5. Ribas A, Puzanov I, Dummer R, et al. Pembrolizumab versus investigator-choice chemotherapy for ipilimumab-refractory melanoma (KEYNOTE-002): a randomised, controlled, phase 2 trial. *Lancet Oncol.* 2015;16(8): 908–918.
6. Motzer RJ, Escudier B, McDermott DF, et al. Nivolumab versus everolimus in advanced renal-cell carcinoma. *N Engl J Med.* 2015;373(19):1803–1813.
7. Reck M, Rodriguez-Abreu D, Robinson AG, et al. Pembrolizumab versus chemotherapy for PD-L1-positive non-small-cell lung cancer. *N Engl J Med.* 2016;375(19): 1823–1833.
8. Robert C, Schachter J, Long GV, et al. Pembrolizumab versus ipilimumab in advanced melanoma. *N Engl J Med.* 2015;372(26):2521–2532.
9. Robert C, Long GV, Brady B, et al. Nivolumab in previously untreated melanoma without BRAF mutation. *N Engl J Med.* 2015;372(4):320–330.
10. Balar AV, Galsky MD, Rosenberg JE, et al. Atezolizumab as first-line treatment in cisplatin-ineligible patients with locally advanced and metastatic urothelial carcinoma: a single-arm, multicentre, phase 2 trial. *Lancet.* 2017;389(10064):67–76.
11. Ferris RL, Blumenschein Jr G, Fayette J, et al. Nivolumab for recurrent squamous-cell carcinoma of the head and neck. *N Engl J Med.* 2016;375(19):1856–1867.
12. Hanahan D, Weinberg RA. Hallmarks of cancer: the next generation. *Cell.* 2011;144(5):646–674.
13. Zhang H, Xu X. Mutation-promoting molecular networks of uncontrolled inflammation. *Tumor Biol.* 2017;39(6): 1010428317701310.
14. Ferlay J, Soerjomataram I, Dikshit R, et al. Cancer incidence and mortality worldwide: sources, methods and major patterns in GLOBOCAN 2012. *Int J Cancer.* 2015; 136(5):E359–E386.
15. Shah MA. Update on metastatic gastric and esophageal cancers. *J Clin Oncol.* 2015;33(16):1760–1769.
16. Cunningham D, Starling N, Rao S, et al. Capecitabine and oxaliplatin for advanced esophagogastric cancer. *N Engl J Med.* 2008;358(1):36–46.
17. Cutsem EV, Moiseyenko VM, Tjulandin S, et al. Phase III study of docetaxel and cisplatin plus fluorouracil compared with cisplatin and fluorouracil as first-line therapy for advanced gastric cancer: a report of the V325 study group. *J Clin Oncol.* 2006;24(31): 4991–4997.
18. The Cancer Genome Atlas Research N. Comprehensive molecular characterization of gastric adenocarcinoma. *Nature.* 2014;513(7517):202–209.
19. Derks S, Liao X, Chiaravalli AM, et al. Abundant PD-L1 expression in epstein-barr virus-infected gastric cancers. *Oncotarget.* 2016;7(22):32925–32932.
20. Falchetti M, Saieva C, Lupi R, et al. Gastric cancer with high-level microsatellite instability: target gene mutations, clinicopathologic features, and long-term survival. *Hum Pathol.* 2008;39(6):925–932.

21. Smyth EC, Wotherspoon A, Peckitt C, et al. Mismatch repair deficiency, microsatellite instability, and survival: an exploratory analysis of the medical research council adjuvant gastric infusional chemotherapy (MAGIC) trial. *JAMA Oncol.* 2017;3(9):1197–1203.

22. Rizvi NA, Hellmann MD, Snyder A, et al. Mutational landscape determines sensitivity to PD-1 blockade in non–small cell lung cancer. *Science.* 2015;348(6230): 124–128.

23. Snyder A, Makarov V, Merghoub T, et al. Genetic basis for clinical response to CTLA-4 blockade in melanoma. *N Engl J Med.* 2014;371(23):2189–2199.

24. Johnson DB, Frampton GM, Rioth MJ, et al. Targeted next generation sequencing identifies markers of response to PD-1 blockade. *Cancer Immunol Res.* 2016;4(11):959–967.

25. Koeppel M, Garcia-Alcalde F, Glowinski F, Schlaermann P, Meyer TF. *Helicobacter pylori* infection causes characteristic DNA damage patterns in human cells. *Cell Rep.* 2015; 11(11):1703–1713.

26. Wu YY, Lin CW, Cheng KS, et al. Increased programmed death-ligand-1 expression in human gastric epithelial cells in Helicobacter pylori infection. *Clin Exp Immunol.* 2010;161(3):551–559.

27. Ohigashi Y, Sho M, Yamada Y, et al. Clinical significance of programmed death-1 ligand-1 and programmed death-1 ligand-2 expression in human esophageal cancer. *Clin Cancer Res.* 2005;11(8):2947–2953.

28. Ralph C, Elkord E, Burt DJ, et al. Modulation of lymphocyte regulation for cancer therapy: a phase II trial of tremelimumab in advanced gastric and esophageal adenocarcinoma. *Clin Cancer Res.* 2010;16(5): 1662–1672.

29. Moehler MH, Cho JY, Kim YH, et al. A randomized, open-label, two-arm phase II trial comparing the efficacy of sequential ipilimumab (ipi) versus best supportive care (BSC) following first-line (1L) chemotherapy in patients with unresectable, locally advanced/metastatic (A/M) gastric or gastro-esophageal junction (G/GEJ) cancer. *J Clin Oncol.* 2016;34(suppl 15):4011.

30. Muro K, Chung HC, Shankaran V, et al. Pembrolizumab for patients with PD-L1-positive advanced gastric cancer (KEYNOTE-012): a multicentre, open-label, phase 1b trial. *Lancet Oncol.* 2016;17(6):717–726.

31. Doi T, Piha-Paul SA, Jalal SI, et al. Safety and antitumor activity of the anti–programmed death-1 antibody pembrolizumab in patients with advanced esophageal carcinoma. *J Clin Oncol.* 2018;36(1):61–67. https:// doi.org/10.1200/JCO.2017.74.9846.

32. Fuchs CS, Doi T, Jang RW-J, et al. KEYNOTE-059 cohort 1: efficacy and safety of pembrolizumab (pembro) monotherapy in patients with previously treated advanced gastric cancer. *J Clin Oncol.* 2017;35(suppl 15):4003.

33. Wainberg ZA, Jalal S, Muro K, et al. LBA28_PRKEYNOTE-059 update: efficacy and safety of pembrolizumab alone or in combination with chemotherapy in patients with advanced gastric or gastroesophageal (G/GEJ) cancer. *Ann Oncol.* 2017;28(suppl 5). https://doi.org/10.1093/annonc/mdx440.020.

34. Janjigian YY, Bendell JC, Calvo E, et al. CheckMate-032: phase I/II, open-label study of safety and activity of nivolumab (nivo) alone or with ipilimumab (ipi) in advanced and metastatic (A/M) gastric cancer (GC). *J Clin Oncol.* 2016;34(suppl 15):4010.

35. Janjigian YY, Ott PA, Calvo E, et al. Nivolumab ± ipilimumab in pts with advanced (adv)/metastatic chemotherapy-refractory (CTx-R) gastric (G), esophageal (E), or gastroesophageal junction (GEJ) cancer: CheckMate 032 study. *J Clin Oncol.* 2017;35(suppl 15):4014.

36. Kudo T, Hamamoto Y, Kato K, et al. Nivolumab treatment for oesophageal squamous-cell carcinoma: an open-label, multicentre, phase 2 trial. *Lancet Oncol.* 2017;18(5):631–639.

37. Kang YK, Boku N, Satoh T, et al. Nivolumab in patients with advanced gastric or gastro-oesophageal junction cancer refractory to, or intolerant of, at least two previous chemotherapy regimens (ONO-4538-12, ATTRACTION-2): a randomised, double-blind, placebo-controlled, phase 3 trial. *Lancet.* 2017;390(10111):2461–2471.

38. Chung HC, Arkenau H-T, Wyrwicz L, et al. Avelumab (MSB0010718C; anti-PD-L1) in patients with advanced gastric or gastroesophageal junction cancer from JAVELIN solid tumor phase Ib trial: analysis of safety and clinical activity. *J Clin Oncol.* 2016;34(suppl 15):4009.

39. Lutzky J, Antonia SJ, Blake-Haskins A, et al. A phase 1 study of MEDI4736, an anti–PD-L1 antibody, in patients with advanced solid tumors. *J Clin Oncol.* 2014;32(suppl 15):3001.

40. Bang Y-J, Muro K, Fuchs CS, et al. KEYNOTE-059 cohort 2: safety and efficacy of pembrolizumab (pembro) plus 5-fluorouracil (5-FU) and cisplatin for first-line (1L) treatment of advanced gastric cancer. *J Clin Oncol.* 2017; 35(suppl 15):4012.

41. Fuchs CS, Tomasek J, Yong CJ, et al. Ramucirumab monotherapy for previously treated advanced gastric or gastro-oesophageal junction adenocarcinoma (REGARD): an international, randomised, multicentre, placebo-controlled, phase 3 trial. *Lancet.* 2014;383(9911):31–39.

42. Wilke H, Muro K, Van Cutsem E, et al. Ramucirumab plus paclitaxel versus placebo plus paclitaxel in patients with previously treated advanced gastric or gastro-oesophageal junction adenocarcinoma (RAINBOW): a double-blind, randomised phase 3 trial. *Lancet Oncol.* 2014;15(11):1224–1235.

43. Terme M, Colussi O, Marcheteau E, Tanchot C, Tartour E, Taieb J. Modulation of immunity by antiangiogenic molecules in cancer. *Clin Dev Immunol.* 2012;2012:492920.

44. Yasuda S, Sho M, Yamato I, et al. Simultaneous blockade of programmed death 1 and vascular endothelial growth factor receptor 2 (VEGFR2) induces synergistic anti-tumour effect in vivo. *Clin Exp Immunol.* 2013;172(3):500–506.

45. Chau I, Penel N, Arkenau HT, et al. Safety and antitumor activity of ramucirumab plus pembrolizumab in treatment naïve advanced gastric or gastroesophageal junction (G/GEJ) adenocarcinoma: preliminary results from a multi- disease phase I study (JVDF). *J Clin Oncol.* 2018; 36(suppl 4):101.

46. Chau I, Bendell JC, Calvo E, et al. Ramucirumab (R) plus pembrolizumab (P) in treatment naive and previously treated advanced gastric or gastroesophageal junction (G/GEJ) adenocarcinoma: a multi-disease phase I study. *J Clin Oncol.* 2017;35(suppl 15):4046.

47. Bang Y-J, Golan T, Lin CC, et al. Interim safety and clinical activity in patients (pts) with locally advanced and unresectable or metastatic gastric or gastroesophageal junction (G/GEJ) adenocarcinoma from a multicohort phase I study of ramucirumab (R) plus durvalumab (D). *J Clin Oncol.* 2018;36(suppl 4):92.

48. Bang YJ, Van Cutsem E, Feyereislova A, et al. Trastuzumab in combination with chemotherapy versus chemotherapy alone for treatment of HER2-positive advanced gastric or gastro-oesophageal junction cancer (ToGA): a phase 3, open-label, randomised controlled trial. *Lancet.* 2010;376(9742):687–697.

49. Catenacci DVT, Park H, Craig Lockhart A, et al. Phase 1b/2 study of margetuximab (M) plus pembrolizumab (P) in advanced HER2+ gastroesophageal junction (GEJ) or gastric (G) adenocarcinoma (GEA). *J Clin Oncol.* 2018;36(suppl 4):140.

50. Huang YH, Zhu C, Kondo Y, et al. CEACAM1 regulates TIM-3-mediated tolerance and exhaustion. *Nature.* 2015;517(7534):386–390.

51. Zhou CJ, Liu B, Zhu KX, et al. The different expression of carcinoembryonic antigen-related cell adhesion molecule 1 (CEACAM1) and possible roles in gastric carcinomas. *Pathol Res Pract.* 2009;205(7):483–489.

52. Setala LP, Tammi MI, Tammi RH, et al. Hyaluronan expression in gastric cancer cells is associated with local and nodal spread and reduced survival rate. *Br J Cancer.* 1999;79(7–8):1133–1138.

53. Clift R, Lee J, Thompson CB, Huang Y. Abstract 641: PEGylated recombinant hyaluronidase PH20 (PEGPH20) enhances tumor infiltrating CD8+ T cell accumulation and improves checkpoint inhibitor efficacy in murine syngeneic breast cancer models. *Cancer Res.* 2017;77(Suppl 13):641.

54. Tureci O, Koslowski M, Helftenbein G, et al. Claudin-18 gene structure, regulation, and expression is evolutionary conserved in mammals. *Gene.* 2011;481(2):83–92.

55. Sahin U, Koslowski M, Dhaene K, et al. Claudin-18 splice variant 2 is a pan-cancer target suitable for therapeutic antibody development. *Clin Cancer Res.* 2008;14(23):7624–7634.

56. Lordick F, Schuler M, Al-Batran SE, et al. 220O Claudin 18.2—a novel treatment target in the multicenter, randomized, phase II FAST study, a trial of epirubicin, oxaliplatin, and capecitabine (EOX) with or without the anti-CLDN18.2 antibody IMAB362 as 1st line therapy in advanced gastric and gastroesophageal junction (GEJ) cancer. *Ann Oncol.* 2016;27(suppl 9):mdw582.001.

57. Al-Batran SE, Zvirbule Z, Lordick F, et al. 664PPhase 1 Study of IMAB362 with immunomodulation in patients with advanced gastric cancer. *Ann Oncol.* 2017;28(suppl 5):mdx369.048.

58. Dewan MZ, Galloway AE, Kawashima N, et al. Fractionated but not single-dose radiotherapy induces an immune-mediated abscopal effect when combined with anti-CTLA-4 antibody. *Clin Cancer Res.* 2009;15(17):5379–5388.

59. Dovedi SJ, Cheadle EJ, Popple AL, et al. Fractionated radiation therapy stimulates antitumor immunity mediated by both resident and infiltrating polyclonal T-cell populations when combined with PD-1 blockade. *Clin Cancer Res.* 2017;23(18):5514–5526.

60. Skolnick AA. Armed with epidemiologic research, China launches programs to prevent liver cancer. *JAMA.* 1996;276(18):1458–1459.

61. Davila JA, Morgan RO, Shaib Y, McGlynn KA, El-Serag HB. Hepatitis C infection and the increasing incidence of hepatocellular carcinoma: a population-based study. *Gastroenterology.* 2004;127(5):1372–1380.

62. El-Serag HB, Kanwal F. Epidemiology of hepatocellular carcinoma in the United States: where are we? Where do we go? *Hepatology.* 2014;60(5):1767–1775.

63. El-Serag HB. Hepatocellular carcinoma. *N Engl J Med.* 2011;365(12):1118–1127.

64. Llovet JM, Ricci S, Mazzaferro V, et al. Sorafenib in advanced hepatocellular carcinoma. *N Engl J Med.* 2008;359(4):378–390.

65. Bruix J, Qin S, Merle P, et al. Regorafenib for patients with hepatocellular carcinoma who progressed on sorafenib treatment (RESORCE): a randomised, double-blind, placebo-controlled, phase 3 trial. *Lancet.* 2017;389(10064):56–66.

66. Jenne CN, Kubes P. Immune surveillance by the liver. *Nat Immunol.* 2013;14(10):996–1006.

67. Harding JJ, El Dika I, Abou-Alfa GK. Immunotherapy in hepatocellular carcinoma: primed to make a difference? *Cancer.* 2016;122(3):367–377.

68. Tagliamonte M, Petrizzo A, Tornesello ML, Ciliberto G, Buonaguro FM, Buonaguro L. Combinatorial immunotherapy strategies for hepatocellular carcinoma. *Curr Opin Immunol.* 2016;39:103–113.

69. Buonaguro L, Petrizzo A, Tagliamonte M, Tornesello ML, Buonaguro FM. Challenges in cancer vaccine development for hepatocellular carcinoma. *J Hepatol.* 2013;59(4):897–903.

70. Thomson AW, Knolle PA. Antigen-presenting cell function in the tolerogenic liver environment. *Nat Rev Immunol.* 2010;10(11):753–766.

71. Pillarisetty VG, Shah AB, Miller G, Bleier JI, DeMatteo RP. Liver dendritic cells are less immunogenic than spleen dendritic cells because of differences in subtype composition. *J Immunol.* 2004;172(2):1009–1017.

72. Schurich A, Khanna P, Lopes AR, et al. Role of the coinhibitory receptor cytotoxic T lymphocyte antigen-4 on apoptosis-Prone CD8 T cells in persistent hepatitis B virus infection. *Hepatology.* 2011;53(5):1494–1503.

73. Nakamoto N, Kaplan DE, Coleclough J, et al. Functional restoration of HCV-specific CD8 T cells by PD-1 blockade is defined by PD-1 expression and compartmentalization. *Gastroenterology.* 2008;134(7):1927–1937, 1937.e1921–1922.

74. Schildberg FA, Hegenbarth SI, Schumak B, Scholz K, Limmer A, Knolle PA. Liver sinusoidal endothelial cells veto CD8 T cell activation by antigen-presenting dendritic cells. *Eur J Immunol.* 2008;38(4):957−967.

75. Knolle PA, Germann T, Treichel U, et al. Endotoxin downregulates T cell activation by antigen-presenting liver sinusoidal endothelial cells. *J Immunol.* 1999;162(3):1401−1407.

76. Heymann F, Peusquens J, Ludwig-Portugall I, et al. Liver inflammation abrogates immunological tolerance induced by Kupffer cells. *Hepatology.* 2015;62(1):279−291.

77. Budhu A, Forgues M, Ye QH, et al. Prediction of venous metastases, recurrence, and prognosis in hepatocellular carcinoma based on a unique immune response signature of the liver microenvironment. *Cancer Cell.* 2006;10(2):99−111.

78. Li M, Sun R, Xu L, et al. Kupffer cells support hepatitis B virus-mediated CD8+ T cell exhaustion via Hepatitis B core antigen-TLR2 interactions in mice. *J Immunol.* 2015;195(7):3100−3109.

79. Prieto J, Melero I, Sangro B. Immunological landscape and immunotherapy of hepatocellular carcinoma. *Nat Rev Gastroenterol Hepatol.* 2015;12(12):681−700.

80. De Luca A, Gallo M, Aldinucci D, et al. Role of the EGFR ligand/receptor system in the secretion of angiogenic factors in mesenchymal stem cells. *J Cell Physiol.* 2011;226(8):2131−2138.

81. Hato T, Goyal L, Greten TF, Duda DG, Zhu AX. Immune checkpoint blockade in hepatocellular carcinoma: current progress and future directions. *Hepatology.* 2014;60(5):1776−1782.

82. Zhang Z, Zhang Y, Sun XX, Ma X, Chen ZN. microRNA-146a inhibits cancer metastasis by downregulating VEGF through dual pathways in hepatocellular carcinoma. *Mol Cancer.* 2015;14:5.

83. Colegio OR, Chu NQ, Szabo AL, et al. Functional polarization of tumour-associated macrophages by tumour-derived lactic acid. *Nature.* 2014;513(7519):559−563.

84. Sangro B, Gomez-Martin C, de la Mata M, et al. A clinical trial of CTLA-4 blockade with tremelimumab in patients with hepatocellular carcinoma and chronic hepatitis C. *J Hepatol.* 2013;59(1):81−88.

85. Crocenzi TS, El-Khoueiry AB, Yau TC, et al. Nivolumab (nivo) in sorafenib (sor)-naive and -experienced pts with advanced hepatocellular carcinoma (HCC): CheckMate 040 study. *J Clin Oncol.* 2017;35(suppl 15):4013.

86. Kudo M. Immune checkpoint blockade in hepatocellular carcinoma: 2017 update. *Liver Cancer.* 2016;6(1):1−12.

87. Zhu AX, Finn RS, Cattan S, et al. KEYNOTE-224: pembrolizumab in patients with advanced hepatocellular carcinoma previously treated with sorafenib. *J Clin Oncol.* 2018;36(suppl 4):209.

88. Wainberg ZA, Segal NH, Jaeger D, et al. Safety and clinical activity of durvalumab monotherapy in patients with hepatocellular carcinoma (HCC). *J Clin Oncol.* 2017;35(suppl 15):4071.

89. Kelley RK, Abou-Alfa GK, Bendell JC, et al. Phase I/II study of durvalumab and tremelimumab in patients with unresectable hepatocellular carcinoma (HCC): phase I safety and efficacy analyses. *J Clin Oncol.* 2017;35(suppl 15):4073.

90. Chen ML, Yan BS, Lu WC, et al. Sorafenib relieves cell-intrinsic and cell-extrinsic inhibitions of effector T cells in tumor microenvironment to augment antitumor immunity. *Int J Cancer.* 2014;134(2):319−331.

91. Alfaro C, Suarez N, Gonzalez A, et al. Influence of bevacizumab, sunitinib and sorafenib as single agents or in combination on the inhibitory effects of VEGF on human dendritic cell differentiation from monocytes. *Br J Cancer.* 2009;100(7):1111−1119.

92. Sprinzl MF, Reisinger F, Puschnik A, et al. Sorafenib perpetuates cellular anticancer effector functions by modulating the crosstalk between macrophages and natural killer cells. *Hepatology.* 2013;57(6):2358−2368.

93. Cabrera R, Ararat M, Xu Y, et al. Immune modulation of effector CD4+ and regulatory T cell function by sorafenib in patients with hepatocellular carcinoma. *Cancer Immunol Immunother.* 2013;62(4):737−746.

94. Houben R, Voigt H, Noelke C, Hofmeister V, Becker JC, Schrama D. MAPK-independent impairment of T-cell responses by the multikinase inhibitor sorafenib. *Mol Cancer Ther.* 2009;8(2):433−440.

95. Shen Y, Wei Y, Wang Z, et al. TGF-beta regulates hepatocellular carcinoma progression by inducing Treg cell polarization. *Cell Physiol Biochem.* 2015;35(4):1623−1632.

96. Schueller G, Kettenbach J, Sedivy R, et al. Heat shock protein expression induced by percutaneous radiofrequency ablation of hepatocellular carcinoma in vivo. *Int J Oncol.* 2004;24(3):609−613.

97. Ali MY, Grimm CF, Ritter M, et al. Activation of dendritic cells by local ablation of hepatocellular carcinoma. *J Hepatology.* 2005;43(5):817−822.

98. Ahmad F, Gravante G, Bhardwaj N, et al. Changes in interleukin-1beta and 6 after hepatic microwave tissue ablation compared with radiofrequency, cryotherapy and surgical resections. *Am J Surg.* 2010;200(4):500−506.

99. Ito F, Ku AW, Bucsek MJ, et al. Immune adjuvant activity of pre-resectional radiofrequency ablation protects against local and systemic recurrence in aggressive murine colorectal cancer. *PLoS One.* 2015;10(11):e0143370.

100. Gravante G, Sconocchia G, Ong SL, Dennison AR, Lloyd DM. Immunoregulatory effects of liver ablation therapies for the treatment of primary and metastatic liver malignancies. *Liver Int.* 2009;29(1):18−24.

101. Liao Y, Wang B, Huang ZL, et al. Increased circulating Th17 cells after transarterial chemoembolization correlate with improved survival in stage III hepatocellular carcinoma: a prospective study. *PLoS One.* 2013;8(4):e60444.

102. Liao J, Xiao J, Zhou Y, Liu Z, Wang C. Effect of transcatheter arterial chemoembolization on cellular immune function and regulatory T cells in patients with hepatocellular carcinoma. *Mol Med Rep.* 2015;12(4):6065−6071.

103. Ikei S, Ogawa M, Beppu T, et al. Changes in IL-6, IL-8, C-reactive protein and pancreatic secretory trypsin inhibitor after transcatheter arterial chemo-embolization therapy for hepato-cellular carcinoma. *Cytokine*. 1992;4(6): 581−584.

104. Ayaru L, Pereira SP, Alisa A, et al. Unmasking of alpha-fetoprotein-specific CD4(+) T cell responses in hepato-cellular carcinoma patients undergoing embolization. *J Immunol*. 2007;178(3):1914−1922.

105. Duffy AG, Ulahannan SV, Fioravanti S, et al. A pilot study of tremelimumab, a monoclonal antibody against CTLA-4, in combination with either transcatheter arterial chemoembolization (TACE) or radiofrequency ablation (RFA) in patients with hepatocellular carcinoma (HCC). *J Clin Oncol*. 2014;32(suppl 15):e15133.

106. Ma Y, Xu YC, Tang L, Zhang Z, Wang J, Wang HX. Cytokine-induced killer (CIK) cell therapy for patients with hepatocellular carcinoma: efficacy and safety. *Exp Hematol Oncol*. 2012;1(1):11.

107. Lee JH, Lee JH, Lim YS, et al. Adjuvant immunotherapy with autologous cytokine-induced killer cells for hepato-cellular carcinoma. *Gastroenterology*. 2015;148(7): 1383−1391.e1386.

108. Xu L, Wang J, Kim Y, et al. A randomized controlled trial on patients with or without adjuvant autologous cytokine-induced killer cells after curative resection for hepatocellular carcinoma. *Oncoimmunology*. 2016;5(3): e1083671.

109. Rizvi S, Gores GJ. Pathogenesis, diagnosis, and management of cholangiocarcinoma. *Gastroenterology*. 2013; 145(6):1215−1229.

110. Keedy AW, Breiman RS, Webb EM, Roberts JP, Coakley FV, Yeh BM. Determinants of second-order bile duct visualization at CT cholangiography in potential living liver donors. *AJR Am J Roentgenol*. 2013;200(5): 1028−1033.

111. Saha SK, Zhu AX, Fuchs CS, Brooks GA. Forty-year trends in cholangiocarcinoma incidence in the U.S.: intrahepatic disease on the rise. *Oncologist*. 2016;21(5): 594−599.

112. Rizvi S, Khan SA, Hallemeier CL, Kelley RK, Gores GJ. Cholangiocarcinoma - evolving concepts and therapeutic strategies. *Nat Rev Clin Oncol*. 2018;15(2):95−111.

113. Jarnagin WR, Fong Y, DeMatteo RP, et al. Staging, resectability, and outcome in 225 patients with hilar cholangiocarcinoma. *Ann Surg*. 2001;234(4):507−517; discussion 517−509.

114. Valle J, Wasan H, Palmer DH, et al. Cisplatin plus gemcitabine versus gemcitabine for biliary tract cancer. *N Engl J Med*. 2010;362(14):1273−1281.

115. Farazi PA, Zeisberg M, Glickman J, Zhang Y, Kalluri R, DePinho RA. Chronic bile duct injury associated with fibrotic matrix microenvironment provokes cholangio-carcinoma in p53-deficient mice. *Cancer Res*. 2006; 66(13):6622−6627.

116. Sirica AE, Gores GJ. Desmoplastic stroma and cholangio-carcinoma: clinical implications and therapeutic targeting. *Hepatology*. 2014;59(6):2397−2402.

117. Thelen A, Scholz A, Weichert W, et al. Tumor-associated angiogenesis and lymphangiogenesis correlate with progression of intrahepatic cholangiocarcinoma. *Am J Gastroenterol*. 2010;105(5):1123−1132.

118. Gani F, Nagarajan N, Kim Y, et al. Program death 1 immune checkpoint and tumor microenvironment: implications for patients with intrahepatic cholangiocarcinoma. *Ann Surg Oncol*. 2016;23(8):2610−2617.

119. Fontugne J, Augustin J, Pujals A, et al. PD-L1 expression in perihilar and intrahepatic cholangiocarcinoma. *Oncotarget*. 2017;8(15):24644−24651.

120. Silva VW, Askan G, Daniel TD, et al. Biliary carcinomas: pathology and the role of DNA mismatch repair deficiency. *Chin Clin Oncol*. 2016;5(5):62.

121. Palmer WC, Patel T. Are common factors involved in the pathogenesis of primary liver cancers? A meta-analysis of risk factors for intrahepatic cholangiocarcinoma. *J Hepatol*. 2012;57(1):69−76.

122. Bang YJ, Doi T, Braud FD, et al. 525 Safety and efficacy of pembrolizumab (MK-3475) in patients (pts) with advanced biliary tract cancer: Interim results of KEYNOTE-028. *Eur J Cancer*. 51:S112.

123. Emens LA, Middleton G. The interplay of immunotherapy and chemotherapy: harnessing potential synergies. *Cancer Immunol Res*. 2015;3(5):436−443.

124. Tran E, Turcotte S, Gros A, et al. Cancer immunotherapy based on mutation-specific CD4+ T cells in a patient with epithelial cancer. *Science*. 2014;344(6184): 641−645.

125. Nakamura H, Arai Y, Totoki Y, et al. Genomic spectra of biliary tract cancer. *Nat Genet*. 2015;47(9):1003−1010.

126. Siegel RL, Miller KD, Jemal A. Cancer statistics, 2017. *CA Cancer J Clin*. 2017;67(1):7−30.

127. Wolfgang CL, Herman JM, Laheru DA, et al. Recent progress in pancreatic cancer. *CA Cancer J Clin*. 2013;63(5): 318−348.

128. Conroy T, Desseigne F, Ychou M, et al. FOLFIRINOX versus gemcitabine for metastatic pancreatic cancer. *N Engl J Med*. 2011;364(19):1817−1825.

129. Von Hoff DD, Ervin T, Arena FP, et al. Increased survival in pancreatic cancer with nab-paclitaxel plus gemcitabine. *N Engl J Med*. 2013;369(18):1691−1703.

130. Nywening TM, Wang-Gillam A, Sanford DE, et al. Targeting tumour-associated macrophages with CCR2 inhibition in combination with FOLFIRINOX in patients with borderline resectable and locally advanced pancreatic cancer: a single-centre, open-label, dose-finding, non-randomised, phase 1b trial. *Lancet Oncol*. 2016;17(5): 651−662.

131. Brahmer JR, Tykodi SS, Chow LQ, et al. Safety and activity of anti-PD-L1 antibody in patients with advanced cancer. *N Engl J Med*. 2012;366(26):2455−2465.

132. Alexandrov LB, Nik-Zainal S, Wedge DC, et al. Signatures of mutational processes in human cancer. *Nature*. 2013; 500(7463):415−421.

133. Salem ME, Xiu J, Weinberg BA, et al. Characterization of tumor mutation burden (TMB) in gastrointestinal (GI) cancers. *J Clin Oncol*. 2017;35(suppl 4):530.

134. Hall MJ, Gowen K, Sanford EM, et al. Evaluation of microsatellite instability (MSI) status in gastrointestinal (GI) tumor samples tested with comprehensive genomic profiling (CGP). *J Clin Oncol.* 2016;34(suppl 4):528.

135. Le DT, Uram JN, Wang H, et al. PD-1 blockade in tumors with mismatch-repair deficiency. *N Engl J Med.* 2015;372(26):2509−2520.

136. Clark CE, Beatty GL, Vonderheide RH. Immunosurveillance of pancreatic adenocarcinoma: insights from genetically engineered mouse models of cancer. *Cancer Lett.* 2009;279(1):1−7.

137. Koido S, Homma S, Takahara A, et al. Current immunotherapeutic approaches in pancreatic cancer. *Clin Dev Immunol.* 2011;2011:267539.

138. Liyanage UK, Moore TT, Joo HG, et al. Prevalence of regulatory T cells is increased in peripheral blood and tumor microenvironment of patients with pancreas or breast adenocarcinoma. *J Immunol.* 2002;169(5):2756−2761.

139. Khaled YS, Ammori BJ, Elkord E. Increased levels of granulocytic myeloid-derived suppressor cells in peripheral blood and tumour tissue of pancreatic cancer patients. *J Immunol Res.* 2014;2014:879897.

140. Markowitz J, Brooks TR, Duggan MC, et al. Patients with pancreatic adenocarcinoma exhibit elevated levels of myeloid-derived suppressor cells upon progression of disease. *Cancer Immunol Immunother.* 2015;64(2):149−159.

141. Katoh H, Watanabe M. Myeloid-derived suppressor cells and therapeutic strategies in cancer. *Mediators Inflamm.* 2015;2015:159269.

142. Takeuchi Y, Nishikawa H. Roles of regulatory T cells in cancer immunity. *Int Immunol.* 2016;28(8):401−409.

143. Feig C, Jones JO, Kraman M, et al. Targeting CXCL12 from FAP-expressing carcinoma-associated fibroblasts synergizes with anti-PD-L1 immunotherapy in pancreatic cancer. *Proc Natl Acad Sci U S A.* 2013;110(50):20212−20217.

144. Mace TA, Ameen Z, Collins A, et al. Pancreatic cancer-associated stellate cells promote differentiation of myeloid-derived suppressor cells in a STAT3-dependent manner. *Cancer Res.* 2013;73(10):3007−3018.

145. Royal RE, Levy C, Turner K, et al. Phase 2 trial of single agent Ipilimumab (anti-CTLA-4) for locally advanced or metastatic pancreatic adenocarcinoma. *J Immunother.* 2010;33(8):828−833.

146. Segal NH, Antonia SJ, Brahmer JR, et al. Preliminary data from a multi-arm expansion study of MEDI4736, an anti-PD-L1 antibody. *J Clin Oncol.* 2014;32(suppl 15):3002.

147. O'Reilly EM, Oh DY, Dhani N, et al. A randomized phase 2 study of durvalumab monotherapy and in combination with tremelimumab in patients with metastatic pancreatic ductal adenocarcinoma (mPDAC): ALPS study. *J Clin Oncol.* 2018;36(suppl 4):217.

148. Uyttenhove C, Pilotte L, Theate I, et al. Evidence for a tumoral immune resistance mechanism based on tryptophan degradation by indoleamine 2,3-dioxygenase. *Nat Med.* 2003;9(10):1269−1274.

149. Munn DH, Shafizadeh E, Attwood JT, Bondarev I, Pashine A, Mellor AL. Inhibition of T cell proliferation by macrophage tryptophan catabolism. *J Exp Med.* 1999;189(9):1363−1372.

150. Witkiewicz A, Williams TK, Cozzitorto J, et al. Expression of indoleamine 2,3-dioxygenase in metastatic pancreatic ductal adenocarcinoma recruits regulatory T cells to avoid immune detection. *J Am Coll Surg.* 2008;206(5):849−854; discussion 854−846.

151. Koblish HK, Hansbury MJ, Bowman KJ, et al. Hydroxyamidine inhibitors of indoleamine-2,3-dioxygenase potently suppress systemic tryptophan catabolism and the growth of Ido-expressing tumors. *Mol Cancer Ther.* 2010;9(2):489−498.

152. Soliman HH, Minton SE, Han HS, et al. A phase I study of indoximod in patients with advanced malignancies. *Oncotarget.* 2016;7(16):22928−22938.

153. Soliman HH, Jackson E, Neuger T, et al. A first in man phase I trial of the oral immunomodulator, indoximod, combined with docetaxel in patients with metastatic solid tumors. *Oncotarget.* 2014;5(18):8136−8146.

154. Jaffee EM, Schutte M, Gossett J, et al. Development and characterization of a cytokine-secreting pancreatic adenocarcinoma vaccine from primary tumors for use in clinical trials. *Cancer J Sci Am.* 1998;4(3):194−203.

155. Jaffee EM, Hruban RH, Biedrzycki B, et al. Novel allogeneic granulocyte-macrophage colony-stimulating factor-secreting tumor vaccine for pancreatic cancer: a phase I trial of safety and immune activation. *J Clin Oncol.* 2001;19(1):145−156.

156. Lutz E, Yeo CJ, Lillemoe KD, et al. A lethally irradiated allogeneic granulocyte-macrophage colony stimulating factor-secreting tumor vaccine for pancreatic adenocarcinoma. A Phase II trial of safety, efficacy, and immune activation. *Ann Surg.* 2011;253(2):328−335.

157. Laheru D, Lutz E, Burke J, et al. Allogeneic granulocyte macrophage colony-stimulating factor-secreting tumor immunotherapy alone or in sequence with cyclophosphamide for metastatic pancreatic cancer: a pilot study of safety, feasibility, and immune activation. *Clin Cancer Res.* 2008;14(5):1455−1463.

158. Thomas AM, Santarsiero LM, Lutz ER, et al. Mesothelin-specific CD8(+) T cell responses provide evidence of in vivo cross-priming by antigen-presenting cells in vaccinated pancreatic cancer patients. *J Exp Med.* 2004;200(3):297−306.

159. Lutz ER, Wu AA, Bigelow E, et al. Immunotherapy converts nonimmunogenic pancreatic tumors into immunogenic foci of immune regulation. *Cancer Immunol Res.* 2014;2(7):616−631.

160. Dieu-Nosjean MC, Antoine M, Danel C, et al. Long-term survival for patients with non-small-cell lung cancer with intratumoral lymphoid structures. *J Clin Oncol.* 2008;26(27):4410−4417.

161. Cipponi A, Mercier M, Seremet T, et al. Neogenesis of lymphoid structures and antibody responses occur in human melanoma metastases. *Cancer Res.* 2012;72(16):3997−4007.

162. Le DT, Lutz E, Uram JN, et al. Evaluation of ipilimumab in combination with allogeneic pancreatic tumor cells transfected with a GM-CSF gene in previously treated pancreatic cancer. *J Immunother*. 2013;36(7):382–389.

163. Soares KC, Rucki AA, Wu AA, et al. PD-1/PD-L1 blockade together with vaccine therapy facilitates effector T-cell infiltration into pancreatic tumors. *J Immunother*. 2015; 38(1):1–11.

164. Le DT, Brockstedt DG, Nir-Paz R, et al. A live-attenuated Listeria vaccine (ANZ-100) and a live-attenuated Listeria vaccine expressing mesothelin (CRS-207) for advanced cancers: phase I studies of safety and immune induction. *Clin Cancer Res*. 2012;18(3):858–868.

165. Nesselhut J, Marx D, Cillien N, et al. Dendritic cells generated with PDL-1 checkpoint blockade for treatment of advanced pancreatic cancer. *J Clin Oncol*. 2015;33(suppl 15):4128.

166. Nesselhut J, Marx D, Lange H, et al. Systemic treatment with anti-PD-1 antibody nivolumab in combination with vaccine therapy in advanced pancreatic cancer. *J Clin Oncol*. 2016;34(Supplement):3092.

167. Strong JE, Coffey MC, Tang D, Sabinin P, Lee PW. The molecular basis of viral oncolysis: usurpation of the RAS signaling pathway by reovirus. *EMBO J*. 1998; 17(12):3351–3362.

168. Prestwich RJ, Errington F, Ilett EJ, et al. Tumor infection by oncolytic reovirus primes adaptive antitumor immunity. *Clin Cancer Res*. 2008;14(22):7358–7366.

169. Gujar SA, Clements D, Dielschneider R, Helson E, Marcato P, Lee PW. Gemcitabine enhances the efficacy of reovirus-based oncotherapy through anti-tumour immunological mechanisms. *Br J Cancer*. 2014;110(1): 83–93.

170. Noonan AM, Farren MR, Geyer SM, et al. Randomized phase 2 trial of the oncolytic virus pelareorep (reolysin) in upfront treatment of metastatic pancreatic adenocarcinoma. *Mol Ther*. 2016;24(6):1150–1158.

171. Mahalingam D, Wang Y, Lu TW, et al. A study of REOLYSIN in combination with gemcitabine in patients with advanced pancreatic adenocarcinoma. *Eur J Cancer*. 2012;48:170–171.

172. Mahalingam D, Goel S, Coffey M, et al. P-175Oncolytic virus therapy in pancreatic cancer: clinical efficacy and pharmacodynamic analysis of REOLYSIN in combination with gemcitabine in patients with advanced pancreatic adenocarcinoma. *Ann Oncol*. 2015;26(suppl 4):iv51.

173. Mahalingam D, Patel S, Nuovo G, et al. The combination of intravenous Reolysin and gemcitabine induces reovirus replication and endoplasmic reticular stress in a patient with KRAS-activated pancreatic cancer. *BMC Cancer*. 2015;15:513.

174. Mahalingam D, Fountzilas C, Moseley JL, et al. A study of REOLYSIN in combination with pembrolizumab and chemotherapy in patients (pts) with relapsed metastatic adenocarcinoma of the pancreas (MAP). *J Clin Oncol*. 2017;35(Supplement):e15753.

175. Plate JM, Plate AE, Shott S, Bograd S, Harris JE. Effect of gemcitabine on immune cells in subjects with adenocarcinoma of the pancreas. *Cancer Immunol Immunother*. 2005;54(9):915–925.

176. Nowak AK, Lake RA, Marzo AL, et al. Induction of tumor cell apoptosis in vivo increases tumor antigen cross-presentation, cross-priming rather than cross-tolerizing host tumor-specific CD8 T cells. *J Immunol*. 2003; 170(10):4905–4913.

177. Galetto A, Buttiglieri S, Forno S, Moro F, Mussa A, Matera L. Drug- and cell-mediated antitumor cytotoxicities modulate cross-presentation of tumor antigens by myeloid dendritic cells. *Anticancer Drugs*. 2003;14(10): 833–843.

178. Hato SV, Khong A, de Vries IJ, Lesterhuis WJ. Molecular pathways: the immunogenic effects of platinum-based chemotherapeutics. *Clin Cancer Res*. 2014;20(11): 2831–2837.

179. Suzuki E, Kapoor V, Jassar AS, Kaiser LR, Albelda SM. Gemcitabine selectively eliminates splenic Gr-1+/CD11b+ myeloid suppressor cells in tumor-bearing animals and enhances antitumor immune activity. *Clin Cancer Res*. 2005;11(18):6713–6721.

180. Vincent J, Mignot G, Chalmin F, et al. 5-Fluorouracil selectively kills tumor-associated myeloid-derived suppressor cells resulting in enhanced T cell-dependent antitumor immunity. *Cancer Res*. 2010;70(8):3052–3061.

181. Takeuchi S, Baghdadi M, Tsuchikawa T, et al. Chemotherapy-derived inflammatory responses accelerate the formation of immunosuppressive myeloid cells in the tissue microenvironment of human pancreatic cancer. *Cancer Res*. 2015;75(13):2629–2640.

182. Eriksson E, Wenthe J, Irenaeus S, Loskog A, Ullenhag G. Gemcitabine reduces MDSCs, tregs and TGFbeta-1 while restoring the teff/treg ratio in patients with pancreatic cancer. *J Transl Med*. 2016;14(1):282.

183. Kalyan A, Kircher SM, Mohindra NA, et al. Ipilimumab and gemcitabine for advanced pancreas cancer: a phase Ib study. *J Clin Oncol*. 2016;34(Supplement):abstr e15747.

184. Wainberg ZA, Hochster HS, George B, et al. Phase I study of nivolumab (nivo) + nab-paclitaxel (nab-P) ± gemcitabine (Gem) in solid tumors: interim results from the pancreatic cancer (PC) cohorts. *J Clin Oncol*. 2017; 35(suppl 4):412.

185. Maleki Vareki S, Chen D, Di Cresce C, et al. Ido downregulation induces sensitivity to pemetrexed, gemcitabine, FK866, and methoxyamine in human cancer cells. *PLoS One*. 2015;10(11):e0143435.

186. Bahary N, Garrido-Laguna I, Wang-Gillam A, et al. Results of the phase Ib portion of a phase I/II trial of the indoleamine 2,3-dioxygenase pathway (Ido) inhibitor indoximod plus gemcitabine/nab-paclitaxel for the treatment of metastatic pancreatic cancer. *J Clin Oncol*. 2016; 34(suppl 4):452.

187. Bahary N, Garrido-Laguna I, Cinar P, et al. Phase 2 trial of the indoleamine 2,3-dioxygenase pathway (Ido) inhibitor indoximod plus gemcitabine/nab-paclitaxel for the treatment of metastatic pancreas cancer: interim analysis. *J Clin Oncol*. 2016;34(Supplement):3020.

188. Triebel F. LAG-3: a regulator of T-cell and DC responses and its use in therapeutic vaccination. *Trends Immunol.* 2003;24(12):619−622.

189. Hannier S, Tournier M, Bismuth G, Triebel F. CD3/TCR complex-associated lymphocyte activation gene-3 molecules inhibit CD3/TCR signaling. *J Immunol.* 1998; 161(8):4058−4065.

190. Fougeray S, Brignone C, Triebel F. A soluble LAG-3 protein as an immunopotentiator for therapeutic vaccines: preclinical evaluation of IMP321. *Vaccine.* 2006;24(26): 5426−5433.

191. Wang-Gillam A, Plambeck-Suess S, Goedegebuure P, et al. A phase I study of IMP321 and gemcitabine as the front-line therapy in patients with advanced pancreatic adenocarcinoma. *Invest New Drugs.* 2013;31(3): 707−713.

192. Duffy AG, Makarova-Rusher OV, Kleiner DE, et al. A pilot study of immune checkpoint inhibition in combination with radiation therapy in patients with metastatic pancreatic cancer. *J Clin Oncol.* 2017;35(suppl 15):e15786.

193. Mantovani A, Sozzani S, Locati M, Allavena P, Sica A. Macrophage polarization: tumor-associated macrophages as a paradigm for polarized M2 mononuclear phagocytes. *Trends Immunol.* 2002;23(11):549−555.

194. Shi C, Pamer EG. Monocyte recruitment during infection and inflammation. *Nat Rev Immunol.* 2011;11(11): 762−774.

195. Highfill SL, Cui Y, Giles AJ, et al. Disruption of CXCR2-mediated MDSC tumor trafficking enhances anti-PD1 efficacy. *Sci Transl Med.* 2014;6(237):237ra267.

196. Steele CW, Karim SA, Leach JD, et al. CXCR2 inhibition profoundly suppresses metastases and augments immunotherapy in pancreatic ductal adenocarcinoma. *Cancer Cell.* 2016;29(6):832−845.

197. Mitchem JB, Brennan DJ, Knolhoff BL, et al. Targeting tumor-infiltrating macrophages decreases tumor-initiating cells, relieves immunosuppression, and improves chemotherapeutic responses. *Cancer Res.* 2013; 73(3):1128−1141.

198. Zhu Y, Knolhoff BL, Meyer MA, et al. CSF1/CSF1R blockade reprograms tumor-infiltrating macrophages and improves response to T-cell checkpoint immunotherapy in pancreatic cancer models. *Cancer Res.* 2014; 74(18):5057−5069.

199. Gunderson AJ, Kaneda MM, Tsujikawa T, et al. Bruton tyrosine kinase-dependent immune cell cross-talk drives pancreas cancer. *Cancer Discov.* 2016;6(3):270−285.

200. Kaneda MM, Cappello P, Nguyen AV, et al. Macrophage PI3Kgamma drives pancreatic ductal adenocarcinoma progression. *Cancer Discov.* 2016;6(8):870−885.

201. Sagiv-Barfi I, Kohrt HE, Czerwinski DK, Ng PP, Chang BY, Levy R. Therapeutic antitumor immunity by checkpoint blockade is enhanced by ibrutinib, an inhibitor of both BTK and ITK. *Proc Natl Acad Sci U S A.* 2015;112(9): E966−E972.

202. Schaller MD, Borgman CA, Cobb BS, Vines RR, Reynolds AB, Parsons JT. pp125FAK a structurally distinctive protein-tyrosine kinase associated with focal adhesions. *Proc Natl Acad Sci U S A.* 1992;89(11): 5192−5196.

203. Jiang H, Hegde S, Knolhoff BL, et al. Targeting focal adhesion kinase renders pancreatic cancers responsive to checkpoint immunotherapy. *Nat Med.* 2016;22(8): 851−860.

204. Stokes JB, Adair SJ, Slack-Davis JK, et al. Inhibition of focal adhesion kinase by PF-562,271 inhibits the growth and metastasis of pancreatic cancer concomitant with altering the tumor microenvironment. *Mol Cancer Ther.* 2011;10(11):2135−2145.

205. Rhim AD, Oberstein PE, Thomas DH, et al. Stromal elements act to restrain, rather than support, pancreatic ductal adenocarcinoma. *Cancer Cell.* 2014;25(6): 735−747.

206. Catenacci DV, Junttila MR, Karrison T, et al. Randomized phase Ib/II study of gemcitabine plus placebo or Vismodegib, a Hedgehog pathway inhibitor, in patients with metastatic pancreatic cancer. *J Clin Oncol.* 2015;33(36): 4284−4292.

207. Archambault PM, Gagnon S, Gagnon MP, et al. Development and validation of questionnaires exploring health care professionals' intention to use wiki-based reminders to promote best practices in trauma. *JMIR Res Protoc.* 2014;3(3):e50.

208. Ozdemir BC, Pentcheva-Hoang T, Carstens JL, et al. Depletion of carcinoma-associated fibroblasts and fibrosis induces immunosuppression and accelerates pancreas cancer with reduced survival. *Cancer Cell.* 2014;25(6):719−734.

209. Schoenberger SP, Toes RE, van der Voort EI, Offringa R, Melief CJ. T-cell help for cytotoxic T lymphocytes is mediated by CD40-CD40L interactions. *Nature.* 1998; 393(6684):480−483.

210. Beatty GL, Chiorean EG, Fishman MP, et al. CD40 agonists alter tumor stroma and show efficacy against pancreatic carcinoma in mice and humans. *Science.* 2011;331(6024):1612−1616.

211. Winograd R, Byrne KT, Evans RA, et al. Induction of T-cell immunity overcomes complete resistance to PD-1 and CTLA-4 blockade and improves survival in pancreatic carcinoma. *Cancer Immunol Res.* 2015;3(4):399−411.

212. Luheshi NM, Coates-Ulrichsen J, Harper J, et al. Transformation of the tumour microenvironment by a CD40 agonist antibody correlates with improved responses to PD-L1 blockade in a mouse orthotopic pancreatic tumour model. *Oncotarget.* 2016;7(14):18508−18520.

213. Quintas-Cardama A, Kantarjian H, Cortes J, Verstovsek S. Janus kinase inhibitors for the treatment of myeloproliferative neoplasias and beyond. *Nat Rev Drug Discov.* 2011;10(2):127−140.

214. Hurwitz HI, Uppal N, Wagner SA, et al. Randomized, double-blind, phase II study of ruxolitinib or placebo in combination with capecitabine in patients with metastatic pancreatic cancer for whom therapy with gemcitabine has failed. *J Clin Oncol.* 2015;33(34):4039−4047.

215. Hurwitz H, Van Cutsem E, Bendell JC, et al. Two randomized, placebo-controlled phase 3 studies of ruxolitinib

(Rux) + capecitabine (C) in patients (pts) with advanced/ metastatic pancreatic cancer (mPC) after failure/intolerance of first-line chemotherapy: JANUS 1 (J1) and JANUS 2 (J2). *J Clin Oncol*. 2017;35(4S):abstract 343.

216. Lu C, Talukder A, Savage NM, Singh N, Liu K. JAK-STAT-mediated chronic inflammation impairs cytotoxic T lymphocyte activation to decrease anti-PD-1 immunotherapy efficacy in pancreatic cancer. *Oncoimmunology*. 2017;6(3):e1291106.

217. Chiappinelli KB, Zahnow CA, Ahuja N, Baylin SB. Combining epigenetic and immunotherapy to combat cancer. *Cancer Res*. 2016;76(7):1683–1689.

218. Kim K, Skora AD, Li Z, et al. Eradication of metastatic mouse cancers resistant to immune checkpoint blockade by suppression of myeloid-derived cells. *Proc Natl Acad Sci U S A*. 2014;111(32):11774–11779.

219. Shakya R, Gonda T, Quante M, et al. Hypomethylating therapy in an aggressive stroma-rich model of pancreatic carcinoma. *Cancer Res*. 2013;73(2):885–896.

220. Missiaglia E, Donadelli M, Palmieri M, Crnogorac-Jurcevic T, Scarpa A, Lemoine NR. Growth delay of human pancreatic cancer cells by methylase inhibitor 5-aza-2'-deoxycytidine treatment is associated with activation of the interferon signalling pathway. *Oncogene*. 2005;24(1):199–211.

221. Patel S, Hurez V, Nawrocki ST, et al. Vorinostat and hydroxychloroquine improve immunity and inhibit autophagy in metastatic colorectal cancer. *Oncotarget*. 2016;7(37):59087–59097.

222. Miller-Ocuin JL, Bahary NS, Singhi AD, et al. Inhibition of autophagy improves pathologic and biomarker response to preoperative gemcitabine/nab-paclitaxel in potentially resectable pancreatic cancer: a phase II randomized controlled trial. *Ann Surg Oncol*. 2017; 24(Supplement):1.

223. Holter S, Borgida A, Dodd A, et al. Germline BRCA mutations in a large clinic-based cohort of patients with pancreatic adenocarcinoma. *J Clin Oncol*. 2015;33(28): 3124–3129.

224. Millis SZ, Abbott BL, Baker EH, et al. Multiplatform molecular profiling of pancreatic adenocarcinomas to identify BRCA1/2 mutations and PD-1/PD-L1 status with therapeutic implications. *J Clin Oncol*. 2015; 33(Supplement):abstract 4124.

225. Waddell N, Pajic M, Patch AM, et al. Whole genomes redefine the mutational landscape of pancreatic cancer. *Nature*. 2015;518(7540):495–501.

226. Kaufman B, Shapira-Frommer R, Schmutzler RK, et al. Olaparib monotherapy in patients with advanced cancer and a germline BRCA1/2 mutation. *J Clin Oncol*. 2015; 33(3):244–250.

227. Lohse I, Borgida A, Cao P, et al. BRCA1 and BRCA2 mutations sensitize to chemotherapy in patient-derived pancreatic cancer xenografts. *Br J Cancer*. 2015;113(3): 425–432.

228. Higuchi T, Flies DB, Marjon NA, et al. CTLA-4 blockade synergizes therapeutically with PARP inhibition in BRCA1-deficient ovarian cancer. *Cancer Immunol Res*. 2015;3(11):1257–1268.

229. Friedlander M, Meniawy T, Markman B, et al. A phase 1b study of the anti-PD-1 monoclonal antibody BGB-A317 (A317) in combination with the PARP inhibitor BGB-290(290) in advanced solid tumors. *J Clin Oncol*. 2017; 35(suppl 15):3013.

230. Siegel RL, Miller KD, Fedewa SA, et al. Colorectal cancer statistics, 2017. *CA Cancer J Clin*. 2017;67(3):177–193.

231. Guinney J, Dienstmann R, Wang X, et al. The consensus molecular subtypes of colorectal cancer. *Nat Med*. 2015; 21(11):1350–1356.

232. Becht E, de Reynies A, Giraldo NA, et al. Immune and stromal classification of colorectal cancer is associated with molecular subtypes and relevant for precision immunotherapy. *Clin Cancer Res*. 2016;22(16): 4057–4066.

233. Boland CR, Goel A. Microsatellite instability in colorectal cancer. *Gastroenterology*. 2010;138(6):2073–2087:e2073.

234. Chung KY, Gore I, Fong L, et al. Phase II study of the anti-cytotoxic T-lymphocyte-associated antigen 4 monoclonal antibody, tremelimumab, in patients with refractory metastatic colorectal cancer. *J Clin Oncol*. 2010;28(21): 3485–3490.

235. Topalian SL, Hodi FS, Brahmer JR, et al. Safety, activity, and immune correlates of anti-PD-1 antibody in cancer. *N Engl J Med*. 2012;366(26):2443–2454.

236. Lipson EJ, Sharfman WH, Drake CG, et al. Durable cancer regression off-treatment and effective reinduction therapy with an anti-PD-1 antibody. *Clin Cancer Res*. 2013; 19(2):462–468.

237. Diaz LA, Marabelle A, Delord J-P, et al. Pembrolizumab therapy for microsatellite instability high (MSI-H) colorectal cancer (CRC) and non-CRC. *J Clin Oncol*. 2017; 35(suppl 15):3071.

238. Overman MJ, McDermott R, Leach JL, et al. Nivolumab in patients with metastatic DNA mismatch repair-deficient or microsatellite instability-high colorectal cancer (CheckMate 142): an open-label, multicentre, phase 2 study. *Lancet Oncol*. 2017;18(9):1182–1191.

239. Overman MJ, Kopetz S, McDermott RS, et al. Nivolumab ± ipilimumab in treatment (tx) of patients (pts) with metastatic colorectal cancer (mCRC) with and without high microsatellite instability (MSI-H): CheckMate-142 interim results. *J Clin Oncol*. 2016;34(suppl 15):3501.

240. Overman MJ, Lonardi S, Wong KYM, et al. Durable clinical benefit with nivolumab plus ipilimumab in DNA mismatch repair-deficient/microsatellite instability-high metastatic colorectal cancer. *J Clin Oncol*. 2018;36(8): 773–779.

241. Liu L, Mayes PA, Eastman S, et al. The BRAF and MEK inhibitors Dabrafenib and Trametinib: effects on immune function and in combination with immunomodulatory antibodies targeting PD-1, PD-L1, and CTLA-4. *Clin Cancer Res*. 2015;21(7):1639–1651.

242. Bendell JC, Kin TW, Goh BC, et al. Clinical activity and safety of cobimetinib (cobi) and atezolizumab in

colorectal cancer (CRC). *J Clin Oncol.* 2016;34(suppl 15): 3502.

243. Tabernero J, Melero I, Ros W, et al. Phase I studies of the novel carcinoembryonic antigen CD3 T-cell bispecific (CEA CD3 TCB) antibody as a single agent and in combination with atezolizumab: preliminary efficacy and safety in patients with metastatic colorectal cancer (mCRC). *J Clin Oncol.* 2017;35(suppl 15):3002.

244. De Vuyst H, Clifford GM, Nascimento MC, Madeleine MM, Franceschi S. Prevalence and type distribution of human papillomavirus in carcinoma and intraepithelial neoplasia of the vulva, vagina and anus: a meta-analysis. *Int J Cancer.* 2009;124(7):1626−1636.

245. Das P, Bhatia S, Eng C, et al. Predictors and patterns of recurrence after definitive chemoradiation for anal cancer. *Int J Radiat Oncol Biol Phys.* 2007;68(3):794−800.

246. de Jong A, van Poelgeest MI, van der Hulst JM, et al. Human papillomavirus type 16-positive cervical cancer is associated with impaired CD4+ T-cell immunity against early antigens E2 and E6. *Cancer Res.* 2004;64(15): 5449−5455.

247. Morris VK, Salem ME, Nimeiri H, et al. Nivolumab for previously treated unresectable metastatic anal cancer (NCI9673): a multicentre, single-arm, phase 2 study. *Lancet Oncol.* 2017;18(4):446−453.

248. Ott PA, Piha-Paul SA, Munster P, et al. Safety and antitumor activity of the anti-PD-1 antibody pembrolizumab in patients with recurrent carcinoma of the anal canal. *Ann Oncol.* 2017;28(5):1036−1041.

249. Cory L, Chu C. ADXS-HPV: a therapeutic Listeria vaccination targeting cervical cancers expressing the HPV E7 antigen. *Hum Vaccin Immunother.* 2014;10(11): 3190−3195.

250. Eng C, Fakih M, Amin M, et al. P2 study of ADXS11-001 Immunotherapy in patients with persistent/recurrent, surgically unresectable locoregional, or metastatic squamous cell anal cancer. *Ann Oncol.* 2017;28(suppl 5): 537P.

251. Spencer KR, Wang J, Silk AW, Ganesan S, Kaufman HL, Mehnert JM. Biomarkers for immunotherapy: current developments and challenges. *Am Soc Clin Oncol Educ Book.* 2016;35:e493−503.

252. Yang JH, Park S, Joung EK, Lee MA, Roh SY, Kim IH. 681PClinical impact of programmed death ligand-1 and -2 expression after platinum based chemotherapy in metastatic gastric cancer. *Ann Oncol.* 2017;28(suppl 5):mdx369.065.

253. Kim MA, Lee HJ, Yang HK, Bang YJ, Kim WH. Heterogeneous amplification of ERBB2 in primary lesions is responsible for the discordant ERBB2 status of primary and metastatic lesions in gastric carcinoma. *Histopathology.* 2011;59(5):822−831.

254. Ayers M, Lunceford J, Nebozhyn M, et al. Relationship between immune gene signatures and clinical response to PD-1 blockade with pembrolizumab (MK-3475) in patients with advanced solid tumors. *J Immunother Cancer.* 2015;3(suppl 2):P80.

255. Le DT, Uram JN, Wang H, et al. PD-1 blockade in mismatch repair deficient non-colorectal gastrointestinal cancers. *J Clin Oncol.* 2016;34(suppl 4):195.

256. George TJ, Frampton GM, Sun J, et al. Tumor mutational burden as a potential biomarker for PD1/PD-L1 therapy in colorectal cancer. *J Clin Oncol.* 2016;34(suppl 15): 3587.

257. Hu ZI, Varghese AM, Shia J, et al. Clinical characterization of pancreatic ductal adenocarcinomas (PDAC) with mismatch repair (MMR) gene mutations. *J Clin Oncol.* 2017;35(suppl 15):e15791.

258. Suh J, Severson E, Hechtman J, et al. 194OHybrid-capture based comprehensive genomic profiling of hepatocellular carcinoma identifies patients who may benefit from targeted therapies and immune checkpoint blockade. *Ann Oncol.* 2017;28(suppl 10):mdx660.001.

259. Beatty GL, O'Hara MH, Nelson AM, et al. Safety and antitumor activity of chimeric antigen receptor modified T cells in patients with chemotherapy refractory metastatic pancreatic cancer. *J Clin Oncol.* 2015;33(suppl 15): 3007.

CHAPTER 5

Cancers of the Head and Neck

AHMAD HANIF, MD • SUMERA KHAN, MD • HONGBIN CHEN, MD, PHD

INTRODUCTION

Cancers of the head and neck represent a heterogeneous group of malignancies with a wide variability in location and histopathology. These include tumors of the oral cavity, pharynx, larynx, nasal cavity, salivary glands, and paranasal sinuses. More than 1 million people worldwide are diagnosed annually, and approximately 64,690 people in the Unites States will be diagnosed with head and neck cancer in 2018 resulting in 13,740 deaths.[1,2] The incidence of head and neck cancers vary with the regional prevalence of risk factors. The main modifiable risk factors are tobacco (smoked or chewed), alcohol, human papillomavirus (HPV) infection for oropharyngeal cancers, and Epstein—Barr virus (EBV) infection for nasopharyngeal cancers.[3] Smoking increases the risk of development of head and neck cancers by 5- to 25-folds, and there are studies suggesting a dose—response relationship.[4—7] Concurrent use of tobacco and alcohol seems to have a synergistic and multiplicative effect on the risk for cancer development.[4,8] Other risk factors include poor dental hygiene, male sex and immunosuppression. Certain environmental and occupational hazards have also been implicated in the pathogenesis of these cancers which include exposure to pesticides, asbestos, dry cleaning agent perchloroethylene, polycyclic aromatic hydrocarbons, plastic and rubber products, and the chemicals handled by textile workers, leather and paint workers, automobile mechanics, and construction workers (cement).[9—13] Prior local irradiation can also predispose to thyroid and salivary glands tumors, although the risk appears to be low and associated with a long latency period.[14]

Infection with HPV is a well-established risk factor for development of oropharyngeal squamous cell carcinoma. HPV is the most common sexually transmitted disease and is a cause of virtually all cervical cancers.[15] In the oropharynx, HPV infects and resides in the lymphoid-rich crypts of tonsils where its replication is facilitated by concurrent inflammation due to other microorganisms.[16] In a case-control study involving 100 patients with newly diagnosed cancer of oropharynx, oral infection with HPV, most frequently HPV16, was significantly associated with oropharyngeal cancer.[17] However, other high-risk HPV types are also found in roughly 10% of oropharyngeal tumors and other head and neck cancers. HPV-positive oropharyngeal carcinomas are usually identified by testing for its surrogate marker p16 protein expression in tumor specimen and show improved response to therapy with better survival when compared with HPV-negative cancers of same site.[18,19] Infection with EBV has been well established as the primary etiologic event in the development of nasopharyngeal carcinoma.[20] EBV infection can be easily identified by serologic testing for IgA antibodies against EBV viral capsid antigen (VCA/IgA) and is being evaluated as a screening tool for high-risk populations such as southern China. Other viruses implicated in the pathogenesis of head and neck cancers are hepatitis C virus and human immunodeficiency virus.[21,22]

A small number of head and neck cancers are familial.[23] The most common abnormalities identified are loss-of-function mutations in the cyclin-dependent kinase inhibitor 2A (CDKN2A) locus leading to ineffective function of tumor suppressor proteins p16INK4A and p14ARF.[24] Mutations of the tumor suppressor gene TP53 also leads to increased predisposition for head and neck cancers among other malignancies (Li—Fraumeni syndrome).[25] Patients with Fanconi anemia are at higher risk of developing a malignancy including head and neck cancer.[26,27] Patients with familial causes of cancer tend to be younger and may present without traditional risk factors of smoking and alcohol. Their management can be complicated owing to increased susceptibility to radiation therapy associated with many of these hereditary syndromes.[28] There is some suggestion of a higher cancer risk with alcohol intake owing to genetic polymorphism of enzymes alcohol dehydrogenase and aldehyde dehydrogenase.[29]

About 90%—95% of head and neck cancers arise from the surface epithelium and are squamous cell carcinomas (squamous cell carcinomas of head and neck, SCCHNs) or one of its variants (lymphoepithelioma, spindle cell carcinoma, verrucous carcinoma, and undifferentiated carcinoma). Other rare histologic subtypes include adenocarcinoma, adenoid cystic carcinoma, lymphomas, sarcomas, and small cell neuroendocrine carcinoma. Management of these tumors depends on the site of origin, pathologic subtype, and extent of the disease. As there is a lack of evidence regarding efficacy of immune checkpoint inhibitors in the management of localized disease, this chapter will mostly focus on the management of metastatic or recurrent disease, not amenable to locally directed treatment options.

MOLECULAR BIOLOGY OF HEAD AND NECK CANCERS

Amplification of epidermal growth factor receptor (EGFR) gene with associated overexpression of EGFR is a common molecular abnormality in head and neck cancers, especially squamous cell carcinoma, and is associated with poor prognosis.[30,31] However, this molecular finding often times does not translate into a clinical benefit with only about a 10% response rate with EGFR-directed therapy.[32] This observation has led to the hypothesis of multiple molecular aberrations working concurrently and driving parallel pathways of cellular activation and inhibition of apoptosis. Many of the molecular alterations identified in head and neck cancers work to deregulate the tumor suppressor function of p53. Mutations, loss of heterozygosity, and methylation of CDKN2A gene are common and believed to be an early event in pathogenesis of SCCHN, which can lead to inactivation of p53.[33–35] Mutation and overexpression of p53 in SCCHN has been found to be associated with better response to induction chemotherapy and radiation, likely owing to inability of tumor cells to repair treatment-induced DNA damage.[36,37] Further studies revealed that coexistence of wild-type and overexpression of Bcl-xL conferred cisplatin resistance secondary to blockage of p53-induced apoptosis by Bcl-xL.[38] Other molecular changes that block the tumor suppressor function of p53 include overexpression of the HPV E6 protein and overexpression or amplification of MDM2.[39–41] The PI3K signaling pathway is also commonly activated owing to mutations involving its two main regulators, PTEN and PIK3CA.[42] Rarely, mutations of HRAS gene can lead to constitutional activation of RAS, RAF, mitogen-activated protein kinase, extracellular signal–related kinase cascade leading to expression of transcription factors, and cellular proliferation.[43] Overall, HPV-positive head and neck cancers have less

number of genetic and molecular abnormalities than HPV-negative tumors.

IMMUNE ESCAPE IN HEAD AND NECK CANCER

Evasion of immune response is a critical step in the development and progression of cancer. Patients with SCCHN are known to have lower absolute counts of T-cells in peripheral blood, leading to the hypothesis that SCCHN is an immunosuppressive disease.[44] They can also have defective natural killer (NK) cell activity leading to impaired immune surveillance.[45,46] Tumor cells can alter human leukocyte antigen class I expression, which interferes recognition by T-cells. Studies have shown that malignant cells in SCCHN produce cytokines, such as transforming growth factor-β, interleukin (IL)-6, and IL-10, which suppress signal transducer and activator of transcription 1 (STAT1) expression, resulting in escape from T-cell–mediated antitumor immunity.[47,48]

Another mechanism used by cancer cells to escape immune response is activation of immune checkpoints. These checkpoints physiologically act as coinhibitory receptors of T-cell activation as part of the immune system's defense mechanism against overactivation during an inflammatory response. One of the most well-studied immune checkpoint pathways involves the interaction between programmed cell death protein 1 (PD-1) on the surface of T-cells and its ligand PD-L1. Multiple studies have documented increased expression of PD-L1 on the surface of SCCHN cells from human tissue samples.[49–54] This high level of PD-L1 expression was observed among all anatomical subtypes of SCCHN ranging from 46% to 100% of tumors across different studies. In addition, PD-L1 was also expressed in the primary, recurrent, and metastatic settings. Interestingly, SCCHN patients who are HPV positive carry a significantly higher expression of PD-L1 compared with HPV-negative patients.[52,55] Cytotoxic T-lymphocyte–associated protein 4 (CTLA-4) is an immune checkpoint receptor expressed by CD4+, CD8+, and regulatory T-cells (Tregs). CTLA-4 belongs to B7 receptor family that binds to stimulatory ligands CD80 and CD86 with higher affinity than CD28, thus inhibiting T-cell activation.[56] Studies have confirmed a higher frequency of head and neck cancer intratumoral Tregs expressing PD-1 and CTLA-4 compared with peripheral blood Tregs.[57] Tregs suppress NK cell, dendritic cell, and B-cell function leading to global immunosuppression.[58,59] Other immune checkpoints expressed in patient with SCCHN include lymphocyte-activation gene-3 (LAG-3), T-cell immunoglobulin mucin protein-3 (TIM-3), and B7-H3.[57,60,61]

SQUAMOUS CELL CARCINOMA OF HEAD AND NECK

SCCHN is the most common type of head and neck cancers. It usually begins as a surface lesion and the spread is dictated by anatomical site of origin. Occasionally, patients may present with squamous cell carcinoma in a cervical lymph node with no apparent site of origin. Even after extensive workup, the primary site of origin remains undiagnosed in about half of these patients and are treated similar to other SCCHNs anatomically related with that nodal group.[62] For localized disease, curative therapy is offered with surgery or radiation with or without combination chemotherapy depending on the site of origin and stage of disease.

The prognosis for recurrent or metastatic SCCHN is poor. When treated with chemotherapy alone, the median survival is 6–9 months.[63] Multiple trials with combination chemotherapy showed higher response rates at the expense of increased toxicity.[64–67] In a large phase III trial, 442 patients were randomized to platinum (cisplatin or carboplatin) and 5-fluorouracil with or without EGFR inhibitor cetuximab for six cycles (EXTREME regimen).[68] Both the progression-free survival (PFS, 5.6 vs. 3 months) and overall survival (OS, 10.1 vs. 7.4 months) were higher in the cetuximab group. This has since become the standard therapy option for eligible patients in metastatic setting. In another randomized trial evaluating the use of EGFR antibody panitumumab with cisplatin and 5-fluorouracil, there was a trend for higher OS in panitumumab group, which was not statistically significant (11.1 vs. 9.0 months, $P = .1403$).[69] It is thus clear that even with combination of chemotherapy and molecularly targeted drugs, response rates and survival statistics for recurrent or metastatic SCCHN remain poor, and there is a clear need for a new class of therapeutic drugs.

Immune checkpoint inhibitors have recently emerged as a new class of immunotherapy drugs with a unique mechanism of action. Preclinical studies evaluating the blockade of PD-1 and PD-L1 concluded that this approach can enhance T-cell activation and results in inhibition of tumor growth.[70,71] Similar results were obtained by blocking CTLA-4.[72] This led to the development of inhibitors of PD-1, PD-L1, and CTLA-4 in humans. Please see Table 5.1 for a list of published trials of immune checkpoint inhibitors in recurrent or metastatic SCCHN. Their use in patients with SCCHN is summarized below.

PD-1 Inhibitors

Pembrolizumab and nivolumab are fully humanized IgG4 monoclonal antibodies against PD-1 receptor.

The first study to demonstrate benefit of pembrolizumab in patients with recurrent or metastatic SCCHN was the open-label phase Ib KEYNOTE-012 trial.[73] In this study, 61 patients with detectable levels of PD-L1 expression (at least 1% as determined by immunohistochemistry) were treated with pembrolizumab 10 mg/kg intravenously every 2 weeks for a maximum of 24 months of treatment. Overall 18% of patients had responses, translating into a median OS of 13 months. Median PFS was 4 months in HPV-positive patients and 2 months in HPV-negative patients. The responses were durable with a median duration of 53 weeks. Sixty-three percent of patients experienced treatment-related side effects, most commonly grade 1–2 pruritus, fatigue, or rash. Severe adverse events (AEs, grade 3–5) occurred in 17% of patients and included fatigue, rash, lymphopenia, atrial fibrillation, diarrhea, liver function tests abnormalities, hyponatremia, and musculoskeletal pain. The degree of PD-L1 expression on tumor cells was associated with improved PFS. This study was subsequently expanded to include 132 patients who were treated with fixed-dose pembrolizumab at 200 mg intravenously every 3 weeks.[74] Patients were included regardless of PD-L1 expression or HPV status. Overall response rate (ORR) was 18% while 20% of patients had stable disease after a median follow up of 9 months. The 6-month PFS and OS rates were 23% and 59%, respectively. Interestingly, PD-L1 positivity on tumor cells (1% or greater) did not correlate with probability of response. However, when tumor-infiltrating immune cells were included in scoring system, a statistically significant increase in ORR was observed for PD-L1–positive ($\geq$1%) versus PD-L1–negative (<1%) patients (22% vs. 4%; $P = .021$). A higher ORR was also observed in patients with HPV-associated SCCHN versus non–HPV-associated disease (32% vs. 14%). In a phase II study (KEYNOTE-055), 171 patients with recurrent or metastatic SCCHN resistant to both platinum and cetuximab were treated with pembrolizumab 200 mg every 3 weeks.[75] The results showed an encouraging ORR of 16% (95% confidence interval, 11%–23%), considering that 75% of patients in this study received two or more prior lines of therapy for metastatic disease. Median PFS was 2.1 months, and OS was 8 months. There was no statistical difference between the response rates in PD-L1–positive and –negative subgroups. In this study, patients had a response to pembrolizumab regardless of HPV status. Median duration of response was 8 months (range, >2 to >12 months; 75% of responses were ongoing at the time of analysis). Based on these results, pembrolizumab was granted accelerated approval by the U.S. Food and

TABLE 5.1

Published Clinical Trials of Checkpoint Inhibitors for Recurrent or Metastatic Squamous Cell Carcinoma of the Head and Neck

Trial	Phase	Patient Population	Treatment	Primary End Point(s)	Primary Outcome(s)/Other Outcomes
Seiwert et al.[73] (KEYNOTE-012)	Ib	60 patients with PD-L1 $\geq$ 1%, with or without prior treatment	Pembrolizumab 10 mg/kg every 2 weeks	Safety	Safety—Well tolerated. 17% of patients had grade $\geq$3 AEs 18% patients had a response
Chow et al.[74] (KEYNOTE-012 expansion cohort)	Ib	132 patients with or without prior treatment	Pembrolizumab 200 mg every 3 weeks	ORR	ORR was 18% (22% vs. 4% in PD-L1+ vs. PD-L1− patients)[a] 6-month PFS was 23% 6-month OS was 59%
Bauml et al.[75] (KEYNOTE-055)	II	171 patients with disease progression on platinum + cetuximab	Pembrolizumab 200 mg every 3 weeks	ORR Safety	ORR—16% (Similar in PD-L1+ and −) Safety—15% of patients had grade $\geq$3 AEs Median PFS = 2.1 months Median OS = 8 months
Ferris et al.[78] (CheckMate 141)	III	361 patients with disease progression on platinum-based chemotherapy	Nivolumab 3 mg/kg versus single-agent chemotherapy	OS	Median OS 7.5 versus 5.1 months favoring nivolumab Median PFS 2.0 versus 2.3 months
Segal et al.[83,84]	I/II	62 patients regardless of prior treatment or PD-L1 status	Durvalumab 10 mg/kg every 2 weeks for 12 months	Safety ORR	[b]Safety—8% of patients had grade $\geq$3 AEs. No deaths ORR—12% in all patients (25% in PD-L1+ patients)

AEs, adverse events; *ORR*, objective response rate; *OS*, overall survival; *PFS*, progression-free survival.

[a] Responses were only significantly different when immune cells were also included in PD-L1 scoring system.

[b] Preliminary results.

Drug Administration (FDA) for treatment of patients with recurrent or metastatic SCCHN with disease progression on or after platinum-containing chemotherapy. The approved dosage of pembrolizumab is 200 mg every 3 weeks, and testing for PD-L1 expression is currently not recommended. There are currently two ongoing phase III trials in recurrent or metastatic SCCHN, the KEYNOTE-040 (NCT02252042) comparing pembrolizumab to standard treatment in platinum-resistant disease and KEYNOTE-048 (NCT02358031) evaluating the first-line use of pembrolizumab, either alone or in combination with chemotherapy.

Nivolumab has also shown antitumor activity in various cancers.[76,77] In the phase III CheckMate 141 trial, 361 patients with recurrent platinum-resistant SCCHN were randomized to receive nivolumab at a dosage of 3 mg/kg every 2 weeks or standard single-agent systemic therapy (methotrexate, docetaxel, or cetuximab).[78] The median age of patients in this trial was 60 years, and most patients (54.8%) received two or more previous lines of therapy. The median OS was significantly longer in nivolumab group compared with standard therapy (7.5 vs. 5.1 months) with no difference in PFS. The ORR was 13.3% in the nivolumab group and 5.8% in the standard-therapy group. Patients treated with nivolumab also experienced less grade 3 or 4 treatment-related AEs than those treated with standard therapy (13.1% vs. 35.1%). The most common grade 3 or 4 AEs with nivolumab were fatigue and anemia. The response to nivolumab was regardless of PD-L1 or HPV status. Based on these results, nivolumab gained FDA approval for treatment of patients with recurrent or metastatic SCCHN with disease progression on or after platinum-containing chemotherapy.

PD-L1 Inhibitors

Inhibitors of PD-L1 such as atezolizumab, durvalumab, and avelumab have produced durable responses in cancers, such as urothelial carcinoma, non–small cell lung cancer (NSCLC), and Merkel cell carcinoma, and have shown an acceptable safety profile.[79–82] Durvalumab is an IgG1 monoclonal antibody to PD-L1 and has shown efficacy in a phase I/II open-label study as monotherapy for multiple solid tumors, including SCCHN.[83,84] The trial included 51 patients with recurrent or metastatic SCCHN in which the ORR to durvalumab monotherapy was 12% (25% in PD-L1–positive patients). Currently, durvalumab is being tested in a phase III clinical trial (NCT02551159) alone and in combination with tremelimumab versus EXTREME regimen (carboplatin or cisplatin + 5-FU + cetuximab) as primary treatment for recurrent or metastatic SCCHN. Other PD-L1 inhibitors are currently in early phase of clinical trials.

Combination Therapy

The rationale for combining an immune checkpoint inhibitor with chemotherapy, another checkpoint inhibitor, or targeted therapy comes from results of animal models or early human trials that showed potentiation of immune response with this approach.

Chemotherapy can increase tumor immunity either by inducing immunogenic cell death or disrupting the mechanisms used by tumor cells for evasion of immune response. The effects depend on the type of drug, dose, and schedule of chemotherapy.[85] There are multiple strategies suggested regarding the optimal combination and sequence of chemotherapy and immune checkpoint inhibitors. One approach calls for upfront debulking of tumor with surgery/chemotherapy followed by immunotherapy for treatment of minimal residual disease. This design can potentiate the antitumor response by reducing tumor bulk, thereby increasing tumor penetration by T-cells, and allow the immunomodulatory effects of chemotherapy before initiating checkpoint inhibitor therapy. There are other studies with concurrent administration of chemotherapy and immunotherapy with synergistic responses. Some chemotherapeutic drugs can induce PD-L1 expression on tumor cells, which can theoretically potentiate the effects of PD-1/PD-L1 inhibitors in the combination setting.[86,87] Combination of chemotherapy with checkpoint inhibitors have produced higher response rates and improvement in PFS in NSCLC,[88] but there is a paucity of published data

with this approach in SCCHN. There are ongoing clinical trials in SCCHN evaluating the combination of pembrolizumab with EXTREME regimen (carboplatin or cisplatin + 5FU + cetuximab) in the first-line setting (NCT02358031) or with docetaxel (NCT02718820) in the second-line setting. A phase I study is evaluating the front-line use of nivolumab in combination with cisplatin and radiation in patients with intermediate- and high-risk locally advanced SCCHN (NCT02764593). Other combination therapies include ongoing phase Ib/II study (NCT03019003) evaluating the combination of hypomethylating agent azacitidine with durvalumab and tremelimumab in patients with SCCHN who have progressed on immune checkpoint inhibitor monotherapy.

Combination of anti–PD-1 or anti–PD-L1 with anti–CTLA-4 antibodies can exert synergistic effects, as these antibodies inhibit distinct immune regulatory points.[89] Preclinical data suggest higher antitumor response with this approach in SCCHN.[90] Combination of PD-1 and CTLA-4 inhibitors has produced higher response rates in metastatic melanoma and NSCLC at the expense of increased toxicity.[91,92] There are several ongoing clinical trials comparing combination of PD-1 and CTLA-4 inhibitors with either standard of care (CheckMate 651) or single-agent immune checkpoint inhibitor (CheckMate 714) in the upfront setting for recurrent or metastatic SCCHN.

Targeted therapies against EGFR have a well-defined role in the treatment of SCCHN. Cetuximab is also known to enhance susceptibility of colon cancer cells to phagocytosis by dendritic cells and enhance the T-cell response.[93] In head and neck cancers, cetuximab promotes activation of NK cells and dendritic cell maturation and induces CTLA-4 expressing Tregs.[94,95] Cetuximab is being evaluated in a phase Ib trial in combination with ipilimumab and radiation therapy in front-line setting for SCCHN (NCT01935921).

Combinations of checkpoint inhibitors with target inhibitors against other immunosuppressive signals such as janus kinase 1, STAT3 pathway, PI3K/Akt pathway, and histone deacetylase are currently in early phases of clinical trials (See Table 5.2).

Immune Checkpoint Inhibitors With Radiotherapy

Radiotherapy can potentiate or dampen the immune response in different situations. In rare cases, local radiotherapy can cause shrinkage of tumor in distant nonirradiated sites, the so-called "abscopal effect."[96] This effect is presumed to be secondary to tumor-antigen release owing to local irradiation, which promotes tumor-specific targeting by adaptive immune system. This has led scientists to combine radiation

TABLE 5.2
Selected Ongoing Phase II and III Clinical Trials of Checkpoint Inhibitors for Squamous Cell Carcinoma of the Head and Neck

Agent	Trial	Phase	Setting	Treatment Arm(s)
Pembrolizumab	NCT02252042	III	R/M (second line)	Versus standard treatment
Pembrolizumab	NCT02358031	III	R/M (Frontline)	With and without EXTREME regimen
Pembrolizumab	NCT02841748	II	Adjuvant	Versus placebo
Pembrolizumab	NCT02641093	II	Adjuvant	With cisplatin and RT
Pembrolizumab	NCT02609503	II	LA (Frontline)	With RT for cisplatin-ineligible patients
Pembrolizumab	NCT02777385 NCT02759575 NCT03040999	II/III	LA (Frontline)	With cisplatin and RT for LA disease
Pembrolizumab	NCT03057613	II	Adjuvant	With postoperative RT
Pembrolizumab	NCT03082534	II	R/M (second line)	With cetuximab
Pembrolizumab	NCT02454179	II	R/M (second line)	With acalabrutinib (BTK inhibitor)
Pembrolizumab	NCT02538510	I/II	R/M[a]	With vorinostat (HDAC inhibitor)
Nivolumab	NCT02823574	II	R/M (Frontline)	With and without ipilimumab
Nivolumab	NCT02741570	III	R/M (Frontline)	With ipilimumab versus EXTREME regimen
Nivolumab	NCT03003637	II	Neoadjuvant	With ipilimumab
Nivolumab	NCT02684253	II	Metastatic	With and without RT
Nivolumab	NCT02335918	II	R/M (second line)	With varlilumab (anti-CD27)
Durvalumab	NCT02207530 NCT01693562	II	R/M (second line)	Monotherapy
Durvalumab	NCT02319044	II	R/M (second line)	With/without tremelimumab versus tremelimumab alone
Durvalumab	NCT03019003	Ib/II	R/M (second line)	In combination with azacitidine and tremelimumab
Durvalumab	NCT03212469	II	R/M (second line)	With tremelimumab and RT
Durvalumab	NCT02551159	III	R/M (Frontline)	With/without tremelimumab versus EXTREME regimen
Durvalumab	NCT03174275	II	Neoadjuvant/adjuvant	With carboplatin and nab-paclitaxel
Durvalumab	NCT02499328	I/II	R/M (second line)	With STAT3 inhibitor (AZD9150) and CXCR2 antagonist (AZD5069)

BTK, Bruton tyrosine kinase; *CXCR*, CXC chemokine receptor; *EXTREME* consists of cetuximab, platinum, and 5-fluorouracil; *HDAC*, histone deacetylase enzyme; *LA*, locally advanced; *R/M*, recurrent/metastatic; *RT*, radiation therapy; *STAT*, signal transducer and activator of transcription.
[a] The trial also included patients with salivary glands cancer and nasopharyngeal carcinoma.

with immunotherapy to further boost the antitumor immune response. In mouse models, radiotherapy has been shown to increase PD-L1 expression on tumor cells, and an abscopal effect was observed when PD-L1 antibody was given with radiotherapy.[97,98] In a small retrospective study of 21 patients with metastatic melanoma with progression on ipilimumab therapy, 11 (52%) patients had an abscopal effect after radiation treatment.[99]

Furthermore, the abscopal effect was only observed in patients who had a local response to radiation. These results have led to clinical trials combining checkpoint inhibitors with radiation in the upfront setting. There is an ongoing phase II trial evaluating the use of pembrolizumab for residual disease after definitive therapy with chemoradiation before surgery (NCT02892201). A randomized phase III trial is analyzing the use of chemoradiation with and without pembrolizumab for locally advanced SCCHN (NCT03040999).

Localized/Locoregional Advanced Disease

Head and neck cancer that is localized (stage I/II) is treated with surgical resection or definitive radiotherapy. Locally advanced disease (stage III/IV) is usually treated with a combination of surgery, radiation, or chemotherapy depending on the site of origin and extent of regional spread.[100,101] Checkpoint inhibitors do not have a defined role yet in the adjuvant or neoadjuvant setting, although multiple clinical trials are underway to explore their efficacy in this capacity either alone or combined with chemoradiation (See Table 5.2 for a list of ongoing trials).

NASOPHARYNGEAL CARCINOMA

Nasopharyngeal carcinoma arises from the lining of nasopharynx. It is uncommon in the Unites States but is endemic in southern China, Southeast Asia, North Africa, and the Arctic. It is usually radiosensitive, and localized disease is most often treated with radiotherapy alone or chemoradiation depending on the stage and extent of tumor.[102,103] Some patients with local recurrence can be treated with surgical resection or reirradiation.[104,105] However, most patients with recurrent or metastatic disease are not eligible for curative techniques. Nasopharyngeal carcinoma not amenable to local-regional therapy is treated with platinum-based chemotherapy combinations. Most recent data from a phase III trial suggest that combination of cisplatin and gemcitabine results in improvement in OS when compared with other chemotherapy combinations.[106] Targeted treatment against EGFR and vascular endothelial growth factor has also shown promise in phase II trials.[107−110]

Preclinical studies on nasopharyngeal carcinomas show a high level of PD-L1 expression on tumor cells and PD-1 expression on tumor-infiltrating lymphocytes.

The PD-L1 expression is also found to be predictive of worse prognosis.[111,112] These observations led to clinical trials of immune checkpoint inhibitors in recurrent and metastatic nasopharyngeal carcinoma. Pembrolizumab has been evaluated in a phase Ib study in which it produced a response in 78% of heavily pretreated patients with metastatic PD-L1−positive nasopharyngeal carcinoma.[113] There are ongoing phase II trials evaluating the use of pembrolizumab (NCT02611960) and nivolumab (NCT02339558) for treatment of metastatic nasopharyngeal carcinoma.

SALIVARY GLANDS CANCER

Salivary gland tumors are rare and can arise from the major salivary glands (parotid, submandibular, and sublingual) or the minor salivary glands scattered throughout the oral cavity, paranasal sinuses, pharynx, and larynx. Most common malignant pathologic types are adenoid cystic carcinoma and mucoepidermoid carcinoma. When possible, surgical resection is the treatment of choice for localized salivary glands malignancies.[114] For localized tumors not feasible for surgical resection, radiotherapy is frequently used. Owing to rarity of these tumors, there is a lack of published data regarding the optimal chemotherapy regimen for treatment of metastatic disease. Most commonly used regimen combines cisplatin with cyclophosphamide and doxorubicin (CAP regimen).[115] The response rates are between 40% and 50% based on retrospective analyses. A phase II trial (NCT03132038) is evaluating the use of nivolumab for recurrent or metastatic salivary gland carcinoma. There are two other phase II trials, which are testing the combination of ipilimumab and nivolumab in this setting. (NCT03146650 and NCT03172624). See Table 5.3 for a list of ongoing clinical trials for salivary glands cancer involving immune checkpoint inhibitors.

TABLE 5.3
Ongoing Clinical Trials of Checkpoint Inhibitors for Non−Squamous Cell Head and Neck Malignancies

Malignancy	Trial	Phase	Setting	Treatment Arm(s)
Salivary gland cancer	NCT02538510	II	R/M	Pembrolizumab with vorinostat (HDAC inhibitor)
Salivary gland cancer	NCT03132038	II	R/M (second line)	Nivolumab
Salivary gland cancer	NCT03172624 NCT03146650	II	R/M (second line)	Nivolumab with ipilimumab
Nasopharyngeal Carcinoma	NCT02611960	II	R/M (second line)	Pembrolizumab versus chemotherapy
Nasopharyngeal Carcinoma	NCT02339558	II	R/M (second line)	Nivolumab with ipilimumab

HDAC, histone deacetylase enzyme; *R/M*, recurrent/metastatic.

CONCLUSION

Immune checkpoint inhibitors have shown promising results in the treatment of head and neck cancers and are established treatment options for recurrent or metastatic SCCHN. Currently pembrolizumab (keytruda) and nivolumab (opdivo) are the only two checkpoint inhibitors with FDA approval for these patients. Ongoing trials will better define their role in the frontline, adjuvant, and neoadjuvant settings. Results of clinical trials testing combination therapies involving checkpoint inhibitors are eagerly awaited. So far, immune checkpoint inhibitors have demonstrated durable responses, but still many people fail to get a response. PD-L1 expression is found to be correlated to response to anti−PD-1 inhibitors in animal models and cancers such as NSCLC.[116,117] However, this association is not significant among other cancers including head and neck cancers. This could be secondary to fluctuations in expression on tumor cells and lack of standardization among various available laboratory assays.[118] Seiwert and colleagues performed various multigene expression signatures on tissue samples from patients in KEYNOTE-012 trial and found that interferon-γ signature, indicating an inflamed phenotype, was a strong predictor of clinical benefit from anti−PD-1 treatment.[119] Recently, in a phase II trial, high microsatellite instability (MSI-high) among different types of cancer, especially metastatic colorectal cancer, was found to be highly predictive of response to checkpoint inhibitors.[120] This has led FDA to grant approval to pembrolizumab for treatment of metastatic disease across all solid cancers with MSI-high that have progressed following prior treatment. However, only about 1% of head and neck cancers express MSI-high.[121] Thus, there is a need to identify further biomarkers in head and neck cancers, which can help in proper patient selection that are likely to get a response from immunotherapy.

REFERENCES

1. Siegel R, Miller K, Jemal A. Cancer statistics. *CA Cancer J Clin.* 2018;68:7−30.
2. Global Burden of Disease Cancer Collaboration, Fitzmaurice C, Allen C, et al. Global, regional, and national cancer incidence, mortality, years of life lost, years lived with disability, and disability-adjusted life-years for 32 cancer groups, 1990 to 2015: a systematic analysis for the global burden of disease study. *JAMA Oncol.* 2017;3:524−548.
3. Sankaranarayanan R, Masuyer E, Swaminathan R, Ferlay J, Whelan S. Head and neck cancer: a global perspective on epidemiology and prognosis. *Anticancer Res.* 1998;18: 4779−4786.
4. Andre K, Schraub S, Mercier M, Bontemps P. Role of alcohol and tobacco in the aetiology of head and neck cancer: a case-control study in the Doubs region of France. *Eur J Cancer B Oral Oncol.* 1995;31B:301−309.
5. Lewin F, Norell SE, Johansson H, et al. Smoking tobacco, oral snuff, and alcohol in the etiology of squamous cell carcinoma of the head and neck: a population-based case-referent study in Sweden. *Cancer.* 1998;82:1367−1375.
6. Blot WJ, McLaughlin JK, Winn DM, et al. Smoking and drinking in relation to oral and pharyngeal cancer. *Cancer Res.* 1988;48:3282−3287.
7. Wyss A, Hashibe M, Chuang SC, et al. Cigarette, cigar, and pipe smoking and the risk of head and neck cancers: pooled analysis in the international head and neck cancer epidemiology consortium. *Am J Epidemiol.* 2013;178: 679−690.
8. Murata M, Takayama K, Choi BC, Pak AW. A nested case-control study on alcohol drinking, tobacco smoking, and cancer. *Cancer Detect Prev.* 1996;20:557−565.
9. Spitz MR. Epidemiology and risk factors for head and neck cancer. *Semin Oncol.* 1994;21:281−288.
10. Guha N, Warnakulasuriya S, Vlaanderen J, Straif K. Betel quid chewing and the risk of oral and oropharyngeal cancers: a meta-analysis with implications for cancer control. *Int J Cancer.* 2014;135:1433−1443.
11. Vaughan TL, Stewart PA, Davis S, Thomas DB. Work in dry cleaning and the incidence of cancer of the oral cavity, larynx, and oesophagus. *Occup Environ Med.* 1997;54: 692−695.
12. Becher H, Ramroth H, Ahrens W, Risch A, Schmezer P, Dietz A. Occupation, exposure to polycyclic aromatic hydrocarbons and laryngeal cancer risk. *Int J Cancer.* 2005;116:451−457.
13. Dietz A, Ramroth H, Urban T, Ahrens W, Becher H. Exposure to cement dust, related occupational groups and laryngeal cancer risk: results of a population based case-control study. *Int J Cancer.* 2004;108:907−911.
14. van der Laan BF, Baris G, Gregor RT, Hilgers FJ, Balm AJ. Radiation-induced tumours of the head and neck. *J Laryngol Otol.* 1995;109:346−349.
15. Walboomers JM, Jacobs MV, Manos MM, et al. Human papillomavirus is a necessary cause of invasive cervical cancer worldwide. *J Pathol.* 1999;189:12−19.
16. Carey T, Prince M. Molecular biology of head and neck cancers. In: DeVita V, Lawrence T, Rosenberg S, eds. *Devita, Hellman, and Rosenberg's Cancer: Principles & Practice of Oncology.* 10th ed. Philadelphia: Wolters Kluwer; 2015:416−417.
17. D'Souza G, Kreimer AR, Viscidi R, et al. Case-control study of human papillomavirus and oropharyngeal cancer. *N Engl J Med.* 2007;356:1944−1956.
18. Fakhry C, Gillison ML. Clinical implications of human papillomavirus in head and neck cancers. *J Clin Oncol.* 2006;24:2606−2611.
19. Salazar CR, Anayannis N, Smith RV, et al. Combined P16 and human papillomavirus testing predicts head and neck cancer survival. *Int J Cancer.* 2014;135:2404−2412.

20. Raghupathy R, Hui EP, Chan AT. Epstein-Barr virus as a paradigm in nasopharyngeal cancer: from lab to clinic. *Am Soc Clin Oncol Educ Book.* 2014:149–153.

21. Mahale P, Sturgis EM, Tweardy DJ, Ariza-Heredia EJ, Torres HA. Association between hepatitis C virus and head and neck cancers. *J Natl Cancer Inst.* 2016;108: djw035.

22. Rabinovics N, Mizrachi A, Hadar T, et al. Cancer of the head and neck region in solid organ transplant recipients. *Head Neck.* 2014;36:181–186.

23. Lacko M, Braakhuis BJ, Sturgis EM, et al. Genetic susceptibility to head and neck squamous cell carcinoma. *Int J Radiat Oncol Biol Phys.* 2014;89:38–48.

24. Sun S, Pollock PM, Liu L, et al. CDKN2A mutation in a non-FAMMM kindred with cancers at multiple sites results in a functionally abnormal protein. *Int J Cancer.* 1997;73:531–536.

25. Frebourg T, Barbier N, Yan YX, et al. Germ-line p53 mutations in 15 families with li-fraumeni syndrome. *Am J Hum Genet.* 1995;56:608–615.

26. Rosenberg PS, Alter BP, Ebell W. Cancer risks in fanconi anemia: findings from the German fanconi anemia registry. *Haematologica.* 2008;93:511–517.

27. Kutler DI, Singh B, Satagopan J, et al. A 20-year perspective on the international fanconi anemia registry (IFAR). *Blood.* 2003;101:1249–1256.

28. Birkeland AC, Auerbach AD, Sanborn E, et al. Postoperative clinical radiosensitivity in patients with fanconi anemia and head and neck squamous cell carcinoma. *Arch Otolaryngol Head Neck Surg.* 2011;137:930–934.

29. Druesne-Pecollo N, Tehard B, Mallet Y, et al. Alcohol and genetic polymorphisms: effect on risk of alcohol-related cancer. *Lancet Oncol.* 2009;10:173–180.

30. Rubin Grandis J, Melhem MF, Gooding WE, et al. Levels of TGF-alpha and EGFR protein in head and neck squamous cell carcinoma and patient survival. *J Natl Cancer Inst.* 1998;90:824–832.

31. Almadori G, Cadoni G, Galli J, et al. Epidermal growth factor receptor expression in primary laryngeal cancer: an independent prognostic factor of neck node relapse. *Int J Cancer.* 1999;84:188–191.

32. Bonner JA, Harari PM, Giralt J, et al. Radiotherapy plus cetuximab for locoregionally advanced head and neck cancer: 5-year survival data from a phase 3 randomised trial, and relation between cetuximab-induced rash and survival. *Lancet Oncol.* 2010;11:21–28.

33. van der Riet P, Nawroz H, Hruban RH, et al. Frequent loss of chromosome 9p21-22 early in head and neck cancer progression. *Cancer Res.* 1994;54:1156–1158.

34. Merlo A, Herman JG, Mao L, et al. 5′ CpG island methylation is associated with transcriptional silencing of the tumour suppressor p16/CDKN2/MTS1 in human cancers. *Nat Med.* 1995;1:686–692.

35. Herman JG, Merlo A, Mao L, et al. Inactivation of the CDKN2/p16/MTS1 gene is frequently associated with aberrant DNA methylation in all common human cancers. *Cancer Res.* 1995;55:4525–4530.

36. Taylor D, Koch WM, Zahurak M, Shah K, Sidransky D, Westra WH. Immunohistochemical detection of p53 protein accumulation in head and neck cancer: correlation with p53 gene alterations. *Hum Pathol.* 1999;30: 1221–1225.

37. Bradford CR, Zhu S, Wolf GT, et al. Overexpression of p53 predicts organ preservation using induction chemotherapy and radiation in patients with advanced laryngeal cancer. department of veterans affairs laryngeal cancer study group. *Otolaryngol Head Neck Surg.* 1995;113:408–412.

38. Kumar B, Cordell KG, D'Silva N, et al. Expression of p53 and bcl-xL as predictive markers for larynx preservation in advanced laryngeal cancer. *Arch Otolaryngol Head Neck Surg.* 2008;134:363–369.

39. Millon R, Muller D, Schultz I, et al. Loss of MDM2 expression in human head and neck squamous cell carcinomas and clinical significance. *Oral Oncol.* 2001;37:620–631.

40. Scheffner M, Werness BA, Huibregtse JM, Levine AJ, Howley PM. The E6 oncoprotein encoded by human papillomavirus types 16 and 18 promotes the degradation of p53. *Cell.* 1990;63:1129–1136.

41. Brown CJ, Lain S, Verma CS, Fersht AR, Lane DP. Awakening guardian angels: drugging the p53 pathway. *Nat Rev Cancer.* 2009;9:862–873.

42. Shao X, Tandon R, Samara G, et al. Mutational analysis of the PTEN gene in head and neck squamous cell carcinoma. *Int J Cancer.* 1998;77:684–688.

43. Anderson JA, Irish JC, Ngan BY. Prevalence of RAS oncogene mutation in head and neck carcinomas. *J Otolaryngol.* 1992; 21:321–326.

44. Kuss I, Hathaway B, Ferris RL, Gooding W, Whiteside TL. Decreased absolute counts of T lymphocyte subsets and their relation to disease in squamous cell carcinoma of the head and neck. *Clin Cancer Res.* 2004;10:3755–3762.

45. Dasgupta S, Bhattacharya-Chatterjee M, O'Malley BW, Chatterjee SK. Inhibition of NK cell activity through TGF-beta 1 by down-regulation of NKG2D in a murine model of head and neck cancer. *J Immunol.* 2005;175: 5541–5550.

46. Bauernhofer T, Kuss I, Henderson B, Baum AS, Whiteside TL. Preferential apoptosis of CD56dim natural killer cell subset in patients with cancer. *Eur J Immunol.* 2003;33:119–124.

47. Leibowitz MS, Srivastava RM, Andrade Filho PA, et al. SHP2 is overexpressed and inhibits pSTAT1-mediated APM component expression, T-cell attracting chemokine secretion, and CTL recognition in head and neck cancer cells. *Clin Cancer Res.* 2013;19:798–808.

48. Leibowitz MS, Andrade Filho PA, Ferrone S, Ferris RL. Deficiency of activated STAT1 in head and neck cancer cells mediates TAP1-dependent escape from cytotoxic T lymphocytes. *Cancer Immunol Immunother.* 2011; 60:525–535.

49. Cho YA, Yoon HJ, Lee JI, Hong SP, Hong SD. Relationship between the expressions of PD-L1 and tumor-infiltrating lymphocytes in oral squamous cell carcinoma. *Oral Oncol.* 2011;47:1148–1153.

50. Hsu MC, Hsiao JR, Chang KC, et al. Increase of programmed death-1-expressing intratumoral CD8 T cells predicts a poor prognosis for nasopharyngeal carcinoma. *Mod Pathol.* 2010;23:1393−1403.
51. Zhang F, Liu Z, Cui Y, Wang G, Cao P. The clinical significance of the expression of costimulatory molecule PD-L1 in nasopharyngeal carcinoma. *Lin Chung Er Bi Yan Hou Tou Jing Wai Ke Za Zhi.* 2008;22:408−410.
52. Ukpo OC, Thorstad WL, Lewis JS. B7-H1 expression model for immune evasion in human papillomavirus-related oropharyngeal squamous cell carcinoma. *Head Neck Pathol.* 2013;7:113−121.
53. Strome SE, Dong H, Tamura H, et al. B7-H1 blockade augments adoptive T-cell immunotherapy for squamous cell carcinoma. *Cancer Res.* 2003;63:6501−6505.
54. Lyford-Pike S, Peng S, Young GD, et al. Evidence for a role of the PD-1:PD-L1 pathway in immune resistance of HPV-associated head and neck squamous cell carcinoma. *Cancer Res.* 2013;73:1733−1741.
55. Badoual C, Hans S, Merillon N, et al. PD-1-expressing tumor-infiltrating T cells are a favorable prognostic biomarker in HPV-associated head and neck cancer. *Cancer Res.* 2013;73:128−138.
56. Wing K, Onishi Y, Prieto-Martin P, et al. CTLA-4 control over Foxp3+ regulatory T cell function. *Science.* 2008;322:271−275.
57. Jie HB, Gildener-Leapman N, Li J, et al. Intratumoral regulatory T cells upregulate immunosuppressive molecules in head and neck cancer patients. *Br J Cancer.* 2013;109:2629−2635.
58. Ralainirina N, Poli A, Michel T, et al. Control of NK cell functions by CD4+CD25+ regulatory T cells. *J Leukoc Biol.* 2007;81:144−153.
59. Ghiringhelli F, Menard C, Terme M, et al. CD4+CD25+ regulatory T cells inhibit natural killer cell functions in a transforming growth factor-beta-dependent manner. *J Exp Med.* 2005;202:1075−1085.
60. Gao X, Zhu Y, Li G, et al. TIM-3 expression characterizes regulatory T cells in tumor tissues and is associated with lung cancer progression. *PLoS One.* 2012;7:e30676.
61. Katayama A, Takahara M, Kishibe K, et al. Expression of B7-H3 in hypopharyngeal squamous cell carcinoma as a predictive indicator for tumor metastasis and prognosis. *Int J Oncol.* 2011;38:1219−1226.
62. Cianchetti M, Mancuso AA, Amdur RJ, et al. Diagnostic evaluation of squamous cell carcinoma metastatic to cervical lymph nodes from an unknown head and neck primary site. *Laryngoscope.* 2009;119:2348−2354.
63. Colevas AD. Chemotherapy options for patients with metastatic or recurrent squamous cell carcinoma of the head and neck. *J Clin Oncol.* 2006;24:2644−2652.
64. Clavel M, Vermorken JB, Cognetti F, et al. Randomized comparison of cisplatin, methotrexate, bleomycin and vincristine (CABO) versus cisplatin and 5-fluorouracil (CF) versus cisplatin (C) in recurrent or metastatic squamous cell carcinoma of the head and neck. A phase III study of the EORTC head and neck cancer cooperative group. *Ann Oncol.* 1994;5:521−526.
65. Jacobs C, Lyman G, Velez-Garcia E, et al. A phase III randomized study comparing cisplatin and fluorouracil as single agents and in combination for advanced squamous cell carcinoma of the head and neck. *J Clin Oncol.* 1992;10:257−263.
66. Gibson MK, Li Y, Murphy B, et al. Randomized phase III evaluation of cisplatin plus fluorouracil versus cisplatin plus paclitaxel in advanced head and neck cancer (E1395): an intergroup trial of the eastern cooperative oncology group. *J Clin Oncol.* 2005;23:3562−3567.
67. Urba S, van Herpen CM, Sahoo TP, et al. Pemetrexed in combination with cisplatin versus cisplatin monotherapy in patients with recurrent or metastatic head and neck cancer: final results of a randomized, double-blind, placebo-controlled, phase 3 study. *Cancer.* 2012;118:4694−4705.
68. Vermorken JB, Mesia R, Rivera F, et al. Platinum-based chemotherapy plus cetuximab in head and neck cancer. *N Engl J Med.* 2008;359:1116−1127.
69. Vermorken JB, Stohlmacher-Williams J, Davidenko I, et al. Cisplatin and fluorouracil with or without panitumumab in patients with recurrent or metastatic squamous-cell carcinoma of the head and neck (SPECTRUM): an open-label phase 3 randomised trial. *Lancet Oncol.* 2013;14:697−710.
70. Brown JA, Dorfman DM, Ma FR, et al. Blockade of programmed death-1 ligands on dendritic cells enhances T cell activation and cytokine production. *J Immunol.* 2003;170:1257−1266.
71. Iwai Y, Ishida M, Tanaka Y, Okazaki T, Honjo T, Minato N. Involvement of PD-L1 on tumor cells in the escape from host immune system and tumor immunotherapy by PD-L1 blockade. *Proc Natl Acad Sci USA.* 2002;99:12293−12297.
72. O'Day SJ, Hamid O, Urba WJ. Targeting cytotoxic T-lymphocyte antigen-4 (CTLA-4): a novel strategy for the treatment of melanoma and other malignancies. *Cancer.* 2007;110:2614−2627.
73. Seiwert TY, Burtness B, Mehra R, et al. Safety and clinical activity of pembrolizumab for treatment of recurrent or metastatic squamous cell carcinoma of the head and neck (KEYNOTE-012): an open-label, multicentre, phase 1b trial. *Lancet Oncol.* 2016;17:956−965.
74. Chow LQ, Haddad R, Gupta S, et al. Antitumor activity of pembrolizumab in biomarker-unselected patients with recurrent and/or metastatic head and neck squamous cell carcinoma: results from the phase ib KEYNOTE-012 expansion cohort. *J Clin Oncol.* 2016;34:3838−3845.
75. Bauml J, Seiwert TY, Pfister DG, et al. Pembrolizumab for platinum- and cetuximab-refractory head and neck cancer: results from a single-arm, phase II study. *J Clin Oncol.* 2017;35:1542−1549.
76. Borghaei H, Paz-Ares L, Horn L, et al. Nivolumab versus docetaxel in advanced nonsquamous non-small-cell lung cancer. *N Engl J Med.* 2015;373:1627−1639.
77. Brahmer J, Reckamp KL, Baas P, et al. Nivolumab versus docetaxel in advanced squamous-cell non-small-cell lung cancer. *N Engl J Med.* 2015;373:123−135.

78. Ferris RL, Blumenschein G, Fayette J, et al. Nivolumab for recurrent squamous-cell carcinoma of the head and neck. *N Engl J Med.* 2016;375:1856–1867.
79. Massard C, Gordon MS, Sharma S, et al. Safety and efficacy of durvalumab (MEDI4736), an anti-programmed cell death ligand-1 immune checkpoint inhibitor, in patients with advanced urothelial bladder cancer. *J Clin Oncol.* 2016;34:3119–3125.
80. Fehrenbacher L, Spira A, Ballinger M, et al. Atezolizumab versus docetaxel for patients with previously treated non-small-cell lung cancer (POPLAR): a multicentre, open-label, phase 2 randomised controlled trial. *Lancet.* 2016;387:1837–1846.
81. Rosenberg JE, Hoffman-Censits J, Powles T, et al. Atezolizumab in patients with locally advanced and metastatic urothelial carcinoma who have progressed following treatment with platinum-based chemotherapy: a single-arm, multicentre, phase 2 trial. *Lancet.* 2016;387:1909–1920.
82. Kaufman HL, Russell J, Hamid O, et al. Avelumab in patients with chemotherapy-refractory metastatic merkel cell carcinoma: a multicentre, single-group, open-label, phase 2 trial. *Lancet Oncol.* 2016;17:1374–1385.
83. Segal NH, Ou SI, Balmanoukian AS, et al. Safety and efficacy of MEDI4736, an anti-PD-L1 antibody, in patients from a squamous cell carcinoma of the head and neck (SCCHN) expansion cohort. *J Clin Oncol.* 2015;33:3011.
84. Segal NH, Hamid O, Hwu W, et al. 1058pda phase i multiarm dose-expansion study of the anti-programmed cell death-ligand-1 (pd-l1) antibody medi4736: preliminary data. *Ann Oncol.* 2014;25:iv365.
85. Chen G, Emens LA. Chemoimmunotherapy: reengineering tumor immunity. *Cancer Immunol Immunother.* 2013;62:203–216.
86. Zhang P, Ma Y, Lv C, et al. Upregulation of programmed cell death ligand 1 promotes resistance response in non-small-cell lung cancer patients treated with neo-adjuvant chemotherapy. *Cancer Sci.* 2016;107:1563–1571.
87. Peng J, Hamanishi J, Matsumura N, et al. Chemotherapy induces programmed cell death-ligand 1 overexpression via the nuclear factor-kappaB to foster an immunosuppressive tumor microenvironment in ovarian cancer. *Cancer Res.* 2015;75:5034–5045.
88. Langer CJ, Gadgeel SM, Borghaei H, et al. Carboplatin and pemetrexed with or without pembrolizumab for advanced, non-squamous non-small-cell lung cancer: a randomised, phase 2 cohort of the open-label KEYNOTE-021 study. *Lancet Oncol.* 2016;17:1497–1508.
89. Das R, Verma R, Sznol M, et al. Combination therapy with anti-CTLA-4 and anti-PD-1 leads to distinct immunologic changes in vivo. *J Immunol.* 2015;194:950–959.
90. Swanson MS, Sinha UK. Rationale for combined blockade of PD-1 and CTLA-4 in advanced head and neck squamous cell cancer-review of current data. *Oral Oncol.* 2015;51:12–15.
91. Larkin J, Chiarion-Sileni V, Gonzalez R, et al. Combined nivolumab and ipilimumab or monotherapy in untreated melanoma. *N Engl J Med.* 2015;373:23–34.
92. Antonia SJ, Lopez-Martin JA, Bendell J, et al. Nivolumab alone and nivolumab plus ipilimumab in recurrent small-cell lung cancer (CheckMate 032): a multicentre, open-label, phase 1/2 trial. *Lancet Oncol.* 2016;17:883–895.
93. Correale P, Botta C, Cusi MG, et al. Cetuximab +/- chemotherapy enhances dendritic cell-mediated phagocytosis of colon cancer cells and ignites a highly efficient colon cancer antigen-specific cytotoxic T-cell response in vitro. *Int J Cancer.* 2012;130:1577–1589.
94. Srivastava RM, Lee SC, Andrade Filho PA, et al. Cetuximab-activated natural killer and dendritic cells collaborate to trigger tumor antigen-specific T-cell immunity in head and neck cancer patients. *Clin Cancer Res.* 2013;19:1858–1872.
95. Jie HB, Schuler PJ, Lee SC, et al. CTLA-4(+) regulatory T cells increased in cetuximab-treated head and neck cancer patients suppress NK cell cytotoxicity and correlate with poor prognosis. *Cancer Res.* 2015;75:2200–2210.
96. Reynders K, Illidge T, Siva S, Chang JY, De Ruysscher D. The abscopal effect of local radiotherapy: using immunotherapy to make a rare event clinically relevant. *Cancer Treat Rev.* 2015;41:503–510.
97. Tang C, Wang X, Soh H, et al. Combining radiation and immunotherapy: a new systemic therapy for solid tumors? *Cancer Immunol Res.* 2014;2:831–838.
98. Deng L, Liang H, Burnette B, et al. Irradiation and anti-PD-L1 treatment synergistically promote antitumor immunity in mice. *J Clin Invest.* 2014;124:687–695.
99. Grimaldi AM, Simeone E, Giannarelli D, et al. Abscopal effects of radiotherapy on advanced melanoma patients who progressed after ipilimumab immunotherapy. *Oncoimmunology.* 2014;3:e28780.
100. Pignon JP, le Maitre A, Maillard E, Bourhis J, MACH-NC Collaborative Group. Meta-analysis of chemotherapy in head and neck cancer (MACH-NC): an update on 93 randomised trials and 17,346 patients. *Radiother Oncol.* 2009;92:4–14.
101. Furness S, Glenny AM, Worthington HV, et al. Interventions for the treatment of oral cavity and oropharyngeal cancer: chemotherapy. *Cochrane Database Syst Rev.* 2011;4:CD006386.
102. Al-Sarraf M, LeBlanc M, Giri PG, et al. Chemoradiotherapy versus radiotherapy in patients with advanced nasopharyngeal cancer: phase III randomized intergroup study 0099. *J Clin Oncol.* 1998;16:1310–1317.
103. Peng G, Wang T, Yang KY, et al. A prospective, randomized study comparing outcomes and toxicities of intensity-modulated radiotherapy vs. conventional two-dimensional radiotherapy for the treatment of nasopharyngeal carcinoma. *Radiother Oncol.* 2012;104:286–293.
104. Chan JY. Surgical salvage of recurrent nasopharyngeal carcinoma. *Curr Oncol Rep.* 2015;17:433.
105. Teo PM, Kwan WH, Chan AT, Lee WY, King WW, Mok CO. How successful is high-dose (> or = 60 gy) reirradiation using mainly external beams in salvaging local failures of nasopharyngeal carcinoma? *Int J Radiat Oncol Biol Phys.* 1998;40:897–913.

106. Zhang L, Huang Y, Hong S, et al. Gemcitabine plus cisplatin versus fluorouracil plus cisplatin in recurrent or metastatic nasopharyngeal carcinoma: a multicentre, randomised, open-label, phase 3 trial. *Lancet*. 2016;388: 1883—1892.
107. Xue C, Huang Y, Huang PY, et al. Phase II study of sorafenib in combination with cisplatin and 5-fluorouracil to treat recurrent or metastatic nasopharyngeal carcinoma. *Ann Oncol*. 2013;24:1055—1061.
108. Lim WT, Ng QS, Ivy P, et al. A phase II study of pazopanib in Asian patients with recurrent/metastatic nasopharyngeal carcinoma. *Clin Cancer Res*. 2011;17:5481—5489.
109. Hui EP, Ma B, Mo F, et al. A phase II study of axitinib in patients with recurrent or metastatic nasopharyngeal carcinoma (NPC). *J Clin Oncol*. 2015;33:6031.
110. Chan AT, Hsu MM, Goh BC, et al. Multicenter, phase II study of cetuximab in combination with carboplatin in patients with recurrent or metastatic nasopharyngeal carcinoma. *J Clin Oncol*. 2005;23:3568—3576.
111. Zhang J, Fang W, Qin T, et al. Co-expression of PD-1 and PD-L1 predicts poor outcome in nasopharyngeal carcinoma. *Med Oncol*. 2015;32:86.
112. Fang W, Zhang J, Hong S, et al. EBV-driven LMP1 and IFN-gamma up-regulate PD-L1 in nasopharyngeal carcinoma: implications for oncotargeted therapy. *Oncotarget*. 2014;5:12189—12202.
113. Hsu C, Lee SH, Ejadi C, et al. Antitumor activity and safety of pembrolizumab in patients with PD-L1-positive nasopharyngeal carcinoma: interim results from a phase 1b study. *Ann Oncol*. 2015;26:93—102.
114. Spiro RH. Salivary neoplasms: overview of a 35-year experience with 2,807 patients. *Head Neck Surg*. 1986;8:177—184.
115. Dreyfuss AI, Clark JR, Fallon BG, Posner MR, Norris CM, Miller D. Cyclophosphamide, doxorubicin, and cisplatin combination chemotherapy for advanced carcinomas of salivary gland origin. *Cancer*. 1987;60:2869—2872.
116. Topalian SL, Hodi FS, Brahmer JR, et al. Safety, activity, and immune correlates of anti-PD-1 antibody in cancer. *N Engl J Med*. 2012;366:2443—2454.
117. Garon EB, Rizvi NA, Hui R, et al. Pembrolizumab for the treatment of non-small-cell lung cancer. *N Engl J Med*. 2015;372:2018—2028.
118. Hirsch FR, McElhinny A, Stanforth D, et al. PD-L1 immunohistochemistry assays for lung cancer: results from phase 1 of the blueprint PD-L1 IHC assay comparison project. *J Thorac Oncol*. 2017;12:208—222.
119. Seiwert TY, Burtness B, Weiss J, et al. Inflamed-phenotype gene expression signatures to predict benefit from the anti-PD-1 antibody pembrolizumab in PD-L1+ head and neck cancer patients. *J Clin Oncol*. 2015;33:6017.
120. Le DT, Uram JN, Wang H, et al. PD-1 blockade in tumors with mismatch-repair deficiency. *N Engl J Med*. 2015;372:2509—2520.
121. Glavac D, Volavsek M, Potocnik U, Ravnik-Glavac M, Gale N. Low microsatellite instability and high loss of heterozygosity rates indicate dominant role of the suppressor pathway in squamous cell carcinoma of head and neck and loss of heterozygosity of 11q14.3 correlates with tumor grade. *Cancer Genet Cytogenet*. 2003;146: 27—32.

CHAPTER 6

Urologic Malignancies

MICHAEL R. HARRISON, MD • MEGAN A. MCNAMARA, MD • TIAN ZHANG, MD •
BRANT A. INMAN, MD, MS

KIDNEY CANCER

INTRODUCTION

Renal cell carcinoma (RCC), the most common type of kidney cancer, is heterogeneous in terms of its histologic, molecular, and clinical features. In the United States in 2017, kidney cancer was estimated to be the 6th most common cancer in men and the 10th most common cancer in women, diagnosed in 65,340 new patients, and leading to 14,970 deaths.[1] Although localized RCC can be cured through surgery, advanced or metastatic RCC (mRCC) is usually incurable. Treatment of mRCC requires systemic therapy; however, mRCC is resistant to traditional cytotoxic chemotherapy. Instead, before 2006, cytokine immunotherapies, such as high-dose interleukin-2 (IL-2) and interferon-alpha (IFNα), became standards of care.[2,3] Research on the role of the von Hippel–Lindau tumor suppressor protein in hereditary RCC syndromes led to the discovery of the importance of vascular endothelial growth factor (VEGF) signaling.[4] This understanding of tumor biology, in turn, resulted in approval from the US Food and Drug Administration (FDA) of multiple targeted therapies inhibiting VEGF signaling (such as sorfenib and sunitinib) beginning in the late 2005.[5] Although these targeted therapies were more broadly applicable and generally more effective than cytokines, early enthusiasm for these agents was tempered by the facts that few complete responses (CRs) were seen and virtually all patients developed resistance. The programmed cell death 1 (PD-1) inhibitor nivolumab was approved for patients with mRCC who have received prior antiangiogenic therapy on November 23, 2015.[6] This approval marked the beginning of a new era of research into immune checkpoint inhibitors (ICIs) in mRCC. This chapter will review the current data for currently approved and selected promising ICIs (including combinations) for treatment of RCC.

BACKGROUND: PRIOR IMMUNOTHERAPIES IN RENAL CELL CARCINOMA

Before 2005, when the first targeted therapy was approved for mRCC, two immunotherapies—IFNα and high-dose bolus IL-2—were the standards of care. IL-2 was discovered in the 1970's and 1980's to stimulate T-cell growth and activation.[7] Subsequently, high-dose IL-2 administration was demonstrated to cause durable remissions in animal models.[8] Based on an analysis of seven phase II studies ($n = 255$ patients), IL-2 was approved in 1992 by the FDA based on durable CRs seen in a small number of patients.[2] IL-2 was administered by 15 min IV (intravenous) infusion at 600,000–720,000 IU/kg every 8 h for up to 14 consecutive doses over 5 days. The overall response rate (ORR) was 14% (90% CI: 10%–19%) with a 9% partial response rate ($n = 24$) and 5% CR rate ($n = 12$). The median duration of response was 19.0 months for partial responders and was not reached for complete responders. These data have been confirmed in a retrospective series at the National Cancer Institute (NCI) and one phase III trial.[9,10] Of note, 4% of patients were judged to have died from treatment-related adverse events (AEs). This rate is believed to be lower when administered at experienced centers.[11] However, IL-2 is only an option for young, healthy patients with certain clinical and pathologic features, such as clear cell histology, a good performance status, the absence of CNS or bone metastases, prior nephrectomy, good cardiopulmonary reserve, and good organ function. As of this writing, the role of high-dose IL-2 is not clear with the advent of combination checkpoint immunotherapy.

Although not FDA-approved, the cytokine IFNα became the de facto standard of care worldwide in the 1990s and early 2000s owing to modest benefits, as well as considerably less toxicity than IL-2. ORR with

IFNα is approximately 10%, with a median overall survival (OS) of 11 months.[12] A meta-analysis demonstrated that IFNα is superior to controls with a pooled overall hazard ratio for death of 0.74 (95% confidence interval [CI] 0.63–0.88) and weighted average median improvement in survival of 3.8 months.[3] As a result, regulatory agencies supported IFNα as the comparator arm in several of the phase III clinical trials that lead to approval of first-line targeted therapies (i.e., sunitinib and temsirolimus).[13,14] A meta-analysis found that IFNα probably increases 1-year overall mortality compared with standard targeted therapies with temsirolimus or sunitinib (RR 1.30, 95% CI 1.13–1.51).[15] Finally, IFNα in combination with the monoclonal antibody against VEGF-A, bevacizumab, versus IFNα was evaluated in two phase III clinical trials (CALGB 90206 and AVOREN).[16,17] Progression-free survival and ORR were higher in the combination arm; however, OS was not significantly improved. This combination regimen was not widely adopted owing to the toxicity profile and the lack of a compelling reason to adopt this subcutaneous and IV regimen over an oral monotherapy regimen. There is currently no role for IFNα in the treatment of mRCC.

SINGLE-AGENT IMMUNE CHECKPOINT INHIBITORS

Given the relative success of cytokine immunotherapies, multiple ICIs have been tested in mRCC. Nivolumab is the only single-agent ICI that is, at the time of this writing, FDA-approved.

Ipilimumab

The anti-CTLA-4 monoclonal antibody ipilimumab (Yervoy) was initially tested in two sequential cohorts (loading dose at 3 mg/kg followed by 1 mg/kg or 3 mg/kg for all doses) in a phase II study of 61 patients with mRCC at the NCI.[18] The response rate was 12.5% (CI: 4%–27%) in the highest dose cohort, but 43% had grade 3 or higher immune-mediated toxicities. Overall, autoimmune AEs were associated with response: response rate was 30% in those with an autoimmune AE and 0% in those without one. Owing to the modest response rate with significant toxicity, ipilimumab was not further developed as single-agent therapy for mRCC.

Nivolumab

This section summarizes the data for the anti-PD-1 monoclonal antibody nivolumab (Opdivo), which was approved on November 23, 2015, for patients with advanced RCC who have received prior antiangiogenic therapy. The phase I study of nivolumab (BMS-936559) was a dose-escalation study from 0.3 mg/kg to 10 mg kg IV every 2 weeks in selected cancers, including 17 patients with RCC, all of whom were treated at the 10 mg/kg dose.[19] The ORR was 12% (2/17) with durations of response of 17 and 4 months. Notably, 41% (7/17) had stable disease for $\geq$24 weeks.

Given these promising results, a randomized phase II dose-ranging study of nivolumab was conducted in patients with advanced clear cell RCC who were previously treated with at least one antiangiogenic agent.[20] One hundred sixty-eight patients were randomized 1:1:1 to receive 0.3 mg/kg, 2 mg/kg, or 10 mg/kg. As measured by progression-free survival (PFS), no dose response was observed: median PFS was 2.7, 4.0, and 4.2 months, respectively ($P = .9$). ORR was 20%, 22%, and 20%. Median time to response was 2.8–3.0 months. Median durations of response were not reached in the first two cohorts and 22.3 months in the 10 mg/kg cohort. Nivolumab was well tolerated; fatigue was the most common AE, and 11% had grade 3 or 4 AEs. A dose of 3 mg/kg was chosen for the phase III study, based on this dose-ranging study as well as other studies in various solid tumors.

In the phase III CheckMate 025 trial, 821 patients with advanced clear cell RCC previously treated with one or two antiangiogenic regimens were randomized 1:1 to receive nivolumab 3 mg/kg IV every 2 weeks or everolimus (a standard of care in this setting at the time) at the FDA-approved dose of 10 mg daily.[6] The primary endpoint of median OS was significantly improved with nivolumab compared with everolimus: 25.0 versus 19.6 months (HR 0.72, $P = .002$). ORR was also better with nivolumab: 25% versus 5% ($P < .001$). However, median PFS was not significantly different: 4.6 versus 4.4 months (HR 0.88, $P = .11$). Nivolumab was well tolerated with more everolimus-treated patients experiencing treatment-related AEs: 19 versus 37%. The most common treatment-related AEs among patients who received nivolumab were fatigue (33%), nausea (14%), and pruritis (14%). Health-related quality of life (QOL) was also improved with nivolumab.[21] Interestingly, benefit for nivolumab was observed regardless of PD-L1 (programmed death-ligand 1) expression (so PD-L1 expression was not predictive); however, PD-L1 positivity was prognostic for poorer survival. In terms of QOL measured by the FKSI-DRS questionnaire, the mean change from baseline in the nivolumab group increased over time and differed significantly from the everolimus group (corresponding to better QOL) at each assessment through week 76 ($P < .05$). Nivolumab was rapidly adopted into the treatment algorithm for mRCC patients after failure of angiogenesis inhibitors.

COMBINATION OR ICI-VEGFI

Ipilimumab Plus Nivolumab

The efficacy of combining CTLA-4 with PD-1 blockade in mRCC was suggested by preclinical work[22] and a large clinical trial in malignant melanoma[23] (which, like mRCC, responds to cytokine immunotherapy). The phase I CheckMate 016 evaluated the safety and efficacy of combinations of nivolumab and ipilimumab at either 1 mg/kg or 3 mg/kg of both drugs.[24] The combination was given as induction every 3 weeks for four doses followed by maintenance single-agent nivolumab every 2 weeks. The nivolumab 3 mg/kg plus ipilimumab 3 mg/kg (N3I3) arm ($n = 6$) had five patients censored for dose-limiting toxicities or other reasons, and the remaining one patient withdrew consent. Forty-seven patients were enrolled on the nivolumab 3 mg/kg plus ipilimumab 1 mg/kg (N3I1) and nivolumab 1 mg/kg plus ipilimumab 3 mg/kg (N1I3) arms. Treatment-naïve patients represented 53% and 47% of patients in the N3I1 and N1I3 arms, respectively. Of pretreated patients, most had had only one prior line of systemic therapy. Grade 3 or 4 treatment-related AEs were observed in 38% and 62% of the N3I1 and N1I3 arms, respectively. With median follow up of 22.3 months, the confirmed ORR was 40% in both arms. Median OS was not reached (95% CI: 26.7-not reached) in the N3I1 arm and 32.6 months (95% CI: 26.0-not reached) in the N1I3 arm. Median PFS was 7.7 months. Responses were ongoing in 42% and 37% of patients on the N3I1 and N1I3 arms, respectively. Based on these promising safety and efficacy results, the phase III CheckMate 214 study (NCT02231749) was launched.

The first results of the phase III CheckMate 214 study were reported at the European Society for Medical Oncology meeting on September 10, 2017 and have now been published.[25,26] Patients with treatment-naïve mRCC ($n = 1096$) with clear cell histology, measurable disease and Karnofsky Performance Status (KPS) $\geq$70 were randomized 1:1 to receive either nivolumab 3 mg/kg plus ipilimumab 1 mg/kg IV every 3 weeks for four cycles followed by nivolumab 3 mg/kg IV every 2 weeks or sunitinib 50 mg by mouth for 4 weeks on therapy followed by 2 weeks off therapy (4/2 schedule). Patients were stratified by IMDC prognostic score[27] (0 vs. 1–2 vs. 3–6) and region (United States vs. Canada/Europe vs. rest of world). The coprimary endpoints in IMDC intermediate- and poor-risk patients were ORR (independent radiographic review committee [IRRC]), PFS (per IRRC), and OS, with overall alpha of 0.05 split among the endpoints.

Secondary endpoints were ORR, PFS, OS, and AE rate in the intention-to-treat (ITT) patients; furthermore, exploratory endpoints included ORR, PFS, and OS in favorable-risk patients. The baseline characteristics of the IMDC intermediate-/poor-risk cohort by treatment arm were similar, with 79% and 21% intermediate and poor risk, respectively. The overall ITT population additionally included 23% favorable risk patients, who had lower rates of PD-L1 expression than the intermediate-/poor-risk patients and the ITT population.

In the IMDC intermediate-/poor-risk group, the coprimary endpoint of ORR was superior with N3I1 versus sunitinib: 42% versus 27% ($P < .0001$), including 9% versus 1% CRs ($P < .0001$).[21] The median duration of response was not reached with N3I1 (95% CI: 21.8 months, not estimable) and 18.2 months with sunitinib (95% CI: 14.8 months, not estimable). The coprimary endpoint of PFS per IRRC numerically favored N3I1 over sunitinib at 11.6 months (95% CI: 8.7−15.5 months) versus 8.4 months (95% CI: 7.0−10.8 months), respectively, although this did not meet the prespecified significance threshold (HR 0.82 [99.1% CI: 0.64−1.05; $P = .0331$]). The coprimary endpoint of median OS was superior in the N3I1 arm versus sunitinib: not reached versus 26.0 months (HR 0.63 [95% CI: 0.44−0.89; $P < .001$]). The secondary endpoints of ORR and OS, but not PFS, were significantly improved in the ITT population. Interestingly, these trends were reversed for exploratory endpoints in the IMDC favorable risk population, favoring sunitinib: confirmed ORR was 29% for N3I1 (95% CI: 21%−28%) compared with 52% for sunitinib (95% CI: 43% −61%; $P = .0002$). Furthermore, median PFS was 15.3 months for N3I1 (95% CI: 9.7−20.3 months) and 25.1 months for sunitinib (20.9 months, not estimable); HR 2.18 (99.1% CI: 1.29−3.68; $P < .0001$). This difference in response characteristics highlights that RCC can have heterogeneous tumor biology, with the IMDC favorable risk portion of mRCC cases likely more dependent on the VEGF-signaling axis and therefore responding preferentially to upfront sunitinib over combination ICI therapy.

Antitumor activity varied by PD-L1 expression level: specifically, higher ORRs were observed in the N3I1-treated versus sunitinib-treated PD-L1 $\geq$1% cohorts. For example, the N3I1-treated, IMDC intermediate-/poor-risk, and PD-L1 $\geq$1% cohort had a 58% ORR and 16% CR rate. PFS was also improved in the N3I1-treated PD-L1 $\geq$1% intermediate-/poor-risk cohort over sunitinib: 22.8 versus 5.9 months (HR 0.48 [0.28−0.82]; $P = .0003$) but not the N3I1-treated PD-L1 <1% intermediate-/poor-risk cohort. These cohorts demonstrate the potential use of the PD-L1 biomarker to be used in selecting patients who may respond better combined upfront ipilimumab−nivolumab therapy; however, an alternative strategy for the biomarker-negative groups is lacking.

The adverse event profile of N3I1 was significant but manageable. Forty-six percent of patients on N3I1 experienced a grade 3−5 AE compared with 63% on sunitinib. There were 22 treatment-related AEs leading to discontinuation compared with 12 with sunitinib, with 7 and 4 treatment-related deaths, respectively. Sixty percent of patients treated with N3I1 required systemic corticosteroids for an AE. The most common immune-mediated AEs were hypothyroidism (19%), rash (17%), hyperthyroidism (12%), and diarrhea/colitis (10%). Grade 3−4 immune-mediated AEs were uncommon individually, with the following as the most common: hepatitis (6%), diarrhea/colitis (5%), adrenal insufficiency (3%), hypophysitis (3%), rash (3%), nephritis (2%), and pneumonitis (2%). Health-related QOL as measured by the FKSI-19 questionnaire demonstrated better symptom control with N3I1 versus sunitinib.

These robust results from the CheckMate 214 trial support the use of N3I1 as the new standard of care for intermediate-/poor-risk patients with mRCC in the front-line setting. Based on these data, the US FDA has granted priority review to a supplemental biologics license application for use of the combination of nivolumab and ipilimumab as a frontline treatment for intermediate- and poor-risk patients with advanced RCC with an action date of April 16, 2018. A phase IIIb/IV trial, CheckMate 920, is evaluating the safety and efficacy of N3I1 on a slightly different dosing schedule than CheckMate 214 and on the same dosing schedule in separate cohorts of N3I1 in nonclear cell histology patients, those with brain metastases, and those with poor performance status (all excluded from CheckMate 214).

Novel combinations of ICIs are also being studied. For example, the randomized phase II FRACTION-RCC study is examining whether nivolumab in combination with modulators of other T-cell checkpoints (e.g., relatlimab, a LAG-3 inhibitor) may be more effective than in combination with ipilimumab in patients with mRCC (NCT02996110). The number of novel combinations with PD-1/PD-L1 targeting antibodies currently in early phase clinical testing is too numerous to list but include epacadostat (indoleamine

2,3-dioxygenase [IDO] inhibitor), CPI-444 (adenosine A2a receptor antagonist), and varlilumab (CD27 agonist).[28−30]

Immune Checkpoint Inhibitor Plus Vascular Endothelial Growth Factor Pathway Inhibition

There is strong rationale to combine ICIs with VEGF signaling pathway inhibitors to improve T-cell infiltration into tumors. VEGF appears to affect dendritic cell maturation from precursors, which may lead to immune escape.[31] In mRCC patients, treatment with the VEGF receptor TKI sunitinib reverses type-1 immunosuppression and decreases regulatory T-cells.[32] Sunitinib can also reverse myeloid-derived suppressor cell (MDSC)−mediated tumor immunosuppression as measured in patient peripheral blood levels.[33] Primary RCC tumors treated with the VEGF-A antibody bevacizumab showed increased infiltration of CD4+ and CD8+ T lymphocytes, as well as CD4+FOXP3+ regulatory T-cells; furthermore, expression of PD-L1 was enhanced. In patients treated with combination anti-VEGF and anti-PD-L1 therapy with bevacizumab and atezolizumab, antigen-specific T-cell migration was improved. Taken together, these data provide a compelling rationale for combining anti-VEGF signaling pathway inhibitors with ICIs.

The existing data suggest that PD-1/PD-L1 inhibitors may combine better with some VEGF pathway inhibitors than others, with more narrow spectrum VEGF inhibitors appearing safer in combination. For example, a phase I/II study of pembrolizumab with the multitargeted VEGFR TKI pazopanib examined combinations with pazopanib at 600 and 800 mg daily and pembrolizumab 2 mg/kg every 2 and 3 weeks (cohort A and B).[34] Even with a 9 week run-in of pazopanib alone (cohort C), there was significant toxicity: 90% of patients in cohorts A and B, as well as 80% of patients in cohort C, experienced grade 3/4 AEs. Hepatotoxicity was the most common dose-limiting toxicity. The pembrolizumab and pazopanib combination is not considered suitable for further development owing to safety issues. Other phase Ib studies of PD-1/PD-L1 inhibitors in mRCC have demonstrated promising preliminary efficacy in the front-line/treatment-naïve setting (Table 6.1). For example, the combination of axitinib 5 mg by mouth twice daily plus pembrolizumab 2 mg/kg IV every 3 weeks demonstrated a 73% ORR (95% CI: 59%−84%) with a tolerable safety profile.[35]

The combination of the PD-L1 inhibitor atezolizumab plus bevacizumab (monoclonal antibody against VEGF-A) is farthest along in clinical testing with results

TABLE 6.1

Selected Early Phase Trials of PD-1/PD-L1 Plus VEGF Inhibitors in mRCC

Combination	N	ORR (%)	CR (%)	PR (%)
Pembrolizumab + axitinib[35]	52	73	8	65
Avelumab + axitinib[36]	54	54.5	3.6	50.9
Pembrolizumab + lenvatinib[37]	30	63.3	0	63.3
Atezolizumab + bevacizumab[38]	101	32	7	25
Nivolumab + tivozanib[39]	14	64.3	0	64.3
Nivolumab + cabozantinib[40]	13	53.9	0	53.9

ORR, overall response rate; *CR*, complete response; *N*, number

publicly presented from randomized phase II and randomized phase III studies. The phase II IMmotion 150 trial randomized 305 treatment-naïve mRCC patients to atezolizumab plus bevacizumab versus atezolizumab versus sunitinib, with crossover on progression allowed on the single-agent arms.[38] In the ITT population, there was no significant difference between median PFS in the atezolizumab plus bevacizumab (11.7 months) versus atezolizumab (6.1 months) versus sunitinib (8.4 months) arms. However, in the PD-L1+ population (defined as PD-L1 expression on $\geq$ 1% of IC), there was a trend toward improved PFS in the atezolizumab plus bevacizumab (14.7 months) versus sunitinib (7.8 months) arm ($P = .095$). Both atezolizumab-containing arms appeared to have a favorable safety profile compared with sunitinib. These data support further testing of the atezolizumab plus bevacizumab combination in the phase III IMmotion 151 trial.

The first results of the IMmotion 151 trial were presented at the 2018 ASCO GU Cancers Symposium on February 10, 2018 in San Francisco, CA.[41] This phase III study randomized 915 patients with treatment-naïve mRCC, clear cell and/or sarcomatoid histology, KPS $\geq$70, and tumor tissue available for PD-L1 staining 1:1 to either the combination of atezolizumab 1200 mg IV every 3 weeks plus bevacizumab 15 mg/kg IV every 3 weeks or sunitinib 50 mg daily for 4 weeks followed by 2 weeks off (4/2 schedule). Patients were stratified by MSKCC risk score,[42] presence of liver metastasis, and PD-L1 status by IHC ($<$1% vs. $\geq$ 1%). The primary analysis of PFS in the PD-L1+ was event triggered (65%, or 236, of PFS events on September 29, 2017), and the first interim OS analysis was conducted with the same cutoff date. The alpha of 0.05 was split between the coprimary endpoints of PFS in PD-L1+ patients (0.04) and OS in the ITT population (0.01). Regarding the coprimary endpoints, median PFS was significantly better with atezolizumab + bevacizumab versus sunitinib in the PD-L1+ cohort: 11.2 versus 7.7 months

(HR 0.74 [95% CI: 0.57–0.96], $P = .02$). However, the data for median OS in the ITT population were immature with only 29% of patients with an OS event, with medians not reached and HR 0.81 (95% CI: 0.63–1.03, $P = .09$). For key secondary endpoints, the atezolizumab + bevacizumab combination demonstrated a 43% ORR in the PD-L1+ cohort and 37% ORR in the ITT population, with CR rates of 9% and 5%, respectively. Median treatment duration was 12.0 months for atezolizumab + bevacizumab and 9.2 months for sunitinib. There were five deaths due to treatment-related AEs in the atezolizumab + bevacizumab arm and one death in the sunitinib arm, with 40% and 54% grade 3–4 AEs, respectively. Sixteen percent of patients on the atezolizumab + bevacizumab arm required treatment with systemic corticosteroids owing to an AE of special interest (defined as rash, hypo- or hyperthyroidism, adrenal insufficiency, LFT abnormalities, colitis, and pneumonitis). The time to symptom interference with activities of daily living per the MD Anderson Symptom Interference Scale was significantly delayed with atezolizumab + bevacizumab versus sunitinib: 11.3 months versus 4.3 months (HR 0.56 [0.46–0.68]). These data support atezolizumab + bevacizumab as a front-line treatment option for patients with PD-L1+ mRCC. At the time of this writing, these data are being discussed with global health authorities such as the US FDA and European Medicines Agency. Multiple other phase III trials of PD-1/PD-L1 inhibitors with anti-VEGF agents are currently accrued and expected to read out in the next 1–2 years (Table 6.2).

Immune Checkpoint Inhibitors as Adjuvant Therapy for High-Risk Localized RCC

Until recently, the standard of care for high-risk localized RCC after nephrectomy was observation; however, sunitinib was recently FDA approved in the adjuvant setting based on improved disease-free

TABLE 6.2
Phase III Trials of Checkpoint Inhibitors in Combination With Anti-VEGF Agents in mRCC

Name	Treatment Arms	Primary Endpoint	ClinicalTrials.gov	Estimated Completion
CLEAR	Pembrolizumab-lenvatinib versus everolimus—lenvatinib versus sunitinib	PFS	NCT02811861	2020
JAVELIN Renal 101	Avelumab—axitinib versus sunitinib	PFS	NCT02684006	2020
KEYNOTE 426	Pembrolizumab—axitinib versus sunitinib	PFS and OS	NCT02853331	2020
CheckMate 9ER	Nivolumab—cabozantinib versus sunitinib	PFS	NCT03141177	2021
PDIGREE (Alliance)	Ipilimumab—nivolumab, followed by nivolumab versus nivolumab—cabozantinib	OS	TBD	2023

OS, overall survival; PFS, progression-free survival; TBD, to be determined

survival (DFS) over placebo in the phase III S-TRAC trial.[43] Multiple adjuvant trials of PD-1/PD-L1 inhibitors are currently ongoing including perioperative (including both neoadjuvant and adjuvant components) adjuvant nivolumab versus observation (PROSPER, NCT03055013), adjuvant pembrolizumab versus placebo (KEYNOTE-564, NCT03142334), adjuvant atezolizumab versus placebo (IMmotion 010, IMmotion 010, NCT03024996) and adjuvant nivolumab plus ipilimumab versus placebo (Check-Mate 914, NCT03138512). All of these trials have DFS (or recurrence-free survival) as the primary endpoint and are expected to read out in approximately 2023–24 or later. It remains to be seen whether accrual will be a challenge given that all of these trials have a placebo arm despite that fact that there is an FDA-approved option (sunitinib).

Challenges

As discussed earlier, the treatment landscape for RCC is rapidly changing and ICIs have become a standard of care in the front-line and VEGF-refractory settings; however, many challenges remain. First, only a small percentage of patients achieve CRs even with ICI—ICI and ICI—VEGF inhibitor combinations. Although PD-L1 positivity had some predictive value in the CheckMate 214 and IMmotion 151 trials, better and more standard biomarkers are clearly needed. Candidates include tumor mutational burden, molecular subtypes, and profiling of tumor-infiltrating lymphocytes.[44] Emerging evidence suggests that the gut microbiome may also affect response to immunotherapy in RCC patients and preclinical evidence demonstrated that fecal transplant could enhance the efficacy of PD-1 blockade in mice.[45] Second, now that nivolumab and ipilimumab have become a front-line standard of care, it will be difficult to integrate other ICI—ICI and ICI—VEGFi therapies into treatment algorithms owing to slightly different trial designs and the fact that sunitinib remains the comparator arm for most phase III CPI-VEGFi trials. The comparator arm now needs to be nivolumab and ipilimumab (or perhaps, cabozantinib based on the CaboSUN trial) and novel clinical trial designs are needed to improve durable complete remission rates and OS, while minimizing treatment-related toxicity.

BLADDER CANCER

Cancer of the urinary bladder will be diagnosed in 81,190 people in 2018, with 17,240 deaths.[1] The most common histology of bladder cancer (BC) is urothelial carcinoma (UC). UC can occur anywhere within the urothelial tract, including the renal pelvis, ureter, bladder, and urethra. Localized BC can be treated with curative intent cystectomy or chemoradiotherapy. However, advanced or metastatic BC is invariably fatal, with a median survival of around 13 months.[46]

Platinum-based chemotherapy is a standard of care for advanced BC, preferably cisplatin if the patient meets eligibility criteria. Until recently, there had been no new drug approvals for BC in approximately 30 years. Several ICIs are presently being developed clinically for use in BC, and these are summarized in this section by target. Note that Table 6.3 summarizes all major trials that have been done using ICIs in BC as well as a multitude of trials that are in progress.

TABLE 6.3
Comparison of the Approved PD-L1/PD-1 Immune Checkpoint Inhibitors for Second-Line Advanced Bladder Cancer

Drug	Alternative Names	Target	Characteristics	Dose	OVERALL				PD-L1+				PD-L1-				Study Type
					ORR (%)	CR (%)	PFS	OS	ORR (%)	CR (%)	PFS	OS	ORR (%)	CR (%)	PFS	OS	
Atezolizumab	Tecentriq MPDL3280A	PD-L1	• Humanized IgG1κ monoclonal antibody • FcγR-binding deficient	1200 mg q 3 weeks	13	3	—	9 months 39% @ 1 year	23	7	—	11 months 46% @ 1 year	—	—	—	—	Phase III
Durvalumab	Imfinzi MEDI4736	PD-L1	• Humanized IgG1κ monoclonal antibody • FcγR-binding deficient	10 mg/kg q 2 weeks	31	—	—	—	46	—	—	—	0	—	—	—	Phase Ib
Avelumab	Bavencio MSB0010718 C	PD-L1	• Humanized IgG1κ monoclonal antibody • FcγR-binding active (can trigger ADCC)	10 mg/kg q 2 weeks	18	11	12 weeks 19% @ 1 year	14 months 54% @ 1 year	54	—	48 weeks 50% @ 1 year	NR 76% @ 1 year	4	—	7 weeks 6% @ 1 year	13 months 56% @ 1 year	Phase Ib
Nivolumab	Opdivo MDX-1106 BMS-936558	PD-1	• Humanized IgG4 monoclonal antibody	3 mg/kg q 2 weeks	20	2	8 weeks	9 months 40% @ 1 year	28	—	6 weeks	11 months	16	—	3 weeks	6 months	Phase Ib
Pembrolizumab	Keytruda Lambrolizumab MK-3476	PD-1	• Humanized IgG4 monoclonal antibody	200 mg q 3 weeks	21	7	8 weeks 17% @ 1 year	10 months 44% @ 1 year	—	—	—	—	22	2	—	—	Phase III

PFS, progression-free survival; ORR, overall response rate; CR, complete response; NR, not reported

PD-L1—TARGETED AGENTS

There are three PD-L1 blocking antibodies that have been tested in clinical trials for the treatment of BC and are now FDA approved: atezolizumab, durvalumab, and avelumab. Although all three block the interaction of PD-L1 with its two receptors, PD-1 and B7.1, they do not block the interaction of PD-L2 with PD-1.[47] The antibodies also have different biological properties and bind to different parts of PD-L1, which may lead to subtle differences in their biological action, which have not yet been fully explored or compared in humans.[48] The PD-L1 and PD-1 antibodies used in BC are summarized in Table 6.3.

Atezolizumab

The first ICI to be FDA approved for use in BC was atezolizumab.[49] Atezolizumab is a fully humanized IgG1 monoclonal antibody and the recommended dosing of atezolizumab is a 1200 mg IV infusion given every 21 days. The volume of distribution of atezolizumab is approximately equal to the plasma volume, and its biodistribution to normal organs includes (in order of accumulation) the spleen, lungs, kidneys, liver, heart, and muscle.[50] The drug first enters tumors at their peripheral borders but then migrates into the hypoxic and acidotic tumor center. Atezolizumab has a dose-dependent nonlinear PK curve, and saturation of PD-L1 receptors by atezolizumab on circulating T-cells occurs in 1—2 days after dosing.[50] Atezolizumab is FcγR-binding deficient, which implies that it cannot bind Fc receptors and lead to antibody-dependent cell-mediated cytotoxicity (ADCC) or complement-mediated cytotoxicity (CMC).[51] Because PD-L1 is highly expressed by a wide variety of normal leukocytes, the fact that atezolizumab is FcγR-binding deficient means that it does not deplete leukocytes, which could lead to deleterious immune suppression. Immunological changes that occur during atezolizumab treatment include increased IFNγ, IL-18, and CXCL11 levels, decreased IL-6 levels, and increased $CD8^+$ T cells. A detailed discussion of the toxicities of ICIs and their management is given in Chapter 11.

Metastatic, second-line, bladder cancer

PCD4989G trial. The first BC patients to receive atezolizumab were treated on this trial, which evaluated the drug in metastatic BC patients who were failed prior platinum-based chemotherapy (i.e., second-line metastatic patients).[52] The objective response rate (ORR) was 43% for BC patients with high/moderate PD-L1 expression and 11% for those with low/absent PD-L1 expression. A CR was noted in 7% of subjects. Of those that responded, 67% had ongoing responses. At 1-year, the PFS was 39% in the high/moderate PD-L1 group and 10% in the low/absent PD-L1 group, suggesting that outcomes were strongly dependent on tumor PD-L1 expression. Median PFS was 6 months in the high/moderate PD-L1 group and 1 month in the low/absent PD-L1 group. Median OS was not reached in the high/moderate PD-L1 group and was 7.6 months in the low/absent PD-L1 group.

IMvigor210 trial (cohort 2). This is a phase II trial of atezolizumab in subjects with locally advanced or metastatic BC and cohort 2 of this trial included subjects that had failed chemotherapy with a platinum-based regimen.[53] Overall, the ORR for cohort 2 was 15% with a CR rate of 5%. As in the PCD4989G trial, the ORR in IMvigor210 was strongly influenced by PD-L1 expression. In the high/moderate PD-L1 group, the ORR was 26% while in the low PD-L1 group it was 11%, and it was 8% in patients without PD-L1—expressing tumors. Median PFS was 2.1 months and median OS was 7.9 months. Based on these results, the US FDA approved atezolizumab for the treatment of BC patients with locally advanced or metastatic UC who (1) have progressed during/after platinum-based chemotherapy or (2) have progressed within 12 months of neoadjuvant or adjuvant treatment with platinum-based chemotherapy.[49] On IMvigor210, 20% of subjects required a treatment interruption for toxicity and 4% discontinued atezolizumab treatment entirely.

IMvigor211 trial. This is a phase III trial where patients with metastatic BC who failed prior platinum-based chemotherapy were randomized to atezolizumab or investigator's choice of second-line chemotherapy, which consisted of vinflunine, docetaxel, or paclitaxel.[54] The trial results were presented in abstract form at the 2017 EACR-AACR-SIC Special Conference on The Challenges of Optimizing Immuno- and Targeted Therapies: From Cancer Biology to the Clinic. This trial was designed to show an OS advantage of atezolizumab over other standard-of-care second-line agents in subjects with high/moderate PD-L1 expression and failed to do so; however, the trial did show a significant difference is median OS (8.6 months for atezolizumab vs. 8.0 months for chemotherapy; HR 0.85 [95% CI: 0.73, 0.99], $P = .038$) for the overall ITT study cohort.[55] The ORR for atezolizumab was 23%

(7% CR) in subjects with high/moderate PD-L1 expression (chemotherapy was 22% with 7% CR) and 13% (3% CR) for the overall population treated with atezolizumab. This trial is seen as a disappointment, and its results are likely due, in part, to vinflunine being a more active second-line agent than anticipated. On the positive side, treatment-related AEs appeared much more favorable in the atezolizumab arm with grade 3/4 AEs occurring in 20% of patients compared with 43% of chemotherapy-treated patients. The most common AEs in the atezolizumab arm were (in order) fatigue, pruritus, decreased appetite, asthenia, diarrhea, and nausea, consistent with the side effects seen in IMvigor210. Death from treatment occurred in 1% of patients in both arms.

Metastatic, first-line, cisplatin-ineligible, bladder cancer

IMvigor210 trial (cohort 1). IMvigor210 also included cohort 1, which consisted of cisplatin-ineligible and chemotherapy-naïve locally advanced and metastatic BC patients.[56] In 119 such patients, the ORR was 23%, including 9% CRs. The median time to first response was 2.1 months, suggesting that atezolizumab efficacy is detectable relatively early in the treatment course for most patients. Only two patients demonstrated a response after 6 months of treatment. Median PFS in cohort 1 was 2.7 months, median OS was 15.9 months, and the 1-year OS rate was 57%. Most patients qualified as cisplatin ineligible based on either decreased renal clearance or poor performance status. Based on this trial, the label for atezolizumab expanded to include an indication for cisplatin-ineligible patients.

Upper tract urothelial carcinomas

Outcomes for UCs of the upper urinary tract (ureter and renal pelvis) were reported for 33 patients that participated in IMvigor210.[56] In these patients, the ORR for atezolizumab was 39% and the median survival was not yet reached, suggesting for the first time that atezolizumab is active in nonbladder UCs.

Response by PD-L1 expression level

All of the trials assessing atezolizumab in BC have found that PD-L1 expression correlates strongly with response to therapy.[52–54,56] However, in BC and other tumors, clinical activity is still observed in tumors that are classified as PD-L1 negative. In the atezolizumab trials, tumor PD-L1 expression was analyzed by the Ventana SP142 immunohistochemistry assay that measures tumor-infiltrating immune cells (IC) PD-L1 expression, which is categorized as high (IC3, ≥10%), moderate (IC2, 5%–10%), low (IC1, 1%–5%), or absent (IC0, <1%). The FDA has approved the Ventana SP142 assay as a companion diagnostic for atezolizumab, and this is the system that has been used in the earlier-discussed trials. It is important to note that the SP142 assay is different than other PD-L1 assays such as the SP263 assay, Dako 28-8 assay, the Dako 22c3 assay, and the Leica E1L3N assay, in that PD-L1 positivity is usually defined with lower thresholds, both on the tumor and on the tumor-infiltrating ICs.[44,57,58]

It is also important to realize that tumor cell PD-L1 expression is strongly correlated with the presence of tumor-infiltrating ICs, which in turn can predict the response of checkpoint inhibitors. The tumor and the immune system interact dynamically to determine PD-L1 levels. Serial biopsies of tumors undergoing atezolizumab treatment demonstrate that PD-L1 expression increases in subjects responding to treatment. There are many challenges of PD-L1 testing, and given that a population of PD-L1–negative patients still respond to atezolizumab, the PD-L1 biomarker is not currently clinically useful to determine which patients should be treated with atezolizumab.

Durvalumab

Durvalumab is a humanized IgG1 monoclonal antibody that, like atezolizumab, blocks the interaction of PD-L1 with its receptors and is FDA approved as a second-line treatment for metastatic BC. Durvalumab is administered as an IV infusion at a dose of 10 mg/kg given every 14 days. To date, only a single trial of durvalumab use in BC has been published and 93% of patients on this trial had disease progression after prior systemic therapy for BC, making this a second-line trial.[59] Of the 61 subjects reported, only 42 were evaluable for efficacy, and the ORR was 31% with a median time to response of 6.3 weeks. In PD-L1–positive patients (defined as >25% expression on the Ventana SP263 assay) the ORR was 46%. PD-L1–negative patients did not experience any objective responses. Although only three patients experienced grade 3 toxicity and no treatment-related deaths were reported, low-grade toxicities were common and included (in order) fatigue, diarrhea, decreased appetite, asthenia, nausea, and fever.

Avelumab

Avelumab is also a humanized IgG1 monoclonal antibody that blocks the interaction of PD-L1 with its receptors and is FDA approved as a second-line treatment for metastatic BC. One major difference between avelumab and the other PD-L1 blockers listed earlier is that it has a functional Fc domain and therefore can trigger ADCC, although it does not appear to deplete leukocyte subsets in vivo.[60] Avelumab is given as a 10 mg/kg IV infusion every 14 days. Only one published clinical trial exists for avelumab use in BC, the JAVELIN solid tumor trial, and on this trial, 44 metastatic patients who had relapsed, refractory, or progressive disease were enrolled following at least one prior line of treatment; cisplatin-ineligible patients were also permitted after protocol amendment.[61] Forty-six percent of patients had ≤1 prior anticancer line of therapy for advanced disease. The overall ORR was 18%, with 11% being CRs, and the median time to response was 13 weeks. In PD-L1−positive tumors (≥5% expression on the Dako 73-10 assay), the ORR was 54%, while in PD-L1−negative tumors, it was 4%. Median PFS was 12 weeks with a 1-year PFS rate of 19%. Median OS was 14 months with a 1-year OS rate of 54%. There were no treatment related mortalities, and the most common grade 3/4 toxicities were (in order) asthenia, decreased appetite, elevated AST, and elevated CPK.

PD-L1−TARGETED AGENTS

There are two PD-1 blocking antibodies that have been tested in clinical trials for the treatment of BC and are now FDA approved: nivolumab and pembrolizumab. Both block the interaction of PD-1 with its two ligands, PD-L1 and PD-L2 (Table 6.3).[47]

Pembrolizumab

Pembrolizumab is a humanized IgG4 monoclonal antibody that blocks the interaction of PD-1 with its ligands and is FDA approved as a second-line treatment for metastatic BC. Pembrolizumab is administered as an IV infusion at a dose of 200 mg every 21 days. There are two published trials of pembrolizumab use in BC.

KEYNOTE-012 (cohort C)

Cohort C of this phase Ib study included subjects with locally advanced or metastatic BC (n = 33), all of whom had undergone prior systemic therapy.[62] Seventy-six percent (n = 25) had received at least one systemic therapy for advanced or metastatic disease; the remaining 24% (n = 8) had received platinum-based therapy in the neoadjuvant or adjuvant setting but progressed within 12 months. There were 27 patients for whom a response was assessable and the

ORR was 26%, with an 11% CR rate. The median time to response was 2 months. For baseline PD-L1−positive tumors (≥1% expression on Dako pharmDx 22C3 assay on biopsy), the ORR was 24% (n = 21) while it was 0% in baseline PD-L1−negative tumors (n = 4). Median PFS was 2 months, with a 1-year PFS rate of 15%. Median OS was 13 months with a 1-year OS rate of 50%. There were no treatment-related mortalities, and the most common toxicities were (in order) fatigue, edema, AST increases, and myalgias.

KEYNOTE-045

This phase III trial was done in the second-line metastatic setting (recurrence or progression after platinum-based chemotherapy) and enrolled 542 patients who were randomized to pembrolizumab or investigator's choice of chemotherapy, which could consist of paclitaxel, docetaxel, or vinflunine.[63] The primary endpoint of this trial was median OS. In all, 266 were assigned to the pembrolizumab arm and the ORR in this arm was 21% with a CR rate of 7%. The median time to response was 2.1 months. PD-L1−positive tumors (≥10% expression on Dako pharmDx 22C3 assay) did not really respond much better with an ORR of 22% and CR rate of 2%. The median PFS was 2.1 months with a 1-year PFS rate of 17%. Impressively, pembrolizumab demonstrated improved median OS at 10.3 months compared with 7.4 months with chemotherapy (HR 0.73, 95% CI 0.59−0.91, $P = .002$). Median duration of response was not reached in the pembrolizumab group (range, 1.6 to 15.6 + months) and, at the time of publication, treatment was ongoing in 36 of the 67 responders (67%) in the pembrolizumab group. One patient died from pembrolizumab-induced pneumonitis and three from causes unrelated to the drug. The most common grade 3/4 toxicities were (in order) pneumonitis, fatigue, diarrhea, colitis, and nephritis.

Nivolumab

Nivolumab is a humanized IgG4 monoclonal antibody that blocks the interaction of PD-1 with its ligands and is FDA-approved as a second-line treatment for metastatic BC. There are two published trials of Nivolumab use in BC. Nivolumab is administered as an IV infusion at a dose of 240 mg every 14 days or 480 mg every 4 weeks.

CheckMate 032 (nivolumab monotherapy arm)

This phase I/II trial enrolled subjects with metastatic BC that had failed prior platinum-based chemotherapy.[64] The trial had two regimens, a nivolumab monotherapy arm and a nivolumab + ipilimumab arm, and only the monotherapy arm has been published. Overall, 78 patients were treated with nivolumab monotherapy and the ORR was 24% with a 6% CR rate. In PD-L1—positive patients (≥1% expression on Dako 28-8 assay), the ORR was still 24% but the CR rate was dramatically higher at 16%. In PD-L1—negative patients, the ORR was 26% but the CR rate was only 2%. The median time to response was 1.5 months. Median PFS was 2.8 months with a 1-year PFS rate of 21%. Median OS was 10 months, and the 1-year OS rate was 46%. There were no treatment-related mortalities, and the most common grade 3/4 toxicities were (in order) elevated lipase, elevated amylase, lymphopenia, neutropenia, dyspnea, rash, and fatigue.

CheckMate 275
This phase II trial also enrolled subjects with metastatic BC that had failed prior platinum-based chemotherapy.[65] Of the 265 subjects for whom outcome was assessable, the ORR was 20% and the CR rate 2%. For PD-L1—positive patients (defined as ≥1% expression on the Dako 28-8 assay), the ORR was 24%, whereas it was only 16% in PD-L1—negative patients. Median OS was 8.7 months, whereas median PFS was 8 weeks. Again, there were no treatment-induced fatalities, and the most common adverse events were (in order) diarrhea, fatigue, liver enzyme changes, and asthenia.

CTLA-4—TARGETED AGENTS
There are two CTLA-4—blocking antibodies that have been tested (or are being tested) in clinical trials for the treatment of BC, but neither is FDA approved in this disease. These antibodies interfere with the ability of two ligands, B7.1 and B7.2, to bind to the CTLA-4 receptor.

Ipilimumab
The first ICI to be tested in humans, as well as in BC, was ipilimumab.[66] Ipilimumab is a fully human IgG1 monoclonal antibody that blocks CTLA-4. In a small trial from MD Anderson Cancer Center, 12 patients who planned to undergo cystectomy for muscle-invasive BC received two doses of ipilimumab 3 weeks apart before surgery, which was done 4 weeks after the last dose. Half the subjects were treated at 3 mg/kg and half at 10 mg/kg. Immunological changes were documented and there was a hint that the treatment might have improved outcomes, but given the small sample size, this was not clear.

Tremelimumab
Tremelimumab is a humanized monoclonal antibody that distinguishes itself from ipilimumab because it is a class IgG2 antibody and therefore it does not fix complement, and its FcγR receptor binding is much less strong.[67] Presently, there are no published studies using tremelimumab for BC. However, trials are underway using tremelimumab in combination with durvalumab (Table 6.4).

OTHER AGENTS
Urelumab
Urelumab is a monoclonal, Fc-deficient, IgG4 antibody whose purpose is to stimulate T-cell costimulation by acting as a 4-1BB (CD137) agonist.[68] Trials are underway in BC in combination with nivolumab, and it appears well tolerated.

MOXR0916
MOXR0916 is a monoclonal antibody whose purpose is to stimulate T-cell costimulation by acting as an OX40 agonist.[69] It is currently being tested in combination with atezolizumab and appears well tolerated.

There are a host of targets to stimulate T-cell activation. These costimulating and coinhibitory signals are being targeted with novel treatment agents. Combined with PD-1—/PD-L1—targeted agents, these new agents have the potential to improve on the response rates that are seen from PD-1/PD-L1 monotherapies above.

PROSTATE CANCER

INTRODUCTION
Prostate cancer is the most common malignancy among American men and the second most common cause of cancer-related mortality.[70] There are currently six FDA-approved treatments for metastatic castrate-resistant prostate cancer (mCRPC), including two cytotoxic chemotherapies (docetaxel, cabazitaxel),[71,72] two second-generation hormonal therapies (enzalutamide, abiraterone),[73-76] a bone-targeting radiopharmaceutical (radium-223),[77] and a cell-based immunotherapy (sipuleucel-T).[78] All of these agents have demonstrated an improvement in OS in randomized phase III trials. Notably, and in contrast to other tumor types, immune checkpoint inhibition in metastatic prostate cancer has had limited success, and there are currently no FDA-approved ICIs for the treatment of prostate cancer.

TABLE 6.4
Selected Clinical Trials of Immune Checkpoint Inhibitors in Bladder Cancer

ClinicalTrials.gov Registry	Acronym	Intervention Arm	Comparator Arm	Phase	N	Primary Endpoint(s)	References
NON–MUSCLE INVASIVE: BCG-UNRESPONSIVE							
NCT02625961	KEYNOTE-57	Pembrolizumab	–	2	260	CR, DFS	
NCT02792192	GU-123	Atezolizumab + BCG	Atezolizumab	2	70	CR, AEs	
MUSCLE INVASIVE: NEOADJUVANT, CISPLATIN-ELIGIBLE							
NCT02736266		Pembrolizumab + Cystectomy	–	2	90	CR	
NCT02862062		Pembrolizumab + Cisplatin + External beam radiation	–	2	30	AEs	
NCT02560636	PLUMMB	Pembrolizumab + External beam radiation		2	34	AEs	
NCT02690558		Pembrolizumab + Gem/Cis + Cystectomy	–	2	39	CR/PR	
NCT02621151		Pembrolizumab + Gemcitabine + External beam radiation	–	2	54	DFS	
		Ipilimumab + Cystectomy	–	1	12	AEs, CR	66
MUSCLE INVASIVE: NEOADJUVANT, CISPLATIN-INELIGIBLE							
NCT02891161	DUART	Durvalumab + External beam radiation	–	2	42	PFS, AEs	
NCT03150836		Durvalumab + Stereotactic radiation	Durvalumab + Tremelimumab + Stereotactic radiation	2	74	PFS, AEs	
NCT02845323		Nivolumab + Urelumab + Cystectomy	Nivolumab + Cystectomy	2	44	Immune	
NCT02812420		Durvalumab + Tremelimumab + Cystectomy	–	1	15	AEs	
MUSCLE INVASIVE: ADJUVANT							
NCT02450331	IMvigor010	Cystectomy + Atezolizumab	Cystectomy	3	700	DFS	
METASTATIC: FIRST LINE, CISPLATIN-ELIGIBLE							
NCT02807636	IMvigor130	Gem/Cis + Atezolizumab	Gem/Cis or atezolizumab	3	1200	PFS, OS, AEs	

NCT number	Study name	Intervention	Comparator	Phase	N	Endpoint	Ref
NCT02603432	JAVELIN 100	Platinum-based chemo + Avelumab maintenance	Platinum-based chemo	3	668	OS	
NCT02500121		Platinum-based chemo + Pembrolizumab maintenance	Platinum-based chemo	2	200	PFS	
METASTATIC: FIRST LINE, CISPLATIN-INELIGIBLE							
NCT02951767	IMvigor210	Atezolizumab	–	2	119	CR/PR	
NCT02335424	KEYNOTE-52	Pembrolizumab	–	2	350	CR/PR	
NCT03029832		Atezolizumab + MOXR0916	Atezolizumab	2	225	PFS, OS	
METASTATIC: SECOND LINE							
NCT02302807	IMvigor211	Atezolizumab	Vinflunine or paclitaxel or docetaxel	3	931	OS	54
NCT02256436	KEYNOTE-45	Pembrolizumab	Vinflunine or paclitaxel or docetaxel	3	542	OS, PFS	
NCT02387996	CheckMate 275	Nivolumab	–	2	386	CR/PR	65
NCT02108652	IMvigor210	Atezolizumab	–	2	310	CR/PR	53,56
NCT02351739	KEYNOTE-143	Pembrolizumab + ACP-196	–	2	75	CR/PR	
NCT02717156		Pembrolizumab + sEphB4-HSA	–	2	60	AEs	
NCT03113266		JS001	–	2	370	CR/PR	
NCT01693562	CD-ON-MEDI4736-1108	Durvalumab	–	1/2	61	AEs, CR/PR	59
NCT01928394	CheckMate 032	Nivolumab	–	1/2	86	AEs, CR/PR	64
NCT02619253		Pembrolizumab + Vorinostat	–	1b	42	AEs	
NCT02437370		Pembrolizumab + Docetaxel	Pembrolizumab + Gemcitabine	1b	38	AEs	
NCT03123055		Atezolizumab + B-701	–	1b	48	AEs	
NCT03138889	PROPEL	Atezolizumab + NKTR-214	–	1b	36	AEs	
NCT01375842	PCD4989G	Atezolizumab	–	1a/b	698	AEs	52
NCT01772004	JAVELIN	Avelumab	–	1b	44	AEs	61
NCT01848834	KEYNOTE-012	Pembrolizumab	–	1b	33	AEs	62

AE, adverse event; CR, complete response; OS, overall survival; PFS, progression-free survival; DFS, disease-free survival; BCG, Bacillus Calmette-Guerin; N, number of subjects

Ipilimumab

Ipilimumab is a fully human IgG1 monoclonal antibody, which blocks CTLA-4, thereby enhancing the antitumor immune response. It is FDA approved for advanced melanoma.

Several trials have investigated ipilimumab in patients with mCRPC. Early phase studies demonstrated acceptable tolerability and durable PSA responses.[79–82] These encouraging results ultimately led to the development of two randomized phase III trials of ipilimumab in mCRPC.[83,84]

In the first study, 799 men with mCRPC who had disease progression following docetaxel chemotherapy were randomized to radiation to a bone metastasis followed by either ipilimumab 10 mg/kg or placebo every 3 weeks for up to four doses. Ipilimumab 10 mg/kg or placebo was continued every 3 months until disease progression, unacceptable toxicity, or death. Radiation was incorporated into the study design because there is preclinical and clinical evidence demonstrating its immunogenic properties. For example, radiation can stimulate an immune response and thus might prime the immune system to respond to CTLA-4 inhibition. Additionally, radiation can induce tumor regression at sites distant from the primary tumor in an immune-mediated process called the abscopal effect.[85,86] Finally, the combination of radiation plus anti-CTLA-4 antibody has been shown to be synergistic in preclinical models[87] and in two case reports of patients with metastatic melanoma.[88,89]

In this study, baseline characteristics were well balanced between the two groups and were representative of advanced prostate cancer, as expected in the post-docetaxel setting. Slightly less than half of the patients in each group were of 70 years of age or older. Approximately two-thirds of patients in each group had five or fewer bone metastases, with the majority of the remaining patients having more than five bone metastases. Visceral metastases were present in about 30% of patients in each group. Median PSA was 138.5 ng/mL in the ipilimumab group and 176.5 ng/mL in the placebo group. Approximately half of patients in each group reported an average daily worst bone pain intensity score of four or more.

After a median follow-up of 9.9 months in the ipilimumab group and 9.3 months in the placebo group, there was no statistically significant difference between groups for the primary endpoint of median OS (11.2 months with ipilimumab vs. 10.0 months with placebo; HR 0.85, 95% CI 0.72–1.00; $P = .053$). Post hoc subgroup analyses suggested that there might

be a survival benefit with ipilimumab in patients with more favorable prognostic features, specifically patients without visceral metastases who have alkaline phosphatase levels less than 1.5 times the upper limit of normal and hemoglobin 110 g/L or higher. PFS was improved among patients treated with ipilimumab compared with placebo (median 4.0 vs. 3.1 months; HR 0.70, 95% CI 0.61–0.82; $P < .0001$). Treatment with ipilimumab was also associated with increased rate of PSA response, defined as proportion of patients with a confirmed reduction of 50% or more at any time (13.1% for ipilimumab and 5.2% for placebo).

50% of patients in the ipilimumab group and 67% of men in the placebo group received all four initial doses of study drug. The most common reasons for not receiving all four initial doses were disease progression or toxicity. Grade 3–4 AEs were more common among patients treated with ipilimumab compared with placebo. The majority of these grade 3–4 AEs were immune related (ipilimumab group 26% vs. placebo group 3%), including diarrhea (ipilimumab group 16% vs. placebo group 2%) and colitis (ipilimumab group 5% vs. placebo group 0). Four patients died owing to toxic effects of ipilimumab.[83]

The second phase III study of ipilimumab in mCRPC built on the subset analyses from the initial phase III trial (discussed earlier), which suggested a benefit with ipilimumab in patients with mCRPC and more favorable prognostic features. In this study, 602 chemotherapy-naïve men with asymptomatic or minimally symptomatic mCRPC and no visceral metastases were randomized to induction treatment with ipilimumab 10 mg/kg or placebo every 3 weeks for up to four doses, followed by maintenance treatment with ipilimumab 10 mg/kg versus placebo every 12 weeks until disease progression or unacceptable toxicity.

Baseline characteristics were well balanced between groups. 75% of patients in both groups had ECOG performance status 0. Hemoglobin was 11 g/dL or higher in 91% of patients in both groups, and alkaline phosphatase was less than 1.5 times the upper limit of normal in more than 80% of patients in both groups. Median PSA was 41.2 ng/mL in the ipilimumab group and 49.5 ng/mL in the placebo group. Bone metastases were present in approximately 80% of patients. Approximately half of patients were asymptomatic and about half were minimally symptomatic.

Unfortunately, there was no improvement in the primary endpoint of median OS observed with ipilimumab compared with placebo (ipilimumab group 28.7 mo vs.

placebo group 29.7 mo, HR 1.11, 95% CI 0.88—1.39, $P = .3667$). A modest PFS benefit (5.6 mo vs. 3.8 mo; HR 0.67, 95% CI 0.55—0.81) and improvement in time to chemotherapy (HR 0.65, 95% CI 0.52—0.83) was associated with ipilimumab treatment.

All four initial doses of study drug were completed by 63% of patients in the ipilimumab group and 88% in the placebo group. The most common reasons for treatment discontinuation were disease progression (49% in ipilimumab group, 78% in placebo group) and toxicity (treatment-related AE leading to drug discontinuation 29% in ipilimumab group, 3% in placebo group). Nine treatment-related deaths occurred owing to ipilimumab.[84]

Given that two large randomized trials conclusively demonstrated that ipilimumab does not improve OS in patients with mCRPC and is associated with considerable toxicity, ipilimumab has not been approved for metastatic prostate cancer.

PD-1/PD-L1 Inhibitors

The PD-1/PD-L1 axis represents another pathway in the immune system that serves to downregulate the immune response. Numerous monoclonal antibodies have been developed against PD-1 and PD-L1 to inhibit this immune checkpoint and stimulate an antitumor immune response. PD-1 or PD-L1 inhibitors are approved, as described earlier, for the treatment of RCC and UC, as well as non—small cell lung cancer, melanoma, Hodgkin lymphoma, and head and neck cancer. Studies are ongoing in prostate cancer and some early clinical trial data, described below, are encouraging.

A phase I study of the PD-1 inhibitor nivolumab demonstrated no objective responses in the 17 patients with mCRPC included in the trial.[90] Subsequently, data emerged demonstrating that PD-L1 expression was increased in patients with mCRPC progressing on enzalutamide compared with enzalutamide responders,[91] suggesting that the enzalutamide-resistant mCRPC population might be more responsive to treatment with PD-1/PD-L1 blockade. A single-institution, single-arm phase II study is currently being conducted to investigate the PD-1 inhibitor pembrolizumab in patients with mCRPC progressing on enzalutamide. In this trial, patients are treated with pembrolizumab 200 mg IV every 3 weeks for four doses, then every 6 weeks until disease progression. Enzalutamide 80—160 mg daily by mouth is continued. This study is ongoing, but the results from the first 10 patients have been published. Marked response was observed in 3 of the 10 patients (ORR 30%) with near complete PSA response in all 3 patients and partial radiographic response in both of the patients with measurable disease. In general, pembrolizumab was well tolerated. One patient developed grade 2 myositis; one patient experienced grade 3 hypothyroidism.[92] Although these data are certainly promising, the final study results and additional clinical trials will be needed to determine the role for pembrolizumab and PD-1/PD-L1 checkpoint inhibition in prostate cancer.

Ongoing Clinical Trials

There are several ongoing and planned clinical trials that will further investigate immune checkpoint blockade in prostate cancer. These studies will largely focus on combination strategies to improve therapeutic efficacy. A few examples include concurrent CTLA-4 plus PD-1/PD-L1 inhibition in mCRPC (NCT02985957), PROST-VAC plus nivolumab and/or ipilimumab in a lead-in cohort of mCRPC then experimental cohorts of patients undergoing radical prostatectomy (NCT02933255), pembrolizumab plus radium-223 in mCRPC (NCT03093428), atezolizumab plus radium-223 in mCRPC (NCT02814669), pembrolizumab plus other therapies (olaparib, docetaxel, enzalutamide) in mCRPC (NCT02861573), and pembrolizumab and cryosurgery in newly diagnosed, oligometastatic prostate cancer (NCT02489357).

DISCLOSURE STATEMENT

Michael R. Harrison: Research Funding (to institution)—Acerta, Argos, Bristol-Myers Squibb, Exelixis, Genentech, Merck, Pfizer; Advisory Board—Argos, AstraZeneca, Bayer, Exelixis, Genentech; Speaker—Exelixis, Genentech; Consultant—Argos, Exelixis, Genentech, Pfizer.

Megan A. McNamara: Research Funding (to institution)—Bayer, Clovis, Agensys, Seattle Genetics, Janssen; Travel: Clovis, Agensys.

Tian Zhang: Research Funding (to institution)—Acerta, Janssen, Novartis, Merrimack, Abbvie/StemCentrx, Pfizer, Merck; Advisory board—Exelixis, Genentech, Sanofi Aventis, Janssen, Pfizer; Speaker—Exelixis, Genentech; Consultant—AstraZeneca, Bayer, Exelixis, Foundation Medicine.

Brant A. Inman: Research Funding (to institution)—Urogen, Abbot Laboratories, Combat Medical, Nucleix, FKD Therapies, Dendreon, Genentech; Consultant—Combat Medical, BioCancell.

REFERENCES

1. Siegel RL, Miller KD, Jemal A. Cancer statistics, 2018. *CA Cancer J Clin.* 2018;68(1):7−30.
2. Fyfe G, Fisher RI, Rosenberg SA, Sznol M, Parkinson DR, Louie AC. Results of treatment of 255 patients with metastatic renal cell carcinoma who received high-dose recombinant interleukin-2 therapy. *J Clin Oncol.* 1995;13(3):688−696.
3. Coppin C, Porzsolt F, Awa A, Kumpf J, Coldman A, Wilt T. Immunotherapy for advanced renal cell cancer. *Cochrane Database Syst Rev.* 2005;(1):CD001425.
4. Kim WY, Kaelin Jr WG. Molecular pathways in renal cell carcinoma−rationale for targeted treatment. *Semin Oncol.* 2006;33(5):588−595.
5. Choueiri TK, Motzer RJ. Systemic therapy for metastatic renal-cell carcinoma. *N Engl J Med.* 2017;376(4):354−366.
6. Motzer RJ, Escudier B, McDermott DF, et al. Nivolumab versus everolimus in advanced renal-cell carcinoma. *N Engl J Med.* 2015;373(19):1803−1813.
7. Smith KA. Interleukin-2: inception, impact, and implications. *Science.* 1988;240(4856):1169−1176.
8. Rosenberg SA, Mule JJ, Spiess PJ, Reichert CM, Schwarz SL. Regression of established pulmonary metastases and subcutaneous tumor mediated by the systemic administration of high-dose recombinant interleukin 2. *J Exp Med.* 1985;161(5):1169−1188.
9. McDermott DF, Regan MM, Clark JI, et al. Randomized phase III trial of high-dose interleukin-2 versus subcutaneous interleukin-2 and interferon in patients with metastatic renal cell carcinoma. *J Clin Oncol.* 2005;23(1):133−141.
10. Klapper JA, Downey SG, Smith FO, et al. High-dose interleukin-2 for the treatment of metastatic renal cell carcinoma: a retrospective analysis of response and survival in patients treated in the surgery branch at the National Cancer Institute between 1986 and 2006. *Cancer.* 2008;113(2):293−301.
11. Clark JI, Wong MKK, Kaufman HL, et al. Impact of sequencing targeted therapies with high-dose Interleukin-2 immunotherapy: an analysis of outcome and survival of patients with metastatic renal cell carcinoma from an on-going observational IL-2 clinical trial: PROCLAIM(SM). *Clin Genitourin Cancer.* 2017;15(1):31−41.e4.
12. Minasian LM, Motzer RJ, Gluck L, Mazumdar M, Vlamis V, Krown SE. Interferon alfa-2a in advanced renal cell carcinoma: treatment results and survival in 159 patients with long-term follow-up. *J Clin Oncol.* 1993;11(7):1368−1375.
13. Motzer RJ, Hutson TE, Tomczak P, et al. Sunitinib versus interferon alfa in metastatic renal-cell carcinoma. *N Engl J Med.* 2007;356(2):115−124.
14. Hudes G, Carducci M, Tomczak P, et al. Temsirolimus, interferon alfa, or both for advanced renal-cell carcinoma. *N Engl J Med.* 2007;356(22):2271−2281.
15. Unverzagt S, Moldenhauer I, Nothacker M, et al. Immunotherapy for metastatic renal cell carcinoma. *Cochrane Database Syst Rev.* 2017;5:CD011673.
16. Rini BI, Halabi S, Rosenberg JE, et al. Bevacizumab plus interferon alfa compared with interferon alfa monotherapy in patients with metastatic renal cell carcinoma: CALGB 90206. *J Clin Oncol.* 2008;26(33):5422−5428.
17. Escudier B, Szczylik C, Hutson TE, et al. Randomized phase II trial of first-line treatment with sorafenib versus interferon Alfa-2a in patients with metastatic renal cell carcinoma. *J Clin Oncol.* 2009;27(8):1280−1289.
18. Yang JC, Hughes M, Kammula U, et al. Ipilimumab (anti-CTLA4 antibody) causes regression of metastatic renal cell cancer associated with enteritis and hypophysitis. *J Immunother.* 2007;30(8):825−830.
19. Brahmer JR, Tykodi SS, Chow LQ, et al. Safety and activity of anti-PD-L1 antibody in patients with advanced cancer. *N Engl J Med.* 2012;366(26):2455−2465.
20. Motzer RJ, Rini BI, McDermott DF, et al. Nivolumab for metastatic renal cell carcinoma: results of a randomized phase II trial. *J Clin Oncol.* 2015;33(13):1430−1437.
21. Cella D, Grunwald V, Nathan P, et al. Quality of life in patients with advanced renal cell carcinoma given nivolumab versus everolimus in CheckMate 025: a randomised, open-label, phase 3 trial. *Lancet Oncol.* 2016;17(7):994−1003.
22. Curran MA, Montalvo W, Yagita H, Allison JP. PD-1 and CTLA-4 combination blockade expands infiltrating T cells and reduces regulatory T and myeloid cells within B16 melanoma tumors. *Proc Natl Acad Sci U S A.* 2010;107(9):4275−4280.
23. Larkin J, Hodi FS, Wolchok JD. Combined nivolumab and ipilimumab or monotherapy in untreated melanoma. *N Engl J Med.* 2015;373(13):1270−1271.
24. Hammers HJ, Plimack ER, Infante JR, et al. Safety and efficacy of nivolumab in combination with ipilimumab in metastatic renal cell carcinoma: the CheckMate 016 study. *J Clin Oncol.* 2017;35(34):3851−3858.
25. Escudier B, Tannir N, McDermott DF, et al. CheckMate 214: efficacy and safety of nivolumab + ipilimumab (N+I) v sunitinib (S) for treatment-naïve advanced or metastatic renal cell carcinoma. *Ann Oncol.* 2017;28(suppl 5):v605−v649.
26. Motzer RJ, Tannir NM, McDermott DF, et al. Nivolumab plus ipilimumab versus sunitinib in advanced renal-cell carcinoma. *N Engl J Med.* 2018;378(14):1277−1290.
27. Heng DY, Xie W, Regan MM, et al. Prognostic factors for overall survival in patients with metastatic renal cell carcinoma treated with vascular endothelial growth factor-targeted agents: results from a large, multicenter study. *J Clin Oncol.* 2009;27(34):5794−5799.
28. Lara P, Bauer TM, Hamid O, et al. Epacadostat plus pembrolizumab in patients with advanced RCC: preliminary phase I/II results from ECHO-202/KEYNOTE-037. *J Clin Oncol.* 2017;35(suppl 15):4515.
29. Fong L, Forde PM, Powderly JD, et al. Safety and clinical activity of adenosine A2a receptor (A2aR) antagonist, CPI-444, in anti-PD1/PDL1 treatment-refractory renal cell (RCC) and non-small cell lung cancer (NSCLC) patients. *J Clin Oncol.* 2017;35(suppl 15):3004.

30. Sanborn RE, Pishvaian MJ, Kluger HM, et al. Clinical results with combination of anti-CD27 agonist antibody, varlilumab, with anti-PD1 antibody nivolumab in advanced cancer patients. *J Clin Oncol.* 2017;35(suppl 15):3007.

31. Gabrilovich DI, Chen HL, Girgis KR, et al. Production of vascular endothelial growth factor by human tumors inhibits the functional maturation of dendritic cells. *Nat Med.* 1996;2(10):1096–1103.

32. Finke JH, Rini B, Ireland J, et al. Sunitinib reverses type-1 immune suppression and decreases T-regulatory cells in renal cell carcinoma patients. *Clin Cancer Res.* 2008;14(20):6674–6682.

33. Ko JS, Zea AH, Rini BI, et al. Sunitinib mediates reversal of myeloid-derived suppressor cell accumulation in renal cell carcinoma patients. *Clin Cancer Res.* 2009;15(6):2148–2157.

34. Chowdhury S, McDermott DF, Voss MH, et al. A phase I/II study to assess the safety and efficacy of pazopanib (PAZ) and pembrolizumab (PEM) in patients (pts) with advanced renal cell carcinoma (aRCC). *J Clin Oncol.* 2017;35(suppl 15):4506.

35. Atkins MB, Plimack ER, Puzanov I, et al. Axitinib in combination with pembrolizumab in patients with advanced renal cell cancer: a non-randomised, open-label, dose-finding, and dose-expansion phase 1b trial. *Lancet Oncol.* 2018;19(3):405–415.

36. Choueiri TK, Larkin JMG, Oya M, et al. First-line avelumab + axitinib therapy in patients (pts) with advanced renal cell carcinoma (aRCC): results from a phase Ib trial. *J Clin Oncol.* 2017;35(suppl 15):4504.

37. Lee C, Makker V, Rasco D, et al. A phase 1b/2 trial of Lenvatinib plus pembrolizumab in patients with renal cell carcinoma. *Ann Oncol.* 2017;28(suppl 5):v295–v329.

38. McDermott DF, Atkins MB, Motzer RJ, et al. A phase II study of atezolizumab (atezo) with or without bevacizumab (bev) versus sunitinib (sun) in untreated metastatic renal cell carcinoma (mRCC) patients (pts). *J Clin Oncol.* 2017;35(suppl 6):431.

39. Escudier B, Barthelemy P, Ravaud A, Negrier S, Needle MN, Albiges L. Tivozanib combined with nivolumab: phase Ib/II study in metastatic renal cell carcinoma (mRCC). *J Clin Oncol.* 2018;36(suppl 6):618.

40. Nadal RM, Mortazavi A, Stein M, et al. Results of phase I plus expansion cohorts of cabozantinib (Cabo) plus nivolumab (Nivo) and CaboNivo plus ipilimumab (Ipi) in patients (pts) with with metastatic urothelial carcinoma (mUC) and other genitourinary (GU) malignancies. *J Clin Oncol.* 2018;36(suppl 6):515.

41. Motzer RJ, Powles T, Atkins MB, et al. IMmotion151: a randomized phase III study of atezolizumab plus bevacizumab vs sunitinib in untreated metastatic renal cell carcinoma (mRCC). *J Clin Oncol.* 2018;36(suppl 6):578.

42. Motzer RJ, Mazumdar M, Bacik J, Berg W, Amsterdam A, Ferrara J. Survival and prognostic stratification of 670 patients with advanced renal cell carcinoma. *J Clin Oncol.* 1999;17(8):2530–2540.

43. Ravaud A. Adjuvant sunitinib in renal-cell carcinoma. *N Engl J Med.* 2017;376(9):893.

44. Zhu J, Armstrong AJ, Friedlander TW, et al. Biomarkers of immunotherapy in urothelial and renal cell carcinoma: PD-L1, tumor mutational burden, and beyond. *J Immunother Cancer.* 2018;6(1):4.

45. Routy B, Le Chatelier E, Derosa L, et al. Gut microbiome influences efficacy of PD-1-based immunotherapy against epithelial tumors. *Science.* 2018;359(6371):91–97.

46. von der Maase H, Hansen SW, Roberts JT, et al. Gemcitabine and cisplatin versus methotrexate, vinblastine, doxorubicin, and cisplatin in advanced or metastatic bladder cancer: results of a large, randomized, multinational, multicenter, phase III study. *J Clin Oncol.* 2000;18(17):3068–3077.

47. Baumeister SH, Freeman GJ, Dranoff G, Sharpe AH. Coinhibitory pathways in immunotherapy for cancer. *Annu Rev Immunol.* 2016;34:539–573.

48. Lee HT, Lee JY, Lim H, et al. Molecular mechanism of PD-1/PD-L1 blockade via anti-PD-L1 antibodies atezolizumab and durvalumab. *Sci Rep.* 2017;7(1):5532.

49. Inman BA, Longo TA, Ramalingam S, Harrison MR. Atezolizumab: a PD-L1-blocking antibody for bladder cancer. *Clin Cancer Res.* 2017;23(8):1886–1890.

50. Deng R, Bumbaca D, Pastuskovas CV, et al. Preclinical pharmacokinetics, pharmacodynamics, tissue distribution, and tumor penetration of anti-PD-L1 monoclonal antibody, an immune checkpoint inhibitor. *mAbs.* 2016;8(3):593–603.

51. Herbst RS, Soria JC, Kowanetz M, et al. Predictive correlates of response to the anti-PD-L1 antibody MPDL3280A in cancer patients. *Nature.* 2014;515(7528):563–567.

52. Powles T, Eder JP, Fine GD, et al. MPDL3280A (anti-PD-L1) treatment leads to clinical activity in metastatic bladder cancer. *Nature.* 2014;515(7528):558–562.

53. Rosenberg JE, Hoffman-Censits J, Powles T, et al. Atezolizumab in patients with locally advanced and metastatic urothelial carcinoma who have progressed following treatment with platinum-based chemotherapy: a single-arm, multicentre, phase 2 trial. *Lancet.* 2016;387(10031):1909–1920.

54. Powles T, Loriot Y, Duran I, et al. IMvigor211: a phase III randomized study examining Atezolizumab vs. Chemotherapy for Platinum-Treated Advanced Urothelial Carcinoma. In: *EACR-AACR-SIC Special Conference 2017: The Challenges of Optimizing Immuno- and Targeted Therapies: From Cancer Biology to the Clinic.* Florence, Italy: 2017.

55. Powles T, Duran I, van der Heijden MS, et al. Atezolizumab versus chemotherapy in patients with platinum-treated locally advanced or metastatic urothelial carcinoma (IMvigor211): a multicentre, open-label, phase 3 randomised controlled trial. *Lancet.* 2018;391(10122):748–757.

56. Balar AV, Galsky MD, Rosenberg JE, et al. Atezolizumab as first-line treatment in cisplatin-ineligible patients with locally advanced and metastatic urothelial carcinoma: a single-arm, multicentre, phase 2 trial. *Lancet.* 2017;389(10064):67–76.

57. Rimm DL, Han G, Taube JM, et al. A prospective, multi-institutional, pathologist-based assessment of 4 immunohistochemistry assays for PD-L1 expression in non-small cell lung cancer. *JAMA Oncol.* 2017;3(8): 1051−1058.

58. Ratcliffe MJ, Sharpe A, Midha A, et al. Agreement between programmed cell death Ligand-1 diagnostic assays across multiple protein expression cutoffs in non-small cell lung cancer. *Clin Cancer Res.* 2017;23(14):3585−3591.

59. Massard C, Gordon MS, Sharma S, et al. Safety and efficacy of durvalumab (MEDI4736), an anti-programmed cell death Ligand-1 immune checkpoint inhibitor, in patients with advanced urothelial bladder cancer. *J Clin Oncol.* 2016;34(26):3119−3125.

60. Donahue RN, Lepone LM, Grenga I, et al. Analyses of the peripheral immunome following multiple administrations of avelumab, a human IgG1 anti-PD-L1 monoclonal antibody. *J Immunother Cancer.* 2017;5:20.

61. Apolo AB, Infante JR, Balmanoukian A, et al. Avelumab, an anti-programmed death-Ligand 1 antibody, in patients with refractory metastatic urothelial carcinoma: results from a multicenter, phase Ib study. *J Clin Oncol.* 2017; 35(19):2117−2124.

62. Plimack ER, Bellmunt J, Gupta S, et al. Safety and activity of pembrolizumab in patients with locally advanced or metastatic urothelial cancer (KEYNOTE-012): a non-randomised, open-label, phase 1b study. *Lancet Oncol.* 2017;18(2):212−220.

63. Bellmunt J, de Wit R, Vaughn DJ, et al. Pembrolizumab as second-line therapy for advanced urothelial carcinoma. *New Engl J Med.* 2017;376(11):1015−1026.

64. Sharma P, Callahan MK, Bono P, et al. Nivolumab monotherapy in recurrent metastatic urothelial carcinoma (CheckMate 032): a multicentre, open-label, two-stage, multi-arm, phase 1/2 trial. *Lancet Oncol.* 2016;17(11): 1590−1598.

65. Sharma P, Retz M, Siefker-Radtke A, et al. Nivolumab in metastatic urothelial carcinoma after platinum therapy (CheckMate 275): a multicentre, single-arm, phase 2 trial. *Lancet Oncol.* 2017;18(3):312−322.

66. Carthon BC, Wolchok JD, Yuan J, et al. Preoperative CTLA-4 blockade: tolerability and immune monitoring in the setting of a presurgical clinical trial. *Clin Cancer Res.* 2010;16(10):2861−2871.

67. Comin-Anduix B, Escuin-Ordinas H, Ibarrondo FJ. Tremelimumab: research and clinical development. *Onco Targets Ther.* 2016;9:1767−1776.

68. Segal NH, Logan TF, Hodi FS, et al. Results from an integrated safety analysis of Urelumab, an agonist anti-CD137 monoclonal antibody. *Clin Cancer Res.* 2017; 23(8):1929−1936.

69. Infante JR, Hansen AR, Pishvaian MJ, et al. A phase Ib dose escalation study of the OX40 agonist MOXR0916 and the PD-L1 inhibitor atezolizumab in patients with advanced solid tumors. *J Clin Oncol.* 2016;34(supp 15):101.

70. Siegel RL, Miller KD, Jemal A. Cancer statistics, 2017. *CA Cancer J Clin.* 2017;67(1):7−30.

71. de Bono JS, Oudard S, Ozguroglu M, et al. Prednisone plus cabazitaxel or mitoxantrone for metastatic castration-resistant prostate cancer progressing after docetaxel treatment: a randomised open-label trial. *Lancet.* 2010; 376(9747):1147−1154.

72. Tannock IF, de Wit R, Berry WR, et al. Docetaxel plus prednisone or mitoxantrone plus prednisone for advanced prostate cancer. *N Engl J Med.* 2004;351(15):1502−1512.

73. Beer TM, Tombal B. Enzalutamide in metastatic prostate cancer before chemotherapy. *N Engl J Med.* 2014; 371(18):1755−1756.

74. Scher HI, Fizazi K, Saad F, et al. Increased survival with enzalutamide in prostate cancer after chemotherapy. *N Engl J Med.* 2012;367(13):1187−1197.

75. de Bono JS, Logothetis CJ, Molina A, et al. Abiraterone and increased survival in metastatic prostate cancer. *N Engl J Med.* 2011;364(21):1995−2005.

76. Ryan CJ, Smith MR, de Bono JS, et al. Abiraterone in metastatic prostate cancer without previous chemotherapy. *N Engl J Med.* 2013;368(2):138−148.

77. Parker C, Nilsson S, Heinrich D, et al. Alpha emitter radium-223 and survival in metastatic prostate cancer. *N Engl J Med.* 2013;369(3):213−223.

78. Kantoff PW, Higano CS, Shore ND, et al. Sipuleucel-T immunotherapy for castration-resistant prostate cancer. *N Engl J Med.* 2010;363(5):411−422.

79. Slovin SF, Higano CS, Hamid O, et al. Ipilimumab alone or in combination with radiotherapy in metastatic castration-resistant prostate cancer: results from an open-label, multicenter phase I/II study. *Ann Oncol.* 2013; 24(7):1813−1821.

80. Madan RA, Mohebtash M, Arlen PM, et al. Ipilimumab and a poxviral vaccine targeting prostate-specific antigen in metastatic castration-resistant prostate cancer: a phase 1 dose-escalation trial. *Lancet Oncol.* 2012; 13(5):501−508.

81. Jochems C, Tucker JA, Tsang KY, et al. A combination trial of vaccine plus ipilimumab in metastatic castration-resistant prostate cancer patients: immune correlates. *Cancer Immunol Immunother.* 2014;63(4):407−418.

82. van den Eertwegh AJ, Versluis J, van den Berg HP, et al. Combined immunotherapy with granulocyte-macrophage colony-stimulating factor-transduced allogeneic prostate cancer cells and ipilimumab in patients with metastatic castration-resistant prostate cancer: a phase 1 dose-escalation trial. *Lancet Oncol.* 2012;13(5):509−517.

83. Kwon ED, Drake CG, Scher HI, et al. Ipilimumab versus placebo after radiotherapy in patients with metastatic castration-resistant prostate cancer that had progressed after docetaxel chemotherapy (CA184-043): a multicentre, randomised, double-blind, phase 3 trial. *Lancet Oncol.* 2014;15(7):700−712.

84. Beer TM, Kwon ED, Drake CG, et al. Randomized, double-blind, phase III trial of ipilimumab versus placebo in asymptomatic or minimally symptomatic patients with metastatic chemotherapy-naive castration-resistant prostate cancer. *J Clin Oncol.* 2017;35(1):40−47.

85. Demaria S, Ng B, Devitt ML, et al. Ionizing radiation inhibition of distant untreated tumors (abscopal effect) is immune mediated. *Int J Radiat Oncol Biol Phys.* 2004; 58(3):862−870.

86. Kaur P, Asea A. Radiation-induced effects and the immune system in cancer. *Front Oncol.* 2012;2:191.

87. Demaria S, Kawashima N, Yang AM, et al. Immune-mediated inhibition of metastases after treatment with local radiation and CTLA-4 blockade in a mouse model of breast cancer. *Clin Cancer Res.* 2005;11(2 Pt 1):728−734.

88. Postow MA, Callahan MK, Barker CA, et al. Immunologic correlates of the abscopal effect in a patient with melanoma. *N Engl J Med.* 2012;366(10):925−931.

89. Stamell EF, Wolchok JD, Gnjatic S, Lee NY, Brownell I. The abscopal effect associated with a systemic anti-melanoma immune response. *Int J Radiat Oncol Biol Phys.* 2013; 85(2):293−295.

90. Topalian SL, Hodi FS, Brahmer JR, et al. Safety, activity, and immune correlates of anti-PD-1 antibody in cancer. *N Engl J Med.* 2012;366(26):2443−2454.

91. Bishop JL, Sio A, Angeles A, et al. PD-L1 is highly expressed in Enzalutamide resistant prostate cancer. *Oncotarget.* 2015;6(1):234−242.

92. Graff JN, Alumkal JJ, Drake CG, et al. Early evidence of anti-PD-1 activity in enzalutamide-resistant prostate cancer. *Oncotarget.* 2016;7(33):52810−52817.

CHAPTER 7

Gynecologic Malignancies

KRISTEN STARBUCK, MD • PAUL MAYOR, MD, MS • EMESE ZSIROS, MD, PHD

INTRODUCTION

Harnessing the immune system to recognize and eliminate cancer has recently become a major focus of cancer research as one of the new treatment modalities for patients with advanced-stage or recurrent disease. Targeted therapies have mostly shown significant clinical benefit in cancers harboring a single dominant mutation, and their antitumor efficacies are generally limited in patients with gynecologic cancers owing to high degree of cancer clonal heterogeneity in these tumors. On the other hand, tumor heterogeneity can induce increased immunogenicity,[1] which is advantageous for other treatment approaches such as immunotherapy.[2]

The role of immunotherapy in gynecologic cancers is an active area of investigation, as the currently available treatment options are only palliative for most patients with advanced-stage or recurrent disease. Several immunotherapy strategies have been tried in this patient population, including cytokines, vaccines, immune modulators, adoptive transfer of endogenous or genetically modified T-cells as well as immune checkpoint inhibitors. As immune checkpoint inhibitors have recently become more widely available, there are numerous ongoing clinical trials to determine the optimal use of these drugs in gynecologic cancers. Ongoing trials include the use of checkpoint inhibitors as single-agent drugs or in combination with other immunotherapy or immune function—enhancing drugs, as well as trials that aim to determine the optimal patient population for these regimens.[3] Here we will review the new emerging data on immune checkpoint inhibitors in the three major gynecologic cancer sites, ovarian, endometrial, and cervical cancers.

OVARIAN CANCER

Every year more than 22,000 women in the United States are diagnosed with epithelial ovarian cancer (EOC). As the fifth most common cancer death for women, it accounts for more than 14,000 deaths each year in the United States,[4] and it is the most lethal gynecologic cancer in the developed world.[5] Owing to its insidious onset, most women present with advanced-stage disease, and standard treatment includes upfront surgery followed by a combination of platinum- and taxane-based chemotherapy.[6] Although most patients respond well to first-line therapy, most women experience recurrence and eventually succumb to the disease; thus, novel approaches to treat ovarian cancer are much needed.

Ovarian cancer is an immunogenic tumor and an ideal cancer type to consider for immunomodulatory approaches among gynecologic malignancies. Several studies investigating the role of immune cells in ovarian cancer demonstrated that over 50% of women with ovarian cancer have CD3+ tumor-infiltrating T-lymphocytes (TILs) within tumor islets, which lead to improved survival in this patient population.[7,8] These TILs are able to recognize tumor-specific antigens,[9-11] undergo oligoclonal expansion in response to tumor antigen challenge,[10] and display tumor-specific cytolytic activity in vitro.[9] Zhang et al. showed that patients with tumors harboring increased TILs had a median progression-free survival (PFS) of 22.4 months, versus 5.8 months in patients without CD3+ TIL infiltration. Overall survival (OS) was similarly improved in patients with T-cell infiltration at 50.3 months versus 18 months in patients without T-cell infiltration.[8] As expected, the 5-year OS for patients whose tumors had increased T-cell infiltration was 38% versus 4.5% for patients without T-cell infiltration. This association persisted even in patients in the most favorable prognostic group, treated with optimal tumor debulking and platinum—taxane combination chemotherapy.

It has been observed that tumor-specific T-cells in the blood and in the tumor microenvironment do not always correlate with tumor control. Even when vaccination with tumor-specific antigens produces specific T-cell responses,[12] regression is not often observed. It has become clear that the type of T-cells present in the tumor microenvironment are important in predicting response[13] and that tumors induce immune tolerance

TABLE 7.1
Classification of Ovarian Cancer by Immunologic Microenvironment

Histologic Subtype	N	% TOTAL FOR HISTOLOGIC SUBTYPE			
		TIL+ PD-L1+ "Adaptive Immune Resistance"	TIL− PD-L1− "Immunologic Ignorance"	TIL− PD-L1+ "Intrinsic Induction"	TIL+ PD-L1− "Tolerance"
High-grade serous	112	57.4	5.1	0	37.4
Low-grade serous	11	0	9.1	0	90.9
Mucinous	30	26.7	16.7	0	56.7
Endometrioid	125	22.4	14.4	1.6	61.6
Clear cell	129	16.4	30.2	0	53.5

N, number of patients; TIL, tumor-infiltrating T-lymphocytes.
Adapted from Webb JR, Milne K, Kroeger DR, Nelson BH. PD-L1 expression is associated with tumor-infiltrating T cells and favorable prognosis in high-grade serous ovarian cancer. *Gynecol Oncol*. 2016;141(2):293−302 and Teng MW, Ngiow SF, Ribas A, Smyth MJ. Classifying cancers based on T-cell infiltration and PD-L1. *Cancer Res*. 2015;75(11):2139−2145.

mechanisms to avoid immune destruction.[14,15] Investigation into immune tolerance strategies found that the presence of CD4+ CD25+ T-regulatory cells (Tregs) promote a tumor-protective environment and confer a poor prognosis.[13,16,17] Murine models have demonstrated that depletion of intratumoral Tregs improves tumor control and improves response to immune-based therapies.[17−19]

More recently, intratumoral CD8+ was compared with CD3+ as a marker for immune cell infiltration and observed to be superior.[20−22] CD8+ correlates with improved disease-specific survival in a large cohort of ovarian cancer patients, especially in those with serous histology.[23,24] It is the only marker able to significantly predict outcome on multivariate analysis.[25] Two recent analyses used data on TILs in tumor specimens to categorize the immune microenvironment in melanomas and ovarian cancer (Table 7.1).[23,26] As molecular profiling of tumors begins to guide therapy in many cancer types, it is probable that characterization of the immune microenvironment will guide selection of patients who are most appropriate for immunotherapy.[27]

Clinical Trials With Immune Checkpoint Inhibitors in Ovarian Cancer

Anti−PD-1 and anti−PD-L1

Most of the data using immune checkpoint inhibitors in patients with gynecologic malignancies come from ovarian cancer patients, as most of the early studies were conducted in this patient population. The first trial to test programmed cell death-1 (PD-1) blockade in ovarian cancer was Brahmer et al. in 2012.[28] This trial included 17 ovarian cancer patients in addition to other solid tumors. In the ovarian cancer cohort, they had one patient with partial response (PR) and two patients with stable disease.[28] They concluded that the response rates of 6%−17% and prolonged stabilization of disease in several patients provided rationale to continue exploring the role of PD-1 blockade. In 2015, Hamanishi et al.[29] reported on their results with nivolumab in 20 ovarian cancer patients. Two patients had a complete response, one patient had a PR, and six patients had stable disease. In some cases, responses were sustained for several months, but the median PFS for all patients was 14 weeks. In this trial, 80% of patients had tumors expressing programmed cell death ligand-1 (PD-L1); however, this did not correlate with response to treatment. Similarly, treatment with pembrolizumab in a phase Ib trial with 26 patients demonstrated an overall response rate (ORR) of 11.5%.[30] Two patients had a complete response, and one patient had a PR; these results were sustained for greater than 6 months. Recently another larger trial using PD-L1 inhibitor avelumab was reported in 2016. This trial included 124 platinum-resistant or -refractory ovarian cancer patients, the largest trial to date. The ORR was similar to previous trials at 11.3%, with 12 PRs and 55 patients with stable disease.[31] Only 6.5% of patients experienced grade 3 or worse adverse events, demonstrating it was well tolerated. This represents a respectable outcome in this heavily pretreated platinum-resistant population, for which there are few alternative therapies. Based on the results of these trials, there are now a large number of ongoing clinical trials with several PD-1 and PD-L1 inhibitors, alone and in combination with other therapies in ovarian cancer (Tables 7.2 and 7.3). The list of completed trials to date using immune checkpoint inhibitors in ovarian cancer can be found in Table 7.2.

Anti—CTLA-4

Anti—CTLA-4 antibodies, which originally had success in treating melanoma, also exhibit activity in ovarian cancer. Clinical benefit of these antibodies as single agents has been limited to a small subset of patients; thus, these limitations necessitate the development of combination strategies that extend therapeutic benefit to a broader range of patients. In the initial report on CTLA-4 inhibition in ovarian cancer, nine patients with recurrent EOC, previously treated with GVAX vaccine (ovarian cancer vaccine transduced with granulocyte-macrophage colony-stimulating factor), were treated with ipilimumab. One PR was reported, lasting in excess of 35 months. Additionally, stable disease was described in three patients and in one patient, lasted greater than 6 months.[32] There is no clinical evidence for tremelimumab or other anti—CTLA-4 antibodies in ovarian cancer yet, and ongoing clinical trials are listed in Table 7.3.

Combination Approaches

Immune checkpoint inhibition holds promise in the treatment of ovarian cancer, as in some cases there have been dramatic responses. However in most cases, monotherapy in patients with relapsed platinum-resistant EOC results in ORRs of 10%—15%; thus, there is a need to develop rational combination approaches. There are several trials currently exploring dual checkpoint inhibitor blockade and other combinatorial approaches. Fully harnessing the power of immune-mediated cytotoxicity requires sufficient T-cell receptor stimulation and the ability to overcome immune escape mechanisms in the tumor microenvironment. Eliciting clinically significant responses will require blockade of several immune pathways simultaneously, as tumors are facile at adapting to selective pressures and monotherapy is usually not sufficient. Preclinical mouse models have been encouraging, as a significant proportion of TILs have dual expression of CTLA-4 and PD-1.[33] Furthermore, functional assays in these models reveal that PD-1 signaling is critical to the suppressive role of tumor-derived Tregs and support the concept that dual-positive PD-1+CTLA-4+ Tregs are responsible for the suppressor function.[33] Dual checkpoint inhibitor treatment with anti—PD-1 and anti—CTLA-4 antibodies resulted in restored T-cell—mediated cytotoxicity, and the response rates in the tumor-bearing

mice were twice as high as those treated with monotherapy.[33] Another important consideration in the T-cell response is the amount of antigen needed to provoke sufficient T-cell receptor signaling, and this has been associated with tumor mutational load.[34] Because of this, adjuvant immunotherapy may work most efficiently when initiated before surgery or neoadjuvant chemotherapy, as these techniques increase exposure to tumor antigens through rapid tumor cell destruction. Chemotherapy, radiation therapy, kinase inhibitors, and epigenetic modulating agents enhance the immunogenicity of the tumor, conceivably leading to increased response rates. Analysis of pre- and postneoadjuvant chemotherapy ovarian cancer specimens revealed increased TILs in two out of three identified immunologic patterns but no change in immunosuppressive cell populations.[35] A preliminary study in triple-negative breast cancer combined nanoparticle albumin-bound paclitaxel with atezolizumab; the confirmed ORR was 41.7%.[36] Investigators noted that the response rate was significantly higher when the combination was given as first-line therapy instead of salvage therapy after recurrence. Research is still needed to further elucidate the mechanisms of shifting tumor microenvironment in response to chemotherapy, and several clinical trials are open to address these questions (Table 7.3).

Of particular interest in ovarian cancer is combination therapy with Poly-ADP ribose polymerase inhibitors (PARP inhibitors) and antiangiogenic agents (especially vascular endothelial growth factor [VEGF]-targeting bevacizumab or VEGF receptor tyrosine kinase inhibitor cediranib). Both classes of inhibitors already have proven benefit in ovarian cancer, have been shown to influence the tumor immune landscape as determined by in vivo models of ovarian cancer, and have demonstrated benefit when combined with checkpoint inhibitors in preclinical studies.[37–40] VEGF inhibitors are particularly effective; they act by normalizing the leaky, abnormal tumor vasculature. Tumor neovasculature is characterized by disruption in the endothelial cells lining blood vessels and abnormal organization of supporting pericytes and the basement membrane. This leads to increased permeability, ascites formation, and increased interstitial pressure within the tumor bed, as well as efflux of tumor cells into lymphatic and vascular pathways.[41–43] VEGF has also been implicated in the downregulation of endothelial adhesion molecules, impaired maturation of dendritic cells, and increased expression of PD-L1.[15,44] Inhibition of these processes can improve both drug delivery and effector T-cell homing to the tumor.[15]

TABLE 7.2
Checkpoint Inhibitor Trials With Results in Ovarian Cancer

Target/Antibody	Trial ID	Population	Phase	N	Results	Median PFS (week)	≥ G3 AE (%)	References
CTLA-4 Ipilimumab		Recurrent EOC, previously treated with GVAX vaccine	I	2	PR 1 (6+ mo.) SD 1 (2+ mo.)	NR	0	Hodi et al.[32]
PD-1 Nivolumab	UMIN000005714	Relapsed platinum-resistant EOC	II	20	CR 2 (11+ mo.) PR 1 (11+ mo.) SD 6 (1 for 11+ mo.)	14.0	40	Hamanishi et al.[29]
PD-1 Pembrolizumab	NCT02054806 (KEYNOTE-028)	Advanced EOC, PD-L1 positive	Ib	26	ORR 11.5% CR 1 (6+ mo.) PR 2 (6+ mo.) SD 8 (2 for 6+ mo.)	NR	3.8	Varga et al.[30]
PD-L1 BMS-936559[a]	NCT00729664	Recurrent EOC	I	17	PR (1; 1.3+ mo.) SD (3; 6+ mo.)	NR	11.7	Brahmer et al.[28]
PD-L1 Avelumab[b]	NCT01772004	Recurrent EOC	Ib	124	PR 12 SD 55	11.3	6.5	Disis (2016)[28a]

AE, adverse events; *ORR*, overall response rate (CR/PR status not provided); *CR*, complete response; *EOC*, epithelial ovarian cancer; *mo.*,months; *N*, number of ovarian cancer patients treated; *NR*, not reported; *PFS*, progressiong-free survival; *PR*, partial response; *SD*, stable disease.
[a] No longer under clinical development.
[b] As of data cutoff date: May 10, 2016.

TABLE 7.3
Ongoing Checkpoint Inhibitor Trials in Ovarian Cancer

Status	Trial ID	Phase	Eligible Population	Intervention
Active, not recruiting	NCT01611558	II	Recurrent platinum-sensitive EOC	Ipilimumab
Active, not recruiting	NCT02674061 (KEYNOTE 100)	I/II	Recurrent EOC with ≤5 prior lines of therapy	Pembrolizumab
Recruiting	NCT01772004 (JAVELIN Solid Tumor)	I	Recurrent/metastatic solid tumors including EOC	Avelumab
Recruiting	NCT02669914	II	Recurrent epithelial cancer (including EOC) with brain metastases	Durvalumab
Recruiting	NCT02498600	II	Recurrent or persistent EOC	Nivolumab +/− ipilimumab
Recruiting	NCT03126110	I	Locally advanced or metastatic solid tumors, including EOC	INCAGN01876 + nivolumab INCAGN01876 + ipilimumab INCAGN01876 + nivolumab + ipilimumab
Recruiting	NCT03026062	I/II	Recurrent, platinum-resistant EOC	Durvalumab and tremelimumab; In combination versus sequentially
Active, not recruiting	NCT01975831	I	Recurrent or refractory EOC, breast, colorectal, RCC, or cervical cancer	Tremelimumab + MEDI4736 (Anti–PD-L1 Ab)
Recruiting	NCT02485990	I/II	Recurrent or persistent EOC	Tremelimumab + olaparib
Recruiting	NCT02657889 (KEYNOTE-162)	I/II	Recurrent EOC	Niraparib + pembrolizumab
Recruiting	NCT02571725	I/II	Recurrent EOC with germline BRCA1/2 mutation	Tremelimumab + olaparib
Recruiting	NCT03101280	I	Advanced, platinum-sensitive EOC	Atezolizumab + rucaparib
Active, not recruiting	NCT02734004	I/II	Recurrent solid tumors (including EOC with germline BRCA1/2 mutation)	Durvalumab + olaparib
Recruiting	NCT02484404	I/II	Advanced or recurrent solid tumors including ovarian cancer	Durvalumab + olaparib Durvalumab + cediranib Durvalumab + olaparib + cediranib
Active, not recruiting	NCT02537444 (KEYNOTE-091)	II	Recurrent, platinum-sensitive EOC	Acalabrutinib +/− pembrolizumab
Listed, not yet recruiting	NCT02953457	I/II	Recurrent or persistent or refractory EOC with germline or somatic BRCA1/2 mutation	Tremelimumab + durvalumab + olaparib
Recruiting	NCT02728830	I	Newly diagnosed EOC or uterine cancer	Pembrolizumab x one dose before primary surgical treatment

Continued

TABLE 7.3
Ongoing Checkpoint Inhibitor Trials in Ovarian Cancer—cont'd

Status	Trial ID	Phase	Eligible Population	Intervention
Recruiting	NCT02520154	II	Stage III/IV EOC with no prior therapy undergoing neoadjuvant chemotherapy	Neoadjuvant paclitaxel/carboplatin + pembrolizumab x three cycles; interval debulking surgery + three additional cycles of chemotherapy + pembrolizumab maintenance if no sign of progression
Recruiting	NCT02726997	I/II	Stage III/IV EOC with no prior therapy undergoing neoadjuvant chemotherapy	Neoadjuvant durvalumab + paclitaxel + carboplatin x three cycles, interval debulking surgery, three more cycles of combination treatment followed by maintenance durvalumab
Listed, not yet recruiting	NCT03126812	II	Stage IV EOC undergoing neoadjuvant chemotherapy	Neoadjuvant paclitaxel + carboplatin + pembrolizumab
Recruiting	NCT02834975	II	Advanced EOC undergoing neoadjuvant chemotherapy	Neoadjuvant paclitaxel + carboplatin + pembrolizumab
Recruiting	NCT03038100	III	Newly diagnosed stage III/IV EOC	Atezolizumab + paclitaxel/carboplatin/bevacizumab Placebo + paclitaxel/carboplatin/bevacizumab
Recruiting	NCT02658214	Ib	Advanced solid tumors including EOC in upfront treatment setting	Durvalumab + tremelimumab + paclitaxel + carboplatin
Recruiting	NCT02718417	III	Newly diagnosed EOC, s/p debulking or eligible for neoadjuvant therapy	Paclitaxel + carboplatin Paclitaxel + carboplatin + maintenance avelumab Paclitaxel + carboplatin + concurrent avelumab + maintenance avelumab
Recruiting	NCT02766582	II	Suboptimally cytoreduced EOC	Carboplatin/weekly paclitaxel/pembrolizumab + 12 months pembrolizumab maintenance
Recruiting	NCT03029598	I/II	Recurrent platinum-resistant EOC; ≥1 previous nonplatinum chemotherapy regimen	Carboplatin + pembrolizumab
Recruiting	NCT02440425	II	Persistent or platinum-resistant EOC after 1 prior line of platinum-based chemotherapy	Weekly paclitaxel + pembrolizumab every 3 weeks starting at day 8
Recruiting	NCT02853318	II	Recurrent/persistent EOC	Pembrolizumab + bevacizumab + oral metronomic cyclophosphamide
Recruiting	NCT02891824	III	Platinum-sensitive nonmucinous EOC	Placebo + bevacizumab + platinum-based chemotherapy Atezolizumab + bevacizumab + platinum-based chemotherapy
Recruiting	NCT02914470	I	Advanced breast and gynecologic cancers (including recurrent EOC)	Carboplatin + cyclophosphamide + atezolizumab

Status	NCT number	Phase	Condition	Treatment/intervention
Recruiting	NCT02608684	II	Recurrent platinum-resistant EOC	Pembrolizumab + gemcitabine + cisplatin
Recruiting	NCT02873962	II	Recurrent EOC	Nivolumab + bevacizumab
Recruiting	NCT02839707	II/III	Platinum-resistant EOC	PEGylated liposomal doxorubicin (PLD) + atezolizumab; PLD + bevacizumab + atezolizumab; PLD + bevacizumab
Recruiting	NCT02580058 (JAVELIN OVARIAN 200)	III	Recurrent, platinum-resistant, or platinum-refractory EOC	PLD; Avelumab; PLD + avelumab
Recruiting	NCT02331251	I/II	Recurrent solid tumors, including EOC	Pembrolizumab + PLD
Recruiting	NCT02865811	II	Platinum-resistant recurrent EOC	Pembrolizumab + PLD
Recruiting	NCT03085225	I	Recurrent platinum-sensitive EOC or soft tissue sarcomas	Durvalumab + trabectedin
Recruiting	NCT02900560	II	Recurrent, platinum-resistant, or platinum-refractory EOC	Azacitidine + pembrolizumab
Recruiting	NCT02811497	II	Recurrent, platinum-resistant EOC, MSS colorectal cancer, ER+, HER2- breast cancer	Azacitidine + durvalumab x three cycles + maintenance durvalumab
Recruiting	NCT02901899	II	Recurrent platinum-resistant EOC	Guadecitabine (DNMT inhibitor SGI-110) + pembrolizumab
Recruiting	NCT02659384	II	Recurrent platinum-resistant EOC	Bevacizumab; Atezolizumab + placebo; Atezolizumab + acetylsalicylic acid; Atezolizumab + bevacizumab + placebo; Atezolizumab + bevacizumab + acetylsalicylic acid
Listed, not yet recruiting	NCT03113487	II	Recurrent platinum-resistant EOC	Modified vaccinia virus ankara vaccine expressing p53 + pembrolizumab
Listed, not yet recruiting	NCT02963831	I/II	Recurrent platinum-resistant or refractory EOC	ONCOS-102 (GM-CSF–encoding adenovirus) + durvalumab
Recruiting	NCT02606305	Ib	Folate receptor α–positive advanced EOC	Mirvetuximab soravtansine (IMGN853) + bevacizumab; IMGN853 + carboplatin; IMGN853 + PLD; IMGN853 + pembrolizumab
Recruiting	NCT02575807	I/II	Recurrent platinum-resistant EOC	CRS-207 (live-attenuated double-deleted Listeria monocytogenes); CRS-207 + epacadostat; CRS-207 + pembrolizumab; CRS-207 + pembrolizumab + epacadostat
Listed, not yet recruiting	NCT03158935	I	Recurrent platinum-resistant EOC	Pembrolizumab in combination with or following adoptive cell therapy + IL-2

Continued

TABLE 7.3
Ongoing Checkpoint Inhibitor Trials in Ovarian Cancer—cont'd

Status	Trial ID	Phase	Eligible Population	Intervention
Recruiting	NCT01174121	II	Recurrent solid tumors including EOC; ≥ 2 prior lines of chemotherapy	Pembrolizumab in combination with Adoptive Cell Therapy + IL-2
Recruiting	NCT02725489	II	Advanced or metastatic EOC, breast, uterine, and cervical cancers	Durvalumab + vigil (autologous tumor cell immunotherapy)
Recruiting	NCT03073525	I	Advanced gynecologic cancers, including EOC without complete response to primary therapy	Vigil then vigil + atezolizumab Atezolizumab then vigil + atezolizumab
Listed, not yet recruiting	NCT03029403	II	Recurrent EOC	Pembrolizumab + DPX-Survivac + oral cyclophosphamide
Recruiting	NCT02298959	II	Metastatic solid tumors including platinum-resistant ovarian cancer	Ziv-aflibercept + pembrolizumab
Recruiting	NCT02452424	I/II	Recurrent or persistent solid tumors, including ovarian cancer	PLX3397 (CSF1R inhibitor) + pembrolizumab
Recruiting	NCT02955251	I	Advanced solid tumor that has progressed on standard therapies	Nivolumab + ABBV-428
Recruiting	NCT03071757	I	Locally advanced or metastatic solid tumors including EOC	Nivolumab + ABBV-368
Recruiting	NCT02335918	I/II	Advanced or metastatic solid tumors including ovarian cancer	Nivolumab + varlilumab (Anti–CD27 Ab)
Recruiting	NCT02526017	I	Advanced or recurrent EOC	Nivolumab + FPA008 (Anti–CSF1R Ab)
Recruiting	NCT02327078	I/II	Advanced or recurrent EOC with 1+ prior platinum-containing regimens	Nivolumab + epacadostat (IDO inhibitor)
Recruiting	NCT02178722	I/II	Recurrent solid tumors including EOC	Pembrolizumab + epacadostat
Recruiting	NCT02431559	I/II	Recurrent or persistent platinum-resistant EOC	Durvalumab + motolimod + PLD
Recruiting	NCT02764333	II	Recurrent or persistent platinum-resistant EOC	Durvalumab + TPIV200 (Multiepitope antifolate receptor vaccine)
Recruiting	NCT03100006	I/II	Recurrent EOC with 2+ prior lines of therapy	Nivolumab + oregovomab
Recruiting	NCT02943317	I	Recurrent platinum-resistant EOC	Durvalumab + defactinib (FAK inhibitor)
Recruiting	NCT02915523	Ib/II	Recurrent or progressive EOC after primary therapy	Avelumab +/− entinostat

Ab, antibody; *DNMT,* DNA methyltransferase; *EOC,* epithelial ovarian cancer; *GM-CSF,* granulocyte-macrophage colony-stimulating factor; *IDO,* indoleamine-pyrrole 2,3-dioxygenase; *IL-2,* interleukin-2; *MSS,* microsatellite stable; *RCC,* renal cell carcinoma.

It has been suggested that BRCA-mutated ovarian cancers are associated with a more immune-responsive molecular subtype,[45] and one study observed markers of higher immunogenicity with an increased CD8+/CD4+ ratio of TILs and higher peritumoral T-cells, supporting the idea that BRCA-mutant tumors might be more responsive to immunotherapy.[45,46] Analysis of the Cancer Genome Atlas (TCGA) Research Network dataset found that the well-established association of increased CD8+ TILs with improved survival was specific to tumors harboring intratumoral plasma cells and did not observe an association between CD8+ infiltration and BRCA1/2 status.[47] Furthermore, they observed synergistic T- and B-cell activity against tumors and were associated with cancer−testis antigen expression. Despite this, preclinical mouse models showed synergy between CTLA-4 inhibitors and PARP inhibitor therapy in ovarian cancer but not with the PD-1/PD-L1 axis and PARP inhibitors,[40] indicating further studies are needed to better elucidate antitumor response profiles in differing tumor subtypes. In human studies, preliminary phase I results with durvalumab/olaparib (NCT02484404) show that the combination has manageable toxicity and is showing activity both in mutated BRCA and wild type BRCA cancers.[48] Several trials are ongoing which combine CTLA-4, PD-1, or PD-L1 inhibitors with PARP inhibitor therapy (Table 7.3).

Lynch syndrome is another genetic alteration associated with EOC. In a European study analyzing the genetic, morphologic, and clinical characteristics of ovarian tumors in Lynch syndrome families, EOC developed at a younger age and had a higher likelihood of nonserous tumors, most commonly endometrioid (35%) and clear cell (17%) histologies.[49] This is meaningful in the context of advanced ovarian clear cell carcinomas (OCCCs), as they tend to have a limited response to chemotherapy and a poor prognosis; thus, alternative strategies are needed. In studying the immunogenicity of OCCC, 10%−15% were found to have high microsatellite instability (MSI-high)[50] and display higher infiltration of CD3+ TILs and PD-1+ TILs compared with corresponding MSI-low tumors.[51] Additionally, OCCC has a similar genomic profile to renal cell carcinoma (RCC); nivolumab was recently approved for the treatment of advanced clear cell renal cancer based on a 25% ORR and a 5-month survival advantage compared with everolimus (ORR of 5%) in the phase III Checkpoint 025 trial.[52] Based on these findings, OCCC may be more responsive to immune-based therapies and provides rationale for checkpoint blockade therapy.

Many distinct combination strategies are being explored in ongoing clinical trials, as listed in Table 7.3. In addition to PARP inhibitors and antiangiogenesis drugs, ongoing trials are testing immune checkpoint inhibitors in combination with agents such as DNA methyltransferase inhibitors, indoleamine-pyrrole 2,3-dioxygenase (IDO) inhibitors, tumor-targeting antibodies, tumor vaccines, oncolytic viral therapy, and adoptive cell therapy, as well as several others. The heterogeneity of ovarian cancer has made successful targeting of recurrent disease challenging; however, this heterogeneity may prove to be beneficial in targeting cancer cells by the immune system. As results of these, trials emerge and the tumor immune microenvironment is more clearly elucidated; combination approaches to immunotherapy will offer a new paradigm for optimal treatment of ovarian cancer and improve patient outcomes.

Measurement of Response to Treatment

Most cancer trials, including immunotherapy trials, commonly use RECIST 1.1 criteria to measure response to treatment.[53] When the primary endpoint is specified as tumor response, which is often the case in early phase trials, patients must have measurable disease to begin the trial. These lesions are measured at each subsequent evaluation to determine the response rate. Immunotherapies exhibit different patterns of response compared with traditional chemotherapies, as it frequently takes several months before response is noted. Tumor lesions may demonstrate early enlargement owing to immune flare at tumor sites before response. Therefore, using traditional RECIST 1.1 criteria can cause inaccurate interpretations of response. The need for new immune-specific response criteria was first addressed by the immune-related response criteria (irRC) in 2009 and was based on World Health Organization (WHO) criteria.[54] An immune-related RECIST (irRECIST) criterion was published in 2013, which combined elements of irRC and RECIST.[55] In 2017, the immune RECIST (iRECIST) criteria were developed, which standardized and validated immune response criteria. It evaluates for response after initial PD based on traditional RECIST criteria, taking into account the immune flare effect and the potential longer timeline for response.[56,57] It has been shown that traditional RECIST 1.1 could underestimate the benefit of pembrolizumab in up to 15% of patients with melanoma; therefore, using irRECIST or iRECIST could be more appropriate in the gynecologic patients receiving immunotherapy as well to prevent premature discontinuation of treatment.[55−58]

Identification of Predictive Biomarkers

As generally the response rate with single agent immune checkpoint inhibitors is not higher than 10%–15%, there is a critical need to identify predictive biomarkers to provide indication of efficacy in this patient population. Molecular characterization of tumors is becoming common, especially in clinical trials using targeted therapies. Deciphering the molecular complexities of tumors through genomic technologies may help determine the best approach to target cancer pathways. Ideally, patients could be matched with therapies based on biomarkers specific to their tumor; however, identification of a biomarker for immunotherapy has been challenging. PD-L1 expression has been associated with response to checkpoint blockade with PD-1 or PD-L1 inhibitors;[59,60] however, responses are still observed in some patients categorized as PD-L1 negative.[29,52,60,61] In a nivolumab trial in ovarian cancer, only 2/16 patients categorized as PD-L1 high had a response to therapy, and 1/4 PD-L1–low patients also had a response.[29] The pattern of PD-L1 expression may also be important; one recent paper described macrophages as the predominant PD-L1–expressing cells in ovarian tumors and, in this setting, were associated with improved prognosis.[23] Discrepancies in observations between studies could be explained by the use of different PD-L1 antibodies, but they also demonstrate the need for further understanding of immune biomarkers. Therefore, the use of PD-L1 in isolation to predict response or survival is insufficient. TIL infiltration has been used in conjunction with PD-L1 in other cancer types as a predictive biomarker.[62–64] For example, in non–small cell lung cancer (NSCLC), the presence of PD-L1 expression on TILs in the tumor microenvironment as opposed to tumor cells themselves predicted response to checkpoint blockade therapy with the PD-L1 inhibitor atezolizumab.[64] Furthermore, another study reported that TIL expression of PD-L1 at the invasive edge of melanomas was associated with response to pembrolizumab.[63] Conversely, a phase I trial including multiple tumor types that examined TIL infiltration did not find an association between TIL infiltration and response to therapy.[65] Examining both TIL infiltration and PD-L1 expression, as well as patterns of expression, might prove beneficial in ovarian cancer; however, novel immune biomarkers and combinations of biomarkers are necessary.

Mutational Load

The number of genetic alterations in a tumor, referred to as mutational load, may contribute to immunogenicity.

Genetic alterations result in the production of neoantigens that are perceived as "foreign" to the immune system and, therefore, provoke an immune response. Tumors characterized by a high mutational burden such as melanoma, NSCLC, and urothelial cancers have shown the highest response rates to checkpoint inhibition with PD-1 and PD-L1 therapy, in contrast to tumors with lower mutational burdens such as pancreatic and prostate cancers.[34] Studies in melanoma have shown that clinical response to checkpoint blockade is correlated with mutational load; however, there are patients with high mutational load who do not respond and some with low mutational load that do respond.[2,66,67]

Mismatch repair (MMR) defects lead to 10–100 times higher mutational load compared with tumors with intact MMR genes. MSI tumors have higher levels of immune checkpoint proteins (CTLA-4, PD-1, LAG3, etc.) and tend to respond better to checkpoint blockade therapy.[68–70] Ovarian cancer patients rarely have germline MMR defects; however, up to 29% of ovarian carcinomas harbor somatic loss of MMR protein expression.[71] It has yet to be determined whether this will predict improved response to checkpoint blockade in patients with MSI-high ovarian cancers.

Functional Assays

Other approaches to identify determinants of response to immunotherapy include functional assays, which aim to measure markers of immune cell function in the tumor microenvironment. This involves intracellular staining to assess markers of T-cell activation or function and interferon-γ signaling versus inhibitory signals such as TGF-β and IL-10. This could give a clear picture of the predominant immune environment (suppressive or responsive), but as of yet, this approach has not been widely tested or validated in association with response.

Human Microbiome

There is growing interest in the association between the human microbiome and the immune system, which has sparked interest in examining the relationship of the microbiome and its role in cancer. Recent evidence from murine models demonstrated that bacterial composition in the gut microbiome contributes to cancer immunotherapy efficacy. Researchers found that response to CTLA-4 blockade was dependent on T-cell responses specific for *Bacteroides thetaiotaomicron* or *B. fragilis*.[72] Tumors in mice that were kept germ-free or treated with antibiotics did not respond to CTLA-4 blockade, whereas mice treated with *B. fragilis* via oral gavage, immunized with *B. fragilis* polysaccharides or treated with *B. fragilis*–specific T-cells responded to CTLA-4 blockade.[72] Another preclinical model showed an association between specific intestinal species and the number of antigen-presenting cells.[73] In one of the first human studies, melanoma patients' baseline gut bacterial "signatures" were found to predict response to anti–PD-1 therapy, implying that modification of the gut microbiome during checkpoint blockade could influence response.[72] These early studies suggest that the gut microbiome contributes to the immune microenvironment, by either activating or suppressing tumor immunity. There are a few early ongoing trials in the ovarian cancer patients as well looking at human microbiome composition in relationship to response to checkpoint inhibitors.

Immune-Related Toxicities in Ovarian Cancer Patients

An important consideration in early phase trials is the side effect profile. Immunotherapies have a distinct toxicity profile compared with traditional chemotherapy. Compared with the bone marrow and gastrointestinal (GI) toxicities usually associated with platinum and taxane compounds, checkpoint inhibitors have more tolerable side effect profiles. These usually stem from boosting the immune system and include rash, diarrhea/colitis, hepatitis, pneumonitis, and endocrinopathies.[74] Because most patients in these trials have a poor prognosis and have had multiple prior lines of chemotherapy, quality of life is of foremost importance. It was noted in a combination trial in melanoma that 53% of patients had grade 3 or 4 adverse events—21% were dose-limiting, but all were reversible.[75] This combination as well as other combination therapies and their toxicities are currently being investigated in gynecologic cancers.

ENDOMETRIAL CANCER

It is estimated in 2017 that approximately 61,380 new cases of endometrial cancer will be diagnosed, making it the most commonly diagnosed cancer of the female genital tract in the United States.[76] The vast majority of these cases will be localized to the uterus at the time of diagnosis conferring an excellent 5-year survival over 95%. However, cases that are diagnosed with regional or distant spread confer a significantly worse 5-year survival of 16%–68% despite current available therapies.[76] For patients with recurrent or distant disease, novel therapies are needed to improve OS.

Predicting outcomes and determining the best treatment strategies for patients diagnosed with endometrial cancer is based on multiple factors including stage of disease and pathologic classification of the tumor.[77] The gold standard of classification for endometrial cancer is based on histologic review. Cancers that arise within the uterine corpus can be grouped pathologically into two broad categories: type I tumors which are low-grade and estrogen-related endometrioid carcinomas whereas type II tumors are nonendometrioid carcinomas of mainly serous or clear cell type.[78] Although these broad categories have existed for many years and can predict outcomes and response rates to traditional therapies, pathologic classification is limited in distinguishing certain high- and low-grade tumors in instances where histologies can be mixed or show no morphologically distinguishing features.[79] There is also significant variability between pathologist when reviewing tumors, which can lead to misclassification and incorrect therapy for patients.[80] In the age of molecular tumor testing, TCGA has developed a classification system based on genomic alterations, which place endometrial cancers into one of four categories: group 1 is endometrioid carcinomas with somatic activating mutations in polymerase ε (POLE) exonuclease and have very high mutation rates, group 2 is endometrioid carcinomas with MSI and MLH-1 promoter hypermethylation and high mutation rates, group 3 is endometrioid carcinomas with low copy number alterations, and group 4 is serous-like tumors with low mutation rates but a high frequency of p53 mutations.[81] Although these classifications have not made their way into clinical practice in a formal manner, they are being used experimentally to predict outcomes and response to therapies. More recently these categories have been used for enrollment of endometrial cancer patients into clinical trials involving immune-based therapies. The rationale behind these enrollment criteria is that group 1 and group 2 tumors have higher somatic mutational load, which results in formation of neoantigens leading to a more prominent lymphocytic infiltration. Therefore, checkpoint inhibition would release some of the inhibitory mechanisms placed on the infiltrating T-cells in the tumor and allow for a more robust immune response against these tumors. Based on this rationale, patients with group 1 or 2 tumors should have more of a response to checkpoint inhibition than patients with group 3 or 4 tumors.[79] Another way to group patients for clinical trial design is based on PD-L1 expression. Although PD-L1 expression is variable across tumor types, it has been shown to have a high level of expression in endometrial tumors (83%–100%).[82] Combining these rationales, of high

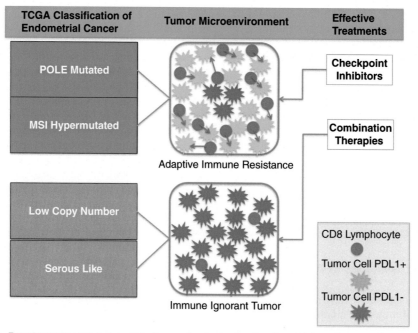

FIG. 7.1 Representative examples of the four molecular types of endometrial carcinoma. *MSI*, microsatellite instability; *TCGA*, the Cancer Genome Atlas.

mutational burden in group 1 and 2 tumors, along with high PD-L1 expression, makes a reasonable foundation for exploring checkpoint inhibition in certain molecular subtypes of endometrial cancer (Fig. 7.1).

Despite the rationale for studying the role of checkpoint inhibition in the treatment of endometrial cancer, current studies with mature data are limited. A phase II trial published in 2015 analyzed the efficacy of pembrolizumab in tumors with MMR deficiencies.[69] The vast majority of patients enrolled in this trial were patients with colorectal tumors; however, two patients with endometrial cancer were enrolled. This study established the concept that MMR-deficient tumors were significantly more responsive to PD-L1 blockade in comparison to MMR-proficient tumors. Of note, the two patients with endometrial cancer enrolled in this study did show a response to therapy. Further evidence from an expanded group of patients in the same trial design was presented as an abstract at the American Society of Clinical Oncology (ASCO) meeting in 2016 and showed that in 29 patients (which included nine patients with endometrial cancer) with noncolorectal MSI-high tumors, there was an overall response rate (ORR) of 48%.[70] Moreover, published in 2016, a study analyzing the effects of nivolumab in heavily pretreated POLE ultramutated and MSH6 hypermutated

endometrial tumors was completed.[83] Although only two patients participated in this study, both patients demonstrated a remarkable clinical response to nivolumab (both had PRs defined by RECIST criteria).[53] Published in May 2017, the KEYNOTE-028 study evaluated the role of pembrolizumab in patients with locally advanced or metastatic endometrial cancer that progressed after standard therapy.[84] In this phase II study, expression of PD-L1 was an inclusion criterion and was defined as membranous staining of at least 1% of tumor and associated inflammatory cells or positive staining in the stroma. Thirty-six patients were enrolled in the trial, and the overall response rate was 13%. These data are summarized in Table 7.4.

The rationale for the use of checkpoint inhibition in patients with endometrial cancer exists; however, clinical outcomes data remain in their infancy. The data, however, reflect the importance of selecting the most appropriate patient who will have the maximum benefit from the use of checkpoint inhibition. ORR in patients with MMR defect tumors are significantly higher than patients enrolled into studies based on more traditional criteria (PD-L1 expression and histology), which may increase the use of TCGA-defined categories when selecting patients for clinical trials (specifically group 1 and group 2 tumors with higher

TABLE 7.4
Completed and Interim Analyses of Trials Using Checkpoint Inhibition in Endometrial Cancer

Phase	Drug Evaluated	Eligibility Criteria	Patients Enrolled (n)	Outcome
II	Pembrolizumab	Tumors with MRD (primarily were colorectal)	n = 41 (two with endometrial cancer)	ORR of 40% for colorectal tumors with MMR defects and 71% for noncolorectal tumors with MMR defects
II	Pembrolizumab	Tumors with MRD	n = 29 (nine with endometrial cancer)	ORR of 48%
Case Report	Nivolumab	POLE ultramutated and MSH6 hypermutated endometrial tumors	n = 2	Partial response in 2/2 patients as defined by RECIST[53]
II	Pembrolizumab	PD-L1−positive endometrial tumors	n = 24	ORR of 13%

ORR, overall response rate; *MMR*, mismatch repair; *MRD*, minimal residual disease; *POLE*, DNA polymerase epsilon.

somatic mutational load). Given the limited but promising results in trials thus far, there are multiple phase I and II studies currently recruiting endometrial cancer patients for checkpoint inhibition alone and in combination with other interventions. These studies are summarized in Table 7.5.

CERVICAL CANCER

Cervical cancer is the fourth most common cancer in women worldwide, with approximately 530,000 cases and 265,000 deaths annually.[5] Although cervical cancer is largely preventable through human papillomavirus (HPV) vaccination campaigns and screening, many women do not have access to these measures, and there are few effective therapies beyond first-line treatment for advanced or recurrent cervical cancer.[85] Platinum-based chemotherapy has been shown to be most active and is now standard in the treatment of advanced or recurrent cervical cancer. However, the prognosis in these patients remains poor, with an estimated survival of approximately 1 year and poor quality of life.[86] Recently, antiangiogenesis therapy with bevacizumab was approved for treatment of advanced cervical cancer; this is the first time in many years any new treatment has shown an improvement in OS.[87] HPV-related cancers are good candidates for immunotherapy, as viral infections produce tumor neoantigens.[88,89] HPV infection provokes an immune response inducing HPV-specific cell-mediated immunity, as well as localized immune-suppressive responses with Tregs.[90] Researchers can take advantage of cell-mediated responses by developing vaccinations,

adoptive cell therapies, and interfering with immuno-suppressive pathways.

Checkpoint Inhibitors in Cervical Cancer
After notable success in melanoma, renewed enthusiasm for immune-based therapy led to preclinical testing and early clinical trials examining the applicability of immune checkpoint inhibitors to other cancers with a high neoantigen load. Analysis of the cervical cancer immune landscape supports further exploration into the use of checkpoint inhibitors in these patients. Initial investigation revealed PD-L1 expression in 95% of cervical intraepithelial neoplasia (CIN) and 80% of cervical squamous cell carcinomas (SCC) but was undetectable in normal cervical epithelium.[91] Expression of PD-1 and PD-L1 has also been correlated with impaired cell-mediated immunity in high-risk HPV and increasing grade of dysplasia.[92,93] Furthermore, a significant proportion of infiltrating CD8+ T-cells in cervical cancer express PD-1, suggesting that PD-1 blockade could have therapeutic potential in cervical cancer.[94] A recent paper by Stevanovic et al. further justifies pursuing PD-1 blockade in HPV-induced cancers.[95] This group of researchers demonstrated preferential expansion of T-cells specific to mutated cancer antigens (neoantigens) rather than typical viral antigens in virally induced cancers. These antigen-specific T-cells were found predominantly in the PD-1−expressing T-cell regions, suggesting that PD-1 blockade may unleash diverse antitumor T-cell reactivity.[95] Therefore, combination therapy with both traditional chemotherapy and checkpoint inhibitors may lead to synergistic effects and improved efficacy.

TABLE 7.5
Ongoing Trials Using Checkpoint Inhibition in Endometrial Cancer

Trial Status	Number	Phase	Trial Name	Eligible Cancers	Planned Intervention
Recruiting	NCT02899793	II	Pembrolizumab in ultramutated and hypermutated endometrial cancer	Endometrial	Pembrolizumab
Recruiting	NCT02630823	I	Pembrolizumab immunotherapy in endometrial carcinoma	Endometrial	Pembrolizumab
Not yet recruiting	NCT02549209	II	Phase II study of pembrolizumab in combination with carboplatin and paclitaxel for advanced or recurrent endometrial adenocarcinoma	Endometrial	Pembrolizumab plus paclitaxel and carboplatin
Recruiting	NCT02606305	Ib	Study of mirvetuximab soravtansine in combination with bevacizumab, carboplatin, PLD, or pembrolizumab in adults with folate receptor-α + advanced EOC, primary peritoneal, fallopian tube, or endometrial cancer	Gynecologic cancers including: endometrial	Pembrolizumab plus mirvetuximab soravtansine, bevacizumab, carboplatin, and/or PLD
Not yet recruiting	NCT03192059	II	Study of pembrolizumab, radiation, and immune modulatory cocktail in cervical/uterine cancer	Cervical and endometrial	Pembrolizumab
Recruiting	NCT02728830	I	A study of pembrolizumab on the tumoral immunoprofile of gynecologic cancers	Gynecologic cancers including endometrial	Pembrolizumab
Recruiting	NCT02646748	I	Pembrolizumab combined with itacitinib (INCB039110) and/or pembrolizumab combined with INCB050465 in advanced solid tumors	Solid tumors	Pembrolizumab plus itacitinib
Recruiting	NCT02628067	II	Study of pembrolizumab (MK-3475) in participants with advanced solid tumors (MK-3475—158/KEYNOTE-158)	Solid tumors	Pembrolizumab
Recruiting	NCT02501096	I/II	Phase Ib trial of lenvatinib plus pembrolizumab in subjects with selected solid tumors	Solid Tumors	Pembrolizumab plus lenvatinib
Recruiting	NCT01174121	II	Immunotherapy using tumor-infiltrating lymphocytes for patients with metastatic cancer	Solid tumors	Pembrolizumab
Recruiting	NCT03126110	I/II	Exploring the safety, tolerability, and efficacy of INCAGN01876 combined with immune therapies in advanced or metastatic malignancies	Solid tumors	Nivolumab plus INCAGN01876 and/or pilimumab
Recruiting	NCT02423954	I/II	Study of nivolumab plus chemotherapy in patients with advanced cancer (NivoPlus)	Multiple solid tumors	Nivolumab plus temsirolimus, irinotecan, and/or capecitabine

TABLE 7.5
Ongoing Trials Using Checkpoint Inhibition in Endometrial Cancer—cont'd

Trial Status	Number	Phase	Trial Name	Eligible Cancers	Planned Intervention
Recruiting	NCT02914470	I	Carboplatin–cyclophosphamide combined with atezolizumab	Gynecologic cancers including: endometrial	Atezolizumab plus carboplatin and/or cyclophosphamide
Recruiting	NCT02912572	II	Study of avelumab in patients with MSS, MSI-H, and POLE-mutated recurrent or persistent endometrial cancer	Endometrial	Avelumab
Recruiting	NCT03015129	II	A study of durvalumab with or without tremelimumab in endometrial cancer	Endometrial	Durvalumab and/or tremelimumab
Recruiting	NCT02725489	II	Pilot study of durvalumab and vigil in advanced women's cancers	Gynecologic cancers including: endometrial	Durvalumab

FRa, Folate receptor-α; *MSI,* microsatellite instability; *MSS,* microsatellite stable; *PLD,* PEGylated liposomal doxorubicin; *POLE,* DNA polymerase epsilon.

Preliminary data from a phase Ib trial of pembrolizumab (KEYNOTE-028) in advanced solid tumors was presented at ASCO in 2016. This study included a cohort of 24 patients with advanced cervical cancer, all heavily pretreated. Eighty-seven percent of patients had PD-L1 expression $\geq$1%. With a median follow-up duration of 48.9 weeks, the effect of pembrolizumab was modest with an ORR of 12.5% (3/24; all PRs). The preliminary 6-month PFS and OS rates were 13% and 66.7%, respectively. The regimen was well tolerated, with 20.8% of patients experiencing grade 3 toxicities, and no patients with grade 4 or 5 toxicities.[96] Based on these results a larger phase II trial was initiated (NCT02628067/KEYNOTE-158) in advanced or metastatic cervical cancer. Preliminary results from KEYNOTE-158 showed similar efficacy; of the first 47 patients enrolled, there were three confirmed and five unconfirmed responses, with an ORR of 17% (95% CI, 8%–31%). For 15 patients with longer follow-up ($\geq$27 weeks vs. $\geq$18 weeks), the ORR was 27% (95% confidence interval (CI) 8%–55%), with three confirmed responses and one unconfirmed response. Although modest, this is considered a good response for a single-agent therapy in patients with refractory cervical cancer.

Nivolumab, which also targets PD-1, is another checkpoint inhibitor being evaluated in cervical cancer. The Checkmate-358 study presented initial results at ASCO 2017 for a small cohort of recurrent cervical, vulvar, and vaginal cancers. Nivolumab demonstrated encouraging clinical activity in cervical cancer, with a 20.8% ORR and a 70.8% disease control rate at the time of data cutoff. The safety profile was reasonable and similar to that seen with nivolumab in other cancer types.

Outcomes from these trials appear promising, considering the universally poor prognosis for patients with recurrent cervical cancer. If these outcomes continue, checkpoint inhibitors will have similar efficacy to that seen with the addition of bevacizumab to chemotherapy in the recurrent setting,[87] the only other significant improvement in cervical cancer treatment in many years. Several other monoclonal antibodies are being evaluated in clinical trials, as well as dual checkpoint inhibitor blockade, and checkpoint inhibition in combination with other therapies. Two trials are evaluating checkpoint inhibitors in addition to chemoradiation in upfront therapy. Rapid tumor destruction during upfront chemoradiation produces an increase in antigen exposure. With localized immune-suppressive mechanisms in place, immune response to the tumor antigens is somewhat impaired. However, if checkpoint blockade is administered during upfront therapy, the immune system has increased capacity to mount a response to the tumor. Future trials will need to address the optimal timing and combination of this class of drugs with other cervical cancer therapies. Lists of completed and ongoing clinical trials in cervical cancer patients are listed in Tables 7.6 and 7.7.

TABLE 7.6
Checkpoint Inhibitor Trials With Results in Cervical Cancer

Target	Drugs	Trial ID	Population	Phase	N	Results	Median PFS (week)	≥ G3 AE (%)	References
PD-1	Nivolumab	NCT02488759 (Checkmate-358)	Recurrent or metastatic cervical, vulvar, or vaginal cancer	I/II	19	Interim analysis: ORR 20.8% Disease control rate: 70.8%	22	12.5%	Hollebecque et al.[95a]
PD-1	Pembrolizumab	NCT02628067 (KEYNOTE-158)	Advanced/recurrent cervical cancer, PD-L1+	II	47	ORR 17%	NR	NR	Schellens et al.[95b]
PD-1	Pembrolizumab	NCT02054806 (KEYNOTE-028)	Advanced/recurrent cervical cancer	Ib	26	ORR 12.5%	NR	20.8%	Frenel et al.[96]

AE, adverse event; *NR*, not reported; *ORR*, overall response rate; *PFS*, progression-free survival.

TABLE 7.7
Ongoing Checkpoint Inhibitor Trials in Cervical Cancer

Status	Trial ID	Phase	Eligible Population	Intervention
Listed, not yet recruiting	NCT03144466 (PAPAYA)	I	Stage IB–IVA cervical cancer; paraaortic lymph node involvement excluded	Pembrolizumab starting 2 weeks before chemoradiation
Recruiting	NCT02635360	II	Advanced cervical cancer	Pembrolizumab + cisplatin + brachytherapy
Active, not recruiting	NCT02257528	II	Recurrent or metastatic cervical cancer	Nivolumab
Active, not recruiting	NCT01975831	I	Recurrent or refractory EOC, RCC, or breast, colorectal, or cervical cancer	Tremelimumab + MEDI4736 (anti–PD-L1 Ab)
Active, not recruiting	NCT01693783	II	Metastatic/recurrent cervical cancer	Ipilimumab
Active, not recruiting	NCT01711515 (GOG 9929)	I	Locally advanced cervical cancer	Ipilimumab after chemoradiation for primary treatment
Recruiting	NCT02379520 (HESTIA)	I	Relapsed HPV-associated cancers, including cervical cancer	HPV-specific T-cells +/− Nivolumab
Recruiting	NCT02291055	I/II	Recurrent/persistent or metastatic cervical cancer	Durvalumab +/− ADXS11–001
Recruiting	NCT02725489	II	Advanced/metastatic cervical cancer	Durvalumab + autologous tumor cell immunotherapy (suppresses TGF-B1/2, expresses GM-CSF)
Recruiting	NCT03073525	I	Advanced gynecologic cancers	Vigil then vigil + atezolizumab atezolizumab then vigil + atezolizumab
Recruiting	NCT02914470	I	Advanced breast and gynecologic cancers (including stage IV cervical cancer)	Carboplatin + cyclophosphamide + atezolizumab
Recruiting	NCT02921269	II	Recurrent, persistent, or metastatic cervical cancer	Atezolizumab + bevacizumab
Recruiting	NCT03074513	II	Refractory cervical cancer	Atezolizumab + bevacizumab
Active, not recruiting	NCT01375842	I	Advanced solid tumors, including cervical cancer	Atezolizumab

Ab, antibody; *EOC,* epithelial ovarian cancer; *GM-CSF,* granulocyte-macrophage colony-stimulating factor; *HCV,* human papillomavirus; *RCC,* renal cell carcinoma.

FUTURE DIRECTIONS

Few advances in medical management have occurred in recent years in the treatment of advanced or recurrent gynecologic malignancies; the prognosis for these patients remains poor, and the treatment remains palliative in most cases. Despite these significant efforts in gynecologic cancers, the role of single-agent checkpoint inhibition has shown very modest effects on disease control in approximately 10%–15% of the patients. Given the low ORR in these tumors, efforts must be made to improve the response rates to checkpoint inhibition. Two approaches to increasing the efficacy of checkpoint inhibition in gynecologic tumors lie in appropriate patient selection for this intervention and the use of combination therapies. In certain disease sites such as endometrial cancer, tumor selection may play a role in improving response rates. Based on the limited data that are available, there appears to be an improved ORR with patients selected using TCGA classification of tumors versus studies selecting for patients based on PD-L1 expression. Selecting the patients who will benefit the most from checkpoint inhibition, based on the genetics of the tumor, will be important in future trials to improve the response rates. In other tumor sites such as ovarian and cervical cancers, the development of appropriate markers for predicting success of checkpoint inhibition is imperative. Currently, the use of PD-1 and PD-L1 immunohistochemical staining has not been reliable in predicting outcomes with checkpoint inhibitors.[97]

There have been significant preclinical data in both endometrial and ovarian cancer tumor models, that combination therapy such as anti–PD-1 inhibition plus a second checkpoint inhibitor (anti–CTLA-4), an antiangiogenic agent (anti-VEGF), PARP inhibitors, or in combination with traditional cytotoxic chemotherapeutic agents.[98] Currently there are multiple trials in each gynecologic disease site using a combination of the aforementioned agents with anti–PD-1 and anti–PD-L1 inhibitors (Tables 7.3, 7.5, and 7.7). To date, no study has been completed in gynecologic cancers using checkpoint inhibitors in combination with another therapy, however, given the strong preclinical rationale as well as improvement in outcomes in other disease sites with combination therapies; this represents a promising strategy to improve patient outcomes with gynecologic malignancies.[99–101] Although combined approaches have shown improved efficacy in other tumor sites, it is important to remember the potential for additive toxicities in gynecologic cancer patients who might be enrolling in these trials. Typically, these patients have been heavily pretreated with traditional cytotoxic chemotherapeutic agents and have a more compromised bone marrow than patients who have enrolled in combination therapies in other disease sites (melanoma and lung cancer patients). Much of the safety data justifying the rationale for the use of these drugs are taken from the melanoma literature, which may not represent the typical gynecologic patient enrolling in a combination therapy clinical trial.

REFERENCES

1. McGranahan N, Furness AJ, Rosenthal R, et al. Clonal neoantigens elicit T cell immunoreactivity and sensitivity to immune checkpoint blockade. *Science (New York, NY)*. 2016;351(6280):1463–1469.
2. Snyder A, Makarov V, Merghoub T, et al. Genetic basis for clinical response to CTLA-4 blockade in melanoma. *N Engl J Med*. 2014;371(23):2189–2199.
3. Hodi FS, Chesney J, Pavlick AC, et al. Combined nivolumab and ipilimumab versus ipilimumab alone in patients with advanced melanoma: 2-year overall survival outcomes in a multicentre, randomised, controlled, phase 2 trial. *Lancet Oncol*. 2016;17(11):1558–1568.
4. Siegel RL, Miller KD, Jemal A. Cancer statistics. *CA Cancer J Clin*. 2017;67(1):7–30.
5. Torre LA, Bray F, Siegel RL, Ferlay J, Lortet-Tieulent J, Jemal A. Global cancer statistics, 2012. *CA Cancer J Clin*. 2015;65(2):87–108.
6. *National Comprehensive Cancer Network (NCCN) Ovarian Cancer Guidelines V1*. 2016.
7. Raspollini MR, Castiglione F, Rossi Degl'innocenti D, et al. Tumour-infiltrating gamma/delta T-lymphocytes are correlated with a brief disease-free interval in advanced ovarian serous carcinoma. *Ann Oncol*. 2005;16(4):590–596.
8. Zhang L, Conejo-Garcia JR, Katsaros D, et al. Intratumoral T cells, recurrence, and survival in epithelial ovarian cancer. *N Engl J Med*. 2003;348(3):203–213.
9. Santin AD, Hermonat PL, Ravaggi A, et al. Phenotypic and functional analysis of tumor-infiltrating lymphocytes compared with tumor-associated lymphocytes from ascitic fluid and peripheral blood lymphocytes in patients with advanced ovarian cancer. *Gynecol Obstet Invest*. 2001;51(4):254–261.
10. Hayashi K, Yonamine K, Masuko-Hongo K, et al. Clonal expansion of T cells that are specific for autologous ovarian tumor among tumor-infiltrating T cells in humans. *Gynecol Oncol*. 1999;74(1):86–92.
11. Dadmarz RD, Ordoubadi A, Mixon A, et al. Tumor-infiltrating lymphocytes from human ovarian cancer patients recognize autologous tumor in an MHC class II-restricted fashion. *Cancer J Sci Am*. 1996;2(5):263–272.
12. Odunsi K, Qian F, Matsuzaki J, et al. Vaccination with an NY-ESO-1 peptide of HLA class I/II specificities induces integrated humoral and T cell responses in ovarian cancer. *Proc Natl Acad Sci USA*. 2007;104(31):12837–12842.
13. Curiel TJ, Coukos G, Zou L, et al. Specific recruitment of regulatory T cells in ovarian carcinoma fosters immune privilege and predicts reduced survival. *Nat Med*. 2004;10(9):942–949.
14. Zou W. Immunosuppressive networks in the tumour environment and their therapeutic relevance. *Nat Rev Cancer*. 2005;5(4):263–274.
15. Motz GT, Coukos G. Deciphering and reversing tumor immune suppression. *Immunity*. 2013;39(1):61–73.
16. Fife BT, Bluestone JA. Control of peripheral T-cell tolerance and autoimmunity via the CTLA-4 and PD-1 pathways. *Immunol Rev*. 2008;224:166–182.
17. Ondondo B, Jones E, Godkin A, Gallimore A. Home sweet home: the tumor microenvironment as a haven for regulatory T cells. *Front Immunol*. 2013;4:197.
18. Litzinger MT, Fernando R, Curiel TJ, Grosenbach DW, Schlom J, Palena C. IL-2 immunotoxin denileukin diftitox reduces regulatory T cells and enhances vaccine-mediated T-cell immunity. *Blood*. 2007;110(9):3192–3201.

19. Steitz J, Bruck J, Lenz J, Knop J, Tuting T. Depletion of CD25(+) CD4(+) T cells and treatment with tyrosinase-related protein 2-transduced dendritic cells enhance the interferon alpha-induced, CD8(+) T-cell-dependent immune defense of B16 melanoma. *Cancer Res.* 2001;61(24):8643–8646.

20. Vermeij R, de Bock GH, Leffers N, et al. Tumor-infiltrating cytotoxic T lymphocytes as independent prognostic factor in epithelial ovarian cancer with wilms tumor protein 1 overexpression. *J Immunother.* 2011;34(6):516–523.

21. Zhang Z, Huang J, Zhang C, et al. Infiltration of dendritic cells and T lymphocytes predicts favorable outcome in epithelial ovarian cancer. *Cancer Gene Ther.* 2015;22(4):198–206.

22. Bachmayr-Heyda A, Aust S, Heinze G, et al. Prognostic impact of tumor infiltrating CD8+ T cells in association with cell proliferation in ovarian cancer patients–a study of the OVCAD consortium. *BMC Cancer.* 2013;13:422.

23. Webb JR, Milne K, Kroeger DR, Nelson BH. PD-L1 expression is associated with tumor-infiltrating T cells and favorable prognosis in high-grade serous ovarian cancer. *Gynecol Oncol.* 2016;141(2):293–302.

24. Milne K, Kobel M, Kalloger SE, et al. Systematic analysis of immune infiltrates in high-grade serous ovarian cancer reveals CD20, FoxP3 and TIA-1 as positive prognostic factors. *PLoS One.* 2009;4(7):e6412.

25. Hamanishi J, Mandai M, Iwasaki M, et al. Programmed cell death 1 ligand 1 and tumor-infiltrating CD8+ T lymphocytes are prognostic factors of human ovarian cancer. *Proc Natl Acad Sci USA.* 2007;104(9):3360–3365.

26. Teng MW, Ngiow SF, Ribas A, Smyth MJ. Classifying cancers based on T-cell infiltration and PD-L1. *Cancer Res.* 2015;75(11):2139–2145.

27. Mahoney KM, Rennert PD, Freeman GJ. Combination cancer immunotherapy and new immunomodulatory targets. *Nat Rev Drug Discov.* 2015;14(8):561–584.

28. Brahmer JR, Tykodi SS, Chow LQ, et al. Safety and activity of anti-PD-L1 antibody in patients with advanced cancer. *N Engl J Med.* 2012;366(26):2455–2465.

28a. Disis ML, Patel MR, Pant S, et al. Avelumab (MSB0010718C; anti-PD-L1) in patients with recurrent/refractory ovarian cancer from the JAVELIN Solid Tumor phase Ib trial: Safety and clinical activity. *J Clin Oncol.* 2016;34(suppl 15):5533–5533.

29. Hamanishi J, Mandai M, Ikeda T, et al. Safety and antitumor activity of anti-PD-1 antibody, nivolumab, in patients with platinum-resistant ovarian cancer. *J Clin Oncol.* 2015;33(34):4015–4022.

30. Varga A, Piha-Paul SA, Ott PA, et al. Antitumor activity and safety of pembrolizumab in patients (pts) with PD-L1 positive advanced ovarian cancer: interim results from a phase Ib study. *J Clin Oncol.* 2015;33(suppl 15):5510.

31. Mary L, Disis MRP, Pant S, et al. Avelumab (MSB0010718C; anti-PD-L1) in patients with recurrent/refractory ovarian cancer from the JAVELIN solid tumor phase Ib trial: safety and clinical activity. *J Clin Oncol.* 2016;34(suppl 15):5533.

32. Hodi FS, Butler M, Oble DA, et al. Immunologic and clinical effects of antibody blockade of cytotoxic T lymphocyte-associated antigen 4 in previously vaccinated cancer patients. *Proc Natl Acad Sci USA.* 2008;105(8):3005–3010.

33. Duraiswamy J, Kaluza KM, Freeman GJ, Coukos G. Dual blockade of PD-1 and CTLA-4 combined with tumor vaccine effectively restores T-cell rejection function in tumors. *Cancer Res.* 2013;73(12):3591–3603.

34. Topalian SL, Taube JM, Anders RA, Pardoll DM. Mechanism-driven biomarkers to guide immune checkpoint blockade in cancer therapy. *Nat Rev Cancer.* 2016;16(5):275–287.

35. Lo CS, Sanii S, Kroeger DR, et al. Neoadjuvant chemotherapy of ovarian cancer results in three patterns of tumor-infiltrating lymphocyte response with distinct implications for immunotherapy. *Clin Cancer Res.* 2017;23(4):925–934.

36. Emens LA, Kok M, Ojalvo LS. Targeting the programmed cell death-1 pathway in breast and ovarian cancer. *Curr Opin Obstet Gynecol.* 2016;28(2):142–147.

37. Ziogas AC, Gavalas NG, Tsiatas M, et al. VEGF directly suppresses activation of T cells from ovarian cancer patients and healthy individuals via VEGF receptor type 2. *Int J Cancer.* 2012;130(4):857–864.

38. Rivera LB, Bergers G. Intertwined regulation of angiogenesis and immunity by myeloid cells. *Trends Immunol.* 2015;36(4):240–249.

39. Huang J, Wang L, Cong Z, et al. The PARP1 inhibitor BMN 673 exhibits immunoregulatory effects in a Brca1(-/-) murine model of ovarian cancer. *Biochem Biophys Res Commun.* 2015;463(4):551–556.

40. Higuchi T, Flies DB, Marjon NA, et al. CTLA-4 blockade synergizes therapeutically with PARP inhibition in BRCA1-deficient ovarian cancer. *Cancer Immunol Res.* 2015;3(11):1257–1268.

41. Cao Z, Shang B, Zhang G, et al. Tumor cell-mediated neovascularization and lymphangiogenesis contrive tumor progression and cancer metastasis. *Biochim Biophys Acta.* 2013;1836(2):273–286.

42. Kobold S, Hegewisch-Becker S, Oechsle K, Jordan K, Bokemeyer C, Atanackovic D. Intraperitoneal VEGF inhibition using bevacizumab: a potential approach for the symptomatic treatment of malignant ascites? *Oncologist.* 2009;14(12):1242–1251.

43. Jain RK. Antiangiogenesis strategies revisited: from starving tumors to alleviating hypoxia. *Cancer Cell.* 2014;26(5):605–622.

44. Curiel TJ, Wei S, Dong H, et al. Blockade of B7-H1 improves myeloid dendritic cell-mediated antitumor immunity. *Nat Med.* 2003;9(5):562–567.

45. Tothill RW, Tinker AV, George J, et al. Novel molecular subtypes of serous and endometrioid ovarian cancer linked to clinical outcome. *Clin Cancer Res.* 2008;14(16):5198–5208.

46. Strickland K, Howitt BE, Rodig SJ, et al. Tumor infiltrating and peritumoral T cells and expression of PD-L1 in BRCA1/2-mutated high grade serous ovarian cancers. *J Clin Oncol.* 2015;33(suppl). abstr 5512.

47. Kroeger DR, Milne K, Nelson BH. Tumor-infiltrating plasma cells are associated with tertiary lymphoid structures, cytolytic T-cell responses, and superior prognosis in ovarian cancer. *Clin Cancer Res.* 2016;22(12):3005–3015.

48. Lee J-M, Zimmer ADS, Lipkowitz S, et al. Phase I study of the PD-L1 inhibitor, durvalumab (MEDI4736; D) in combination with a PARP inhibitor, olaparib (O) or a VEGFR inhibitor, cediranib (C) in women's cancers (NCT02484404). *J Clin Oncol.* 2016;34. abstr 3015.

49. Tan DS, Miller RE, Kaye SB. New perspectives on molecular targeted therapy in ovarian clear cell carcinoma. *Br J Cancer.* 2013;108(8):1553–1559.

50. Cai KQ, Albarracin C, Rosen D, et al. Microsatellite instability and alteration of the expression of hMLH1 and hMSH2 in ovarian clear cell carcinoma. *Hum Pathol.* 2004;35(5):552–559.

51. Strickland K, Howitt BE, Rodig SJ, Matulonis UA, Konstantinopoulos P. Immunogenicity of clear cell ovarian cancer: association with ARID1A loss, microsatellite instability and endometriosis. *J Clin Oncol.* 2016;34. abstr 5514.

52. Motzer RJ, Rini BI, McDermott DF, et al. Nivolumab for metastatic renal cell carcinoma: results of a randomized phase II trial. *J Clin Oncol.* 2015;33(13):1430–1437.

53. Eisenhauer EA, Therasse P, Bogaerts J, et al. New response evaluation criteria in solid tumours: revised RECIST guideline (version 1.1). *Eur J Cancer.* 2009;45(2): 228–247.

54. Wolchok JD, Hoos A, O'Day S, et al. Guidelines for the evaluation of immune therapy activity in solid tumors: immune-related response criteria. *Clin Cancer Res.* 2009; 15(23):7412–7420.

55. Nishino M, Giobbie-Harder A, Gargano M, Suda M, Ramaiya NH, Hodi FS. Developing a common language for tumor response to immunotherapy: immune-related response criteria using unidimensional measurements. *Clin Cancer Res.* 2013;19(14):3936–3943.

56. Hodi FS, Hwu WJ, Kefford R, et al. Evaluation of immune-related response criteria and RECIST v1.1 in Patients with advanced melanoma treated with pembrolizumab. *J Clin Oncol.* 2016;34(13):1510–1517.

57. Seymour L, Bogaerts J, Perrone A, et al. iRECIST: guidelines for response criteria for use in trials testing immunotherapeutics. *Lancet Oncol.* 2017; 18(3):e143–e152.

58. Ades F, Yamaguchi N. WHO, RECIST, and immune-related response criteria: is it time to revisit pembrolizumab results? *Ecancermedicalscience.* 2015;9:604.

59. Topalian SL, Hodi FS, Brahmer JR, et al. Safety, activity, and immune correlates of anti-PD-1 antibody in cancer. *N Engl J Med.* 2012;366(26):2443–2454.

60. Garon EB, Rizvi NA, Hui R, et al. Pembrolizumab for the treatment of non-small-cell lung cancer. *N Engl J Med.* 2015;372(21):2018–2028.

61. Robert C, Long GV, Brady B, et al. Nivolumab in previously untreated melanoma without BRAF mutation. *N Engl J Med.* 2015;372(4):320–330.

62. Balkwill FR, Capasso M, Hagemann T. The tumor microenvironment at a glance. *J Cell Sci.* 2012;125(Pt 23): 5591–5596.

63. Tumeh PC, Harview CL, Yearley JH, et al. PD-1 blockade induces responses by inhibiting adaptive immune resistance. *Nature.* 2014;515(7528):568–571.

64. Herbst RS, Soria JC, Kowanetz M, et al. Predictive correlates of response to the anti-PD-L1 antibody MPDL3280A in cancer patients. *Nature.* 2014;515(7528):563–567.

65. Taube JM, Klein A, Brahmer JR, et al. Association of PD-1, PD-1 ligands, and other features of the tumor immune microenvironment with response to anti-PD-1 therapy. *Clin Cancer Res.* 2014;20(19):5064–5074.

66. Rizvi NA, Hellmann MD, Snyder A, et al. Cancer immunology. Mutational landscape determines sensitivity to PD-1 blockade in non-small cell lung cancer. *Science (New York, NY).* 2015;348(6230):124–128.

67. Van Allen EM, Miao D, Schilling B, et al. Genomic correlates of response to CTLA-4 blockade in metastatic melanoma. *Science (New York, NY).* 2015;350(6257): 207–211.

68. Llosa NJ, Cruise M, Tam A, et al. The vigorous immune microenvironment of microsatellite instable colon cancer is balanced by multiple counter-inhibitory checkpoints. *Cancer Discov.* 2015;5(1):43–51.

69. Le DT, Uram JN, Wang H, et al. PD-1 blockade in tumors with mismatch-repair deficiency. *N Engl J Med.* 2015; 372(26):2509–2520.

70. Diaz LAUJ, Wang H, Bartlett B, et al. Programmed death-1 blockade in mismatch repair deficient cancer independent of tumor histology. *J Clin Oncol.* 2016;34(suppl 15): 3003. abstr 3003.

71. Xiao X, Melton DW, Gourley C. Mismatch repair deficiency in ovarian cancer — molecular characteristics and clinical implications. *Gynecol Oncol.* 2014;132(2): 506–512.

72. Vetizou M, Pitt JM, Daillere R, et al. Anticancer immunotherapy by CTLA-4 blockade relies on the gut microbiota. *Science (New York, NY).* 2015;350(6264): 1079–1084.

73. Botticelli A, Zizzari I, Mazzuca F, et al. Cross-talk between microbiota and immune fitness to steer and control response to anti PD-1/PDL-1 treatment. *Oncotarget.* 2017;8(5):8890–8899.

74. Kumar V, Chaudhary N, Garg M, Floudas CS, Soni P, Chandra AB. Current diagnosis and management of immune related adverse events (irAEs) induced by immune checkpoint inhibitor therapy. *Front Pharmacol.* 2017;8:49.

75. Wolchok JD, Kluger H, Callahan MK, et al. Nivolumab plus ipilimumab in advanced melanoma. *N Engl J Med.* 2013;369(2):122–133.

76. Institute NC. *Cancer of the Endometrium. Cancer Stat Facts;* 2017. https://seer.cancer.gov/statfacts/html/corp.html.

77. Huijgens A, Mertens H. Factors predicting recurrent endometrial cancer. *Facts Views Vis ObGyn.* 2013;5(3): 179–186.

78. Bokhman JV. Two pathogenetic types of endometrial carcinoma. *Gynecol Oncol.* 1983;15(1):10−17.
79. Piulats JM, Guerra E, Gil-Martin M, et al. Molecular approaches for classifying endometrial carcinoma. *Gynecol Oncol.* 2017;145(1):200−207.
80. Gilks CB, Oliva E, Soslow RA. Poor interobserver reproducibility in the diagnosis of high-grade endometrial carcinoma. *Am J Surg Pathol.* 2013;37(6):874−881.
81. Network TCGAR. Integrated genomic characterization of endometrial carcinoma. *Nature.* 2013;497(7447):67−73.
82. Vanderstraeten A, Luyten C, Verbist G, Tuyaerts S, Amant F. Mapping the immunosuppressive environment in uterine tumors: implications for immunotherapy. *Cancer Immunol Immunother.* 2014;63(6):545−557.
83. Santin AD, Bellone S, Buza N, et al. Regression of chemotherapy-resistant polymerase ε (POLE) ultra-mutated and MSH6 hyper-mutated endometrial tumors with nivolumab. *Clin Cancer Res.* 2016;22(23): 5682−5687.
84. Ott PA, Bang YJ, Berton-Rigaud D, et al. Safety and antitumor activity of pembrolizumab in advanced programmed death ligand 1-positive endometrial cancer: results from the KEYNOTE-028 study. *J Clin Oncol.* 2017;35(34):3823−3829. https://doi.org/10.12 00/JCO.2017.72.5069.
85. *Comprehensive Cervical Cancer Control: A Guide to Essential Practice.* 2nd ed. Geneva; 2014.
86. Monk BJ, Sill MW, McMeekin DS, et al. Phase III trial of four cisplatin-containing doublet combinations in stage IVB, recurrent, or persistent cervical carcinoma: a Gynecologic Oncology Group study. *J Clin Oncol.* 2009;27(28): 4649−4655.
87. Tewari KS, Sill MW, Long 3rd HJ, et al. Improved survival with bevacizumab in advanced cervical cancer. *N Engl J Med.* 2014;370(8):734−743.
88. Alexandrov LB, Nik-Zainal S, Wedge DC, et al. Signatures of mutational processes in human cancer. *Nature.* 2013; 500(7463):415−421.
89. Schumacher TN, Schreiber RD. Neoantigens in cancer immunotherapy. *Science (New York, NY).* 2015; 348(6230):69−74.
90. Deligeoroglou E, Giannouli A, Athanasopoulos N, et al. HPV infection: immunological aspects and their utility in future therapy. *Infect Dis Obstet Gynecol.* 2013;2013: 540850.
91. Mezache L, Paniccia B, Nyinawabera A, Nuovo GJ. Enhanced expression of PD L1 in cervical intraepithelial neoplasia and cervical cancers. *Mod Pathol.* 2015; 28(12):1594−1602.
92. Yang W, Song Y, Lu YL, Sun JZ, Wang HW. Increased expression of programmed death (PD)-1 and its ligand PD-L1 correlates with impaired cell-mediated immunity in high-risk human papillomavirus-related cervical intra-epithelial neoplasia. *Immunology.* 2013;139(4):513−522.
93. Crafton SM, Salani R. Beyond chemotherapy: an overview and review of targeted therapy in cervical cancer. *Clin Ther.* 2016;38(3):449−458.
94. Karim R, Jordanova ES, Piersma SJ, et al. Tumor-expressed B7-H1 and B7-DC in relation to PD-1+ T-cell infiltration and survival of patients with cervical carcinoma. *Clin Cancer Res.* 2009;15(20):6341−6347.
95. Stevanovic S, Pasetto A, Helman SR, et al. Landscape of immunogenic tumor antigens in successful immunotherapy of virally induced epithelial cancer. *Science (New York, NY).* 2017;356(6334):200−205.
95a. Hollebecque A, Meyer T, Moore, et al. An open-label, multicohort, phase I/II study of nivolumab in patients with virus-associated tumors (CheckMate 358): efficacy and safety in recurrent or metastatic (R/M) cervical, vaginal, and vulvar cancers. *J Clin Oncol.* 2017; 35(suppl 15):5504−5504.
95b. Schellens JHM, Marabelle A, Zeigenfuss, et al. Pembrolizumab for previously treated advanced cervical squamous cell cancer: preliminary results from the phase 2 KEYNOTE-158 study. *J Clin Oncol.* 2017; 35(suppl 15):5514−5514.
96. Frenel JS, Tourneau CL, O'Neil BH, et al. Pembrolizumab in patients with advanced cervical squamous cell cancer: preliminary results from the phase Ib KEYNOTE-028 study. *J Clin Oncol.* 2016;34(suppl 15):5515.
97. Meng X, Huang Z, Teng F, Xing L, Yu J. Predictive biomarkers in PD-1/PD-L1 checkpoint blockade immunotherapy. *Cancer Treat Rev.* 2015;41(10):868−876.
98. Weber J. Immune checkpoint proteins: a new therapeutic paradigm for cancer—preclinical background: CTLA-4 and PD-1 blockade. *Semin Oncol.* 2010;37(5):430−439.
99. Hammers HJ, Plimack ER, Infante JR, et al. Safety and efficacy of nivolumab in combination with ipilimumab in metastatic renal cell carcinoma: the CheckMate 016 study. *J Clin Oncol.* 2016;0(0); JCO.2016.2072.1985.
100. Hellmann MD, Rizvi NA, Goldman JW, et al. Nivolumab plus ipilimumab as first-line treatment for advanced non-small-cell lung cancer (CheckMate 012): results of an open-label, phase 1, multicohort study. *Lancet Oncol.* 2017;18(1):31−41.
101. Larkin J, Chiarion-Sileni V, Gonzalez R, et al. Combined nivolumab and ipilimumab or monotherapy in untreated melanoma. *N Engl J Med.* 2015;373(1):23−34.

CHAPTER 8

Breast Cancer

MEGAN KRUSE, MD • JAME ABRAHAM, MD, FACP

INTRODUCTION

Breast cancer is the most common cancer in women in the United States and represents the second leading cause of death from cancer.[1] Approximately 230,000 new cases of breast cancer occur in the United States each year with over 40,000 deaths due to breast cancer.[2] Current treatment paradigms for breast cancer are based on cellular protein expression of hormone receptors (HRs) (estrogen receptor [ER] and progesterone receptor [PR]) and human epidermal growth factor receptor 2 (HER2). The expression patterns of these cellular markers result in three distinct clinical phenotypes: HR positive, HER2 positive, and those who are negative for all three markers or so-called triple-negative breast cancer (TNBC). Treatment of HR-positive breast cancer includes endocrine therapy to block the effect of estrogen on tumor cell proliferation. Several HER2-directed therapies are available to treat HER2-positive breast cancer and have resulted in improved survival in this subtype of breast cancer.[3,4] TNBC is treated with traditional cytotoxic chemotherapy, as no specific targeted therapies are available.

Although there are many effective treatments for breast cancer, a significant number of patients ultimately experience relapse of disease with associated morbidity or mortality. This has prompted continued interest and investigation into new treatment strategies. Given the success of immune-based therapies in other cancers and the generally favorable side effect profile, which is distinctly different from chemotherapy, immune checkpoint inhibitors are being actively investigated in all phases of breast cancer treatment. The following sections of this chapter will discuss the rationale for immune checkpoint inhibitors in treatment of breast cancer and summarize the existing data in this setting.

MUTATIONAL BURDEN/TUMOR-ASSOCIATED ANTIGENS IN BREAST CANCER

In a basic sense, the immune system is built on the ability to distinguish between self and nonself. This recognition is based on immune cells being exposed to antigens that can be differentially expressed on normal cells of the body and cancer cells. The antigens on cancer cells can be tumor-associated antigens such as aberrantly expressed self-antigens, mutated self-antigens, and tumor-specific antigens. It has been demonstrated that a higher number of "neoantigens," which are foreign to the immune system, are associated with presence of tumor-infiltrating lymphocytes (TILs) and improved response to immune checkpoint therapy.[5,6] Breast cancer overall is known to have low to moderate mutational burden; however, it is known that the mutational load varies by breast cancer subtype.[7]

SIGNIFICANCE OF TUMOR-INFILTRATING LYMPHOCYTES IN BREAST CANCER

TILs are an important component of the tumor microenvironment and have received much attention owing to potential prognostic and predictive power in breast cancer.[8-11] An international working group proposed a standardized manner of TIL categorization in which the percentage of tumor stroma (rather than tumor itself) occupied by TILs is reported.[12] The information that TILs provide seems to be subtype dependent. It has been demonstrated that TILs are highly prevalent in aggressive subtypes such as TNBC and HER2-positive disease.[13] It is in these same subtypes that TILs appear to be prognostic.[9,10] In the early stage breast cancer setting, the presence of TILs has been shown to correlate with pathologic complete response (pCR) following neoadjuvant chemotherapy for TNBC and risk for distant recurrence in those TNBC patients receiving adjuvant chemotherapy.[14,15] Stromal TILs are generally less prominent in luminal breast cancers, and their impact on disease outcome and prognosis is less substantial.[13,16] Interestingly, one retrospective study of invasive lobular carcinoma suggested that increased TILs was associated with poor prognosis, although this finding did not reach statistical significance.[17]

PROGRAMMED DEATH-LIGAND 1 [PD-L1] PD-L1 EXPRESSION IN BREAST CANCER

High PD-L1 expression in breast cancer has been associated with a variety of negative prognostic factors including high grade, HR negativity, high proliferative index, and increased tumor size.[18] It has also been reported that PD-L1 is more frequently expressed in inflammatory breast cancers (IBCs) compared with non-IBCs.[19] Quantification of PD-L1 expression has been evaluated in multiple breast cancer studies; however, it is difficult to compare across clinical trials, as the reporting and categorization of PD-L1 expression has not been standardized. Overall, PD-L1 expression is reported to be present in 20%–30% of breast cancers with the absolute percentage varying based on the type of assay performed.[20] For example, in recent clinical trials where assessment of PD-L1 expression was done with an immunohistochemistry (IHC) assay (such as that used in melanoma or lung cancer), 58% of TNBC cases were "positive" for PD-L1 while 19% of HR-positive cases were "positive."[21,22] In contrast, RNA sequencing (RNA-seq) data obtained from The Cancer Genome Atlas (TCGA) database showed that 19% of TNBC cases were considered "PD-L1 expressing."[23] Although the absolute numbers may vary, it is clear that there is a trend toward greater PD-L1 expression in TNBC when compared with HR-positive disease. This likely accounts, in part, for the degree of interest in use of immune checkpoint inhibitors in the TNBC setting.

As will be detailed in the following sections that describe specific studies of immune checkpoint inhibition in breast cancer, the correlation between PD-L1 expression and response to PD-1/PD-L1 inhibitors is not a perfect one. Although higher PD-L1 expression is often associated with response to these agents, response does not appear to be linear and can also occur in patients whose tumors do not express PD-L1 (Table 8.1).

PD-L1 AND PD-1 INHIBITOR STUDIES IN METASTATIC BREAST CANCER

Atezolizumab

Atezolizumab, an anti-PD-L1 monoclonal antibody, was first studied in metastatic TNBC in a multicenter phase I study presented by Emens et al. at the AACR 2015 national meeting. This study enrolled 27 patients with metastatic TNBC in an expansion cohort. These patients were treated with atezolizumab at doses of 15 mg/kg, 20 mg/kg, or 1200 mg (flat dose) IV every 3 weeks.[24] All patients were screened for PD-L1 expression on tumor-infiltrating immune cells; however, there was not a PD-L1 expression criteria for inclusion in the study. Of the patients in this study, 85% were heavily pretreated, having received ≥4 prior chemotherapy regimens (in the combined neoadjuvant, adjuvant, and metastatic settings). Of the 54 patients who were enrolled and evaluable for safety, 25 were evaluable for efficacy. Unconfirmed RECIST objective response was reported for 24% of patients, including three partial responses (PRs) and two complete responses (CRs). All of those who had a response were determined to be PD-L1 positive (had either 2+ or 3+ PD-L1 expression by IHC). Of note, pseudoprogression occurred in three patients, all of whom ultimately had a decrease in tumor size.

A larger phase I study presented at the AACR 2017 national meeting, reported a 10% objective response rate in 112 patients with metastatic TNBC who were treated with single-agent atezolizumab in the metastatic setting.[25] Those patients who received atezolizumab in the first-line setting (n = 19) had a response rate of 26% while pretreated patients (n = 93, exposed to ≥2 prior therapies) had a response rate of 7%. Those expressing PD-L1 at >5% on immune cells had a response rate of 13% compared with 8% in those with <5% PD-L1 expression on immune cells. The majority of responders (9/11) were found to have PD-L1 expression >5% at the time of study entry. In addition, the median duration of response in this trial was 21 months, and 30% of patients experienced overall disease control (objective response and stable disease combined).

This report represents the largest cohort of metastatic breast cancer (MBC) patients treated with immune checkpoint inhibitor therapy and is the first to comment on overall survival outcomes in breast cancer patients treated with such therapy. Interestingly, the overall survival of those patients who responded to therapy (as per RECIST v 1.1 criteria) was 100% at both 1 year and 2 years while the overall survival in nonresponders was 33% and 11% at these same time points, respectively. These data again suggest that while immune checkpoint inhibitors produce a disease response in a minority of patients, those who do respond can have potentially durable response with resulting improved survival. In a metastatic TNBC population, this is particularly significant as the median survival in this setting remains in the range of 9–12 months with presently available therapies.

The combination of immune checkpoint inhibitor therapy with chemotherapy has been of interest in many malignancies with the rationale that use of traditional cytotoxic chemotherapy will result in cell death and exposure of the immune system to multiple tumor antigens. This antigenic stimulation may then enhance the efficacy of immune checkpoint agents. In breast

TABLE 8.1
Trials With Reported Results for Immune Checkpoint Inhibition in Breast Cancer

Intervention	Study Design	Study Population	PD-L1 Expression Criteria	Results	Reference
Atezolizumab	Phase I	Metastatic TNBC n = 27	All patients screened Not used as inclusion criteria	ORR 24% All patients evaluable for response were PD-L1+	24
Atezolizumab	Phase I	Metastatic TNBC n = 112	All patients screened Not used as inclusion criteria	ORR 10% overall ORR 13% with PD-L1 expression >5%, 8% with PD-L1 expression <5% 100% 1 and 2 year survival in responders	25
Nab-paclitaxel ± atezolizumab	Phase I	Metastatic TNBC n = 24	All patients screened Not used as inclusion criteria	ORR 42% No correlation between PD-L1 expression and response	26
Pembrolizumab (KEYNOTE-012)	Phase I	Metastatic TNBC n = 32	PD-L1 ≥ 1% in all enrolled patients	ORR 18.5% Increasing probability of response with increasing PD-L1 expression	21
Pembrolizumab (KEYNOTE-086)	Phase II	Metastatic TNBC Cohort A = previously treated patients n = 170 Cohort B = untreated patients n = 52	Cohort A = no PD-L1 requirement Cohort B = PD-L1 positive (≥1% CPS)	Cohort A overall ORR 5% ORR 9.5% in PD-L1+ patients, 4.7% in PD-L1− patients in Cohort A Cohort B ORR 23%	28
Pembrolizumab (KEYNOTE-028)	Phase I	ER+/HER2− MBC n = 25	No requirement for inclusion	ORR 12%	22

Continued

TABLE 8.1
Trials With Reported Results for Immune Checkpoint Inhibition in Breast Cancer—cont'd

Intervention	Study Design	Study Population	PD-L1 Expression Criteria	Results	Reference
Pembrolizumab with trastuzumab (KEYNOTE-014)	Phase II	HER2+ MBC	All patients screened PD-L1 ≥ 1% considered positive	ORR 15.2% in PD-L1 + patients, 0% in PD-L1− patients	29
Pembrolizumab with anthracycline- and taxane-based neoadjuvant chemotherapy (I-SPY 2)	Phase II	Neoadjuvant HR +/HER−; TNBC n = 69	No requirement for inclusion	pCR 28% HR+ pCR 74% TNBC	30
Avelumab (JAVELIN)	Phase I	MBC n = 168 58 TNBC 72 HR+/HER2− 26 HER2+ 12 unknown subtype	All patients screened No requirement for inclusion	ORR 4.8% ORR in TNBC patients highest at 8.6% ORR 33% in PD-L1 ≥10% versus 2.4% in PD-L1 ≤10%	31
Tremelimumab with exemestane	Phase I	Postmenopausal HR+ MBC n = 26	Not evaluated	42% stable disease ≥ 12 weeks	32

ER, estrogen receptor; *HER2*, human epidermal growth factor receptor 2; *HR*, hormone receptor; *MBC*, metastatic breast cancer; *ORR*, objective response rate; *pCR*, pathologic complete response; *TNBC*, triple negative breast cancer.

cancer, this concept was initially explored in a phase Ib trial of atezolizumab in combination with nab-paclitaxel in patients with metastatic TNBC treated with three or fewer prior lines of therapy in the metastatic setting.[26] These patients received atezolizumab at a dose of 800 mg on days 1 and 15 with nab-paclitaxel 125 mg/m^2 on days 1, 8, and 15 of a 28 day cycle. A confirmed objective response rate of 42% was achieved in 24 patients who were evaluable for treatment response. In this population of 24 patients, 4% had CR, 67% had PR, and 21% had stable disease. Importantly, at 6 months of follow-up, 6 of 12 responders remained on therapy with evidence of continued therapeutic benefit. This finding adds to the growing body of evidence that durable responses do occur with checkpoint inhibitor therapy in multiple malignancies. Interestingly, 87% of patients had received prior taxane-based chemotherapy. Moreover, consistent with prior reports, this study found no correlation between degree of response and PD-L1 expression. Neutropenia was the most common treatment-related adverse event, 41% of which was grade 3 or 4, in the 32 patients who were evaluable for safety.

Given the promising results of this trial, a global phase III multicenter, double-blind, placebo-controlled trial of atezolizumab/nab-paclitaxel versus placebo/nab-paclitaxel is currently underway in first-line treatment of metastatic TNBC.[27] This study is expected to enroll 900 patients who will be randomized in a 1:1 fashion to either atezolizumab (840 mg) or placebo on days 1 and 15 of a 28-day cycle with nab-paclitaxel at a dose of 100 mg/m^2 given on days 1, 8, and 15. The patients will be stratified by prior taxane chemotherapy (in the neoadjuvant or adjuvant setting) and by the presence of liver metastases. The primary endpoints of the trial are progression-free survival and overall survival.

Pembrolizumab

The KEYNOTE-012 study is a phase Ib study of pembrolizumab, an anti-PD-1 monoclonal antibody, in patients with metastatic TNBC, gastric cancer, urothelial cancer, and head and neck cancer. The study was non-randomized, and all patients included in the study had PD-L1 expression in stroma of ≥1%.[21] A total of 111 patients were screened for PD-L1 expression in this study, and 59% of these patients were deemed "positive" for PD-L1 expression as per the prespecified criteria for PD-L1 expression. All of the 32 breast cancer patients enrolled were evaluable for safety. The primary efficacy endpoint of this study was objective response rate. Efficacy was assessed in all patients who received

at least one dose of pembrolizumab and had a least one postbaseline scan or came off study before the first follow-up scan owing to evidence of progressive disease or treatment-related adverse event. The study population was heavily pretreated with half of patients having received at least three prior lines of therapy for metastatic disease and a quarter of patients receiving at least five prior lines of therapy.

In the 27 patients who were evaluable for efficacy, the objective response rate was 18.5%, consisting of one CR and four PRs. An additional seven patients had stable disease for a disease control rate (defined as the sum of CR, PR, and stable disease for ≥24 weeks) of 25.9%. The median duration of response was 17 weeks for the cohort, and three of the five patients with RECIST defined response remained on pembrolizumab for ≥1 year at the time of data cutoff. In an exploratory analysis, it was found that there was increasing probability of response and decreased likelihood of progression with increasing expression of PD-L1 (one-sided p value of .28 for objective response rate and .12 for progression-free survival).

With respect to safety, 56% of patients in the TNBC cohort of KEYNOTE-012 experienced treatment-related adverse events with 16% of patients experiencing a grade 3 or higher adverse event. The grade 3 events included anemia, aseptic meningitis, lymphopenia, headache, and pyrexia. The more common adverse events observed are consistent with other reports of pembrolizumab including fatigue, arthralgia, myalgia, and nausea. Immune-related adverse events were also assessed in this cohort with one case each of grade 3 colitis, grade 3 hepatitis, and grade 2 hypothyroidism.

In the subsequent KEYNOTE-086 phase II trial, the efficacy of pembrolizumab was again evaluated in patients with metastatic TNBC. This study divided patients into two cohorts. Cohort A consisted of patients with previously treated metastatic TNBC regardless of tumor PD-L1 expression. Cohort B included patients with previously untreated metastatic TNBC with positive tumor PD-L1 expression, defined as ≥1% PD-L1 expression using the combined positive score (CPS), which is calculated by taking the total number of PD-L1−positive cells on IHC (including tumor cells, lymphocytes, macrophages) out of the total number of tumor cells × 100.[28] The preliminary results of cohort A were presented at the 2017 American Society of Clinical Oncology meeting. A total of 170 patients were enrolled in this cohort with 62% classified as PD-L1 positive. With a median follow-up of 10.9 months, the overall objective response rate was 5%, including one CR (occurred in a PD-L1−positive patient) and seven PRs. When stable disease for ≥24 weeks was included in the clinical benefit definition, the clinical benefit rate for the entire study population was nearly 8% (9.5% in the PD-L1–positive patients and 4.7% in the PD-L1–negative patients). An early evaluation of the cohort B data was also presented for comparison, and in those 52 previously untreated, PD-L1–positive patients, the objective response rate was 23%. Of note, the safety profile for pembrolizumab in this population was very similar to that reported for the phase I study with no new signals of concern identified.

While the above studies focused primarily on metastatic TNBC patients, the phase IB KEYNOTE-028 study of pembrolizumab monotherapy enrolled multiple advanced solid tumor malignancies including 25 HR-positive, HER2-negative MBC patients.[22] This study reported a 12% objective response rate and 20% clinical benefit rate among the breast cancer patients and suggests that use of PD-L1 inhibitors are also of interest in HR-positive breast cancers, as the magnitude of benefit and toxicity profile are likely similar to that seen in metastatic TNBC patients.

The KEYNOTE-014 (PANACEA) study was presented at the 2017 San Antonio Breast Cancer Symposium and reported on the activity of pembrolizumab in combination with trastuzumab in patients with HER2-positive advanced breast cancer that previously progressed on trastuzumab therapy.[29] The primary aim of this phase II study was the assessment of efficacy and safety of the combination of pembrolizumab and trastuzumab in PD-L1–expressing (defined as ≥1%) HER2-positive advanced breast cancer, although there were PD-L1–negative patients included for comparison. Overall, 52 patients were enrolled in this study consisting of 40 PD-L1–positive patients and 12 PD-L1–negative patients.

The ORR in the PD-L1–positive cohort was 15.2% with disease control rate (objective responses plus stable disease) of 24%, whereas the PD-L1–negative cohort had an ORR of 0%. Patients in the PD-L1–positive cohort had a median duration of disease control of 11.1 months, and five patients continued on therapy without disease progression at the time of presentation of the data. The 12-month overall survival was noted to be significantly different between the PD-L1-positive and PD-L1-negative cohorts at 65% and 12%, respectively ($P = .0006$). The investigators also sought to find predictive biomarkers for response to pembrolizumab-containing therapy and found that a stromal TILs cutoff of ≥5% was worthy of further study, as the ORR for patients with stromal TILs ≥5% was 39%

compared with 5% in those with TILs <5%. The same relationship was found for disease control rate where the difference was 47% compared with 5% for TILs ≥5% and <5%, respectively.

Avelumab

The JAVELIN study investigated the use of the anti-PD-L1 antibody avelumab in patients with multiple cancers including locally advanced breast cancer/MBC. The breast cancer patients in this trial were unselected, meaning the population included patients with HR-positive, HER2-positive, and triple-negative disease.[31] The patients in this study were screened for PD-L1 expression; however, there was no specific cutoff for enrollment in the study. A total of 168 patients were included in the study with 58 patients having triple-negative disease, 72 having HR-positive/HER2-negative disease, and 26 patients having HER2-positive disease. Disease of unknown subtype was present in 12 patients. The overall response rate for the study population was 4.8% (8/168) with TNBC patients having a response rate of 8.6% compared with 2.8% in the HR-positive patients. The responses observed consisted of one CR and seven PRs. An additional 23% of patients in the study were reported to have stable disease after a median follow-up of 10 months. There also appeared to be greater efficacy in those patients with "positive" PD-L1 expression (defined as PD-L1 expression of ≥10% on immune cells) with 33% of patients with PD-L1–positive disease having a response comparable with only 2.4% of those with PD-L1–negative disease ($P = .001$). PD-L1 expression on tumor cells was also analyzed using cutoffs of ≥1%, ≥5%, and ≥25%; however, these categorizations had no impact on efficacy of avelumab in this population.

In terms of toxicity, 68.5% of patients in this study experienced a treatment-related adverse event with 14% of these events being grade 3 in nature. The most common toxicities (all grade) observed were fatigue, nausea, infusion-related reactions, and diarrhea. Immune-related adverse events were experienced by a lower number of patients with events including hypothyroidism (5%), autoimmune hepatitis (2%), pneumonitis (2%), and thrombocytopenia (1%). In total, approximately 5% of patients discontinued study treatment for reasons other than disease progression, so although treatment-related adverse events were common, they seemed to be manageable, as only a minority of patients actually discontinued treatment for this reason.

CTLA-4 Inhibitor Therapy in Metastatic Breast Cancer

The anti-CTLA4 monoclonal antibody tremelimumab was studied in combination with exemestane in a phase I study of postmenopausal women with metastatic HR-positive breast cancer. This study enrolled patients in a standard 3 + 3 design with dose escalation of tremelimumab according to two schedules (either tremelimumab on day 1 of a 28-day cycle or day 1 of a 90-day cycle) with exemestane 25 mg daily.[32] The study was designed such that the maximum tolerated dose (MTD) was identified as the dose level where <33% of patients experienced dose-limiting toxicities (DLTs). The maximum duration of therapy was 1 year in the absence of disease progression or DLT, and patients who had stable disease or better were eligible for continued treatment with tremelimumab.

A total of 26 patients were enrolled in this study in the United States and Canada. The treatment was found to be safely tolerated, although diarrhea (46%), pruritus (42%), constipation (23%), and fatigue (23%) were the commonly encountered treatment-related adverse events. Notably, one serious adverse event occurred in which a patient experienced diarrhea, fever, and dehydration that required hospitalization and administration of an anti-TNFα antibody for symptom control. The MTD was determined to be 6 mg/kg every 90 days in combination with exemestane 25 mg daily. From an efficacy standpoint, stable disease for ≥12 weeks was the best treatment response achieved, and 42% of patients met criteria for this. The response to treatment was not associated with dose or schedule of tremelimumab.

NEOADJUVANT BREAST STUDIES

Pembrolizumab has also been studied in the neoadjuvant setting as part of the I-SPY 2 trial. This phase II study has multiple arms testing various investigational drugs in the newly diagnosed stage II—III breast cancer preoperative setting and is designed to identify potentially active drugs in a faster, more efficient way than traditional clinical trials. The results of the I-SPY 2 arm investigating pembrolizumab in combination with standard neoadjuvant chemotherapy were presented at the American Society of Clinical Oncology 2017 annual meeting. The primary endpoint of this study is pathologic complete response (pCR), defined as no residual breast cancer identified in the breast and axillary lymph nodes at the time of surgical evaluation. The patients in this study had newly diagnosed invasive breast cancer with tumor size ≥2.5 cm on clinical exam or ≥2 cm on imaging. Although all receptor

profiles (HR positive/HER2 negative, HR negative/HER2 negative, HR positive/HER2 positive, and triple negative) were included in this study, the presented results were for only the HER2-negative patients.[30] Importantly, patients are grouped into "signatures," which take into account receptor profile as well as MammaPrint risk group. Patients with HR positive disease that had "low risk" mammaprint results were not included in the randomization but rather were included in a "low risk" registry. All patients in this study received weekly paclitaxel for 12 cycles followed by 4 cycles of doxorubicin/cyclophosphamide with random assignment to pembrolizumab or no pembrolizumab (which was added to the weekly paclitaxel portion of therapy if given). This study uses Bayesian modeling to estimate mean pCR rate by signature and to determine the probability that experimental arm is superior to the control arm per signature. Reported results also include the probability of success of the experimental arm in a 300-patient phase III trial.

At the time of presentation, 69 patients had been treated with pembrolizumab on this protocol, 46 of whom had completed surgery. The actual pCR rate was 28% for HR-positive/HER2-negative patients treated with pembrolizumab and 74% for TNBC patients treated with pembrolizumab compared with pCR of 15% and 19%, for those that did not receive pembrolizumab respectively. The estimated pCR rate for the HR+ group was 34% and for the TNBC group was 62%. Finally, the predictive probability of success of the pembrolizumab combination therapy in a phase III trial was >99% for the TNBC cohort and 88% for the HR+ cohort. Pembrolizumab is actually the first agent to "graduate" for HR+ patients in the I-SPY 2 trial, and results of the confirmatory phase III trial will be highly anticipated, particularly in light of the historically low pCR response to neoadjuvant therapy in HR+ patients.

CONCLUSION

Despite considerable excitement about the use of immune checkpoint inhibitors in all cancers, none of the aforementioned agents have been approved for use in the breast cancer space, and results of the few reported trials are mixed. The reported response rates are generally low, although each study includes patients who have durable responses, which keeps the hope for these agents alive (Table 8.1). It is difficult to choose a target population for immunotherapy studies in breast cancer, as no clear biomarker for response has been found. It should be noted that many of the reported studies are immune checkpoint inhibitor monotherapy studies.

TABLE 8.2
Select Ongoing/Upcoming Trials of Immune Checkpoint Inhibitors in Breast Cancer

Agent	Study Design	Study Population	PD-L1 Expression	Intervention	ClinicalTrials.gov Identifier
METASTATIC BREAST CANCER TRIALS					
Nivolumab	Phase I	HER2− MBC	All	Nab-paclitaxel + nivolumab	NCT02309177
Nivolumab	Phase II	HER2+ MBC	All	Nivolumab + ipilimumab	NCT02892734
Atezolizumab	Phase II	Metastatic lobular carcinoma	All	Atezolizumab + carboplatin	NCT03147040
Atezolizumab	Phase III	Metastatic TNBC	All	Atezolizumab or placebo + nab-paclitaxel	NCT02425891
Atezolizumab	Phase II	HER2+ MBC	All	Atezolizumab + paclitaxel + trastuzumab + pertuzumab	NCT03125928
Pembrolizumab	Phase II	HER2− MBC	All	Pembrolizumab + gemcitabine	NCT03025880
Pembrolizumab	Phase II	Metastatic TNBC	All	Pembrolizumab + carboplatin/nab-paclitaxel	NCT03121352
Pembrolizumab	Phase II	HR+ MBC	All	Eribulin versus eribulin + pembrolizumab	NCT03051659
Pembrolizumab	Phase II	HR+ MBC	All	Pembrolizumab + palliative radiation	NCT03051672
Pembrolizumab	Phase II	HR+ MBC	All	Pembrolizumab +letrozole and palbociclib	NCT02778685
Pembrolizumab	Phase I/II	HR+ MBC	All	Pembrolizumab +exemestane and luprolide	NCT02990845
Pembrolizumab	Phase Ib	HER2+ MBC	All	Pembrolizumab + TDM-1	NCT03032107

Drug	Phase	Disease	PD-L1 status	Regimen	NCT number
Pembrolizumab	Phase Ib/II	Trastuzumab-refractory advanced HER2+ BC	All for Phase I PD-L1 + for Phase II	Trastuzumab + pembrolizumab	NCT02129556
NEOADJUVANT BREAST CANCER TRIALS					
Pembrolizumab	Phase Ib	TNBC	All	Pembrolizumab + chemotherapy (six different regimens)	NCT02622074
Durvalumab	II	TNBC	All	Durvalumab or placebo followed by taxane/anthracycline based chemotherapy	NCT02685059
Atezolizumab	Phase II	TNBC	All	Paclitaxel/carboplatin ± atezolizumab	NCT02883062
ADJUVANT BREAST CANCER TRIALS					
Pembrolizumab	Phase II	HR+ IBC with no pCR after chemotherapy	All	Pembrolizumab + endocrine therapy	NCT02971748
Pembrolizumab	Phase III	TNBC	All	Pembrolizumab (or placebo) + taxane/anthracycline/platinum chemotherapy preoperatively then pembrolizumab (or placebo) continued as adjuvant therapy	NCT03036488

BC, breast cancer; *HER2*, human epidermal growth factor receptor 2; *HR*, hormone receptor; *IBC*, inflammatory breast cancer; *MBC*, metastatic breast cancer; *pCR*, pathologic complete response; *TNBC*, triple negative breast cancer.

Many upcoming trials are investigating immune checkpoint inhibitors with chemotherapy, and the results of these studies are of great interest (Table 8.2).

REFERENCES

1. Division of Cancer Prevention and Control, Centers for Disease Control and Prevention. Breast Cancer Statistics. https://www.cdc.gov/cancer/breast/statistics/index.htm.
2. American Cancer Society. Breast Cancer Facts and Figures 2015–2016. https://www.cancer.org/content/dam/cancer-org/research/cancer-facts-and-statistics/breast-cancer-facts-and-figures/breast-cancer-facts-and-figures-2015-2016.pdf.
3. Romond EH, Perez EA, Bryant J, et al. Trastuzumab plus adjuvant chemotherapy for operable HER2-positive breast cancer. *N Engl J Med.* 2005;353(16):1673–1684.
4. Swain SM, Kim SB, Cortes J, et al. Pertuzumab, trastuzumab, and docetaxel for HER2-positive metastatic breast cancer (CLEOPATRA study): overall survival results from a randomized, double-blind, placebo-controlled, phase 3 study. *Lancet Oncol.* 2013;14(6):461–471.
5. Brown SD, Rl Warren, Gibb EA, et al. Neo-antigens predicted by tumor genome meta-analysis correlate with increased patient survival. *Genome Res.* 2014;24:743–750.
6. Alexandrov LB, Nik-Zainal S, Wedge DC, et al. Signatures of mutational processes in human cancer. *Nature.* 2013; 500:415–421.
7. Schumacher TN, Schreiber RD. Neoantigens in cancer immunotherapy. *Science.* 2015;348(6230):69–74.
8. Marme F. Immunotherapy in breast cancer. *Oncol Res Treat.* 2016;39:335–346.
9. Loi S, Sirtaine N, Piette F, et al. Prognostic and predictive value of tumor-infiltrating lymphocytes in a phase III randomized adjuvant breast cancer trial in node-positive breast cancer comparing the addition of docetaxel to doxorubicin with doxorubicin- based chemotherapy: BIG 02-98. *J Clin Oncol.* 2013;31(7):860–867.
10. Adams S, Gray RJ, Demaria S, et al. Prognostic value of tumor-infiltrating lymphocytes in triple-negative breast cancers from two phase III randomized adjuvant breast cancer trials: ECOG 2197 and ECOG 1199. *J Clin Oncol.* 2014;32(27):2959–2966.
11. Loi S, Michiels S, Salgado R, et al. Tumor infiltrating lymphocytes are prognostic in triple negative breast cancer and predictive for trastuzumab benefit in early breast cancer: results from the FinHER trial. *Ann Oncol.* 2014;25(8): 1544–1550.
12. Salgado R, Denkert C, Demaria S, et al. The evaluation of tumor-infiltrating lymphocytes (TILs) in breast cancer: recommendations by an International TILs Working Group 2014. *Ann Oncol.* 2015;26:259–271.
13. Pusztai L, Karn T, Safonov A, Abu-Khalaf MM, Bianchini G. New strategies in breast cancer: immunotherapy. *Clin Cancer Res.* 2016;22(9):2105–2110.
14. Loi S, Drubay D, Adams S, et al. Pooled individual patient data analysis of tumor infiltrating lymphocytes (TILs) in

15. Dushyanthen S, Beavis PA, Savas P, et al. Relevance of tumor-infiltrating lymphocytes in breast cancer. *BMC Med.* 2015;13:202.
16. Bianchini G, Qi Y, Alvarez RH, et al. Molecular anatomy of breast cancer stroma and its prognostic value is estrogen receptor-positive and −negative cancers. *J Clin Oncol.* 2010;28:4316–4323.
17. Desmedt C, Salgado R, Buisseret L, et al. Characterization of lymphocytic infiltration in invasive lobular breast cancer. In: *San Antonio Breast Cancer Symposium, San Antonio, TX.* 2015. Abstract S1-02.
18. Sabatier R, Finetti P, Mamessier E, et al. Prognostic and predictive value of PDL1 expression in breast cancer. *Oncotarget.* 2015;6:5449–5464.
19. Bertucci F, Finetti P, Colpaert C, et al. PDL1 expression in inflammatory breast cancer is frequent and predicts for the pathological response to chemotherapy. *Oncotarget.* 2015; 6:13506–13519.
20. Wimberly H, Brown JR, Schalper K, et al. PD-L1 expression correlates with tumor-infiltrating lymphocytes and response to neoadjuvant chemotherapy in breast cancer. *Cancer Immunol Res.* 2015;3:326–332.
21. Nanda R, Chow L, Dees EC, et al. Pembrolizumab in patients with advanced triple-negative breast cancer: phase Ib KEYNOTE-012 study. *J Clin Oncol.* 2016;34(21): 2460–2467.
22. Rugo H, DeLord J-P, Im S-A, et al. Preliminary efficacy and safety of pembrolizumab (MK-3475) in patients with PD-L1-positive, estrogen receptor positive (ER+)/HER2-negative advanced breast cancer enrolled in KEYNOTE-028. In: *Abstract Presented at: San Antonio Breast Cancer Symposium, San Antonio, TX.* 2015. Abstract S5-07.
23. Mittendorf EA, Philips AV, Meric-Bernstam F, et al. PD-L1 expression in triple-negative breast cancer. *Cancer Immunol Res.* 2014;2:361–370.
24. Emens LA, Braiteh FS, Cassier P, et al. Inhibition of PD-L1 by MPDL3280A leads to clinical activity in patients. In: *AACR Annual Meeting, Philadelphia, PA.* 2015. Abstract 2859.
25. Schmid P, Cruz C, Braiteh FS, et al. Atezolizumab in metastatic triple-negative breast cancer: long-term clinical outcomes and biomarker analyses. In: *Abstract Presented at: AACR Annual Meeting, Washington, DC.* 2015. Abstract 2986.
26. Adams S, Robinson Diamond J, Hamilton EP, et al. Phase Ib trial of atezolizumab in combination with nab-paclitaxel in patients with metastatic triple-negative breast cancer (mTNBC). In: *Abstract Presented at: ASCO Annual Meeting, Chicago, IL.* 2016. Abstract 1009.
27. Emens LA, Adams S, Loi S, et al. Impassion130: a phase III randomized trial of atezolizumab with nab-paclitaxel for first-line treatment of patients with metastatic triple-negative breast cancer (mTNBC). In: *Abstract Presented at:*
primary triple negative breast cancer (TNBC) treated with antracycline-based chemotherapy. In: *San Antonio Breast Cancer Symposium, San Antonio, TX.* 2015. Abstract S1-03.

ASCO Annual Meeting, Chicago, IL. 2016. Abstract TPS1104.

28. Adams S, Schmid P, Rugo H, et al. A phase 2 study of pembrolizumab (pembro) monotherapy for previously treated metastatic triple negative breast cancer (mTNBC): KEYNOTE-086 cohort A. In: *Abstract Presented at: ASCO Annual Meeting, Chicago, IL.* 2017. Abstract 1008.

29. Loi S, Giobbe-Hurder A, Gombos A, et al. Phase Ib/II study evaluating safety and efficacy of pembrolizumab and trastuzumab in patients with trastuzumab-resistant HER2-positive metastatic breast cancer: results from the PANACEA (IBCSG 45-3/BIG4-13/KEYNOTE-014) study. In: *Abstract Presented at: San Antonio Breast Cancer Symposium, San Antonio, TX.* 2017. Oral Session: General Session 2.

30. Nanda R, Liu MC, Yau C, et al. Pembrolizumab plus standard neoadjuvant therapy for high-risk breast cancer (BC): results from I-SPY 2. In: *Abstract Presented at: ASCO Annual Meeting, Chicago, IL.* 2017. Abstract 506.

31. Dirix LY, Takacs I, Nikolinakos P, et al. Avelumab, an anti-PD-L1 antibody, in patients with locally advanced or metastatic breast cancer: a phase Ib JAVELIN solid tumor trial. In: *Abstract Presented at: San Antonio Breast Cancer Symposium, San Antonio, TX.* 2015. Abstract S1-04.

32. Vonderheide RH, LoRusso PM, Khalil M, et al. Tremelimumab in combination with exemestane in patients with advanced breast cancer and treatment associated modulation of inducible costimulator expression on patient T cells. *Clin Cancer Res.* 2010;16(13):3485−3494.

CHAPTER 9

Hematologic Malignancies

YAZEED SAWALHA, MD • ANJALI ADVANI, MD

INTRODUCTION

As therapy with the immune checkpoint inhibitors has revolutionized the treatment of several types of solid tumors in recent years, there is great enthusiasm to incorporate these agents in the treatment paradigm of hematologic malignancies. Harnessing the immune system to fight malignant cells is not a novel concept in the treatment of hematologic malignancies. Interferon (IFN)-α was long used for the treatment of several types of lymphoma and leukemia. Rituximab, the first monoclonal antibody approved for use in cancer in 1997 and the backbone of therapy for several types of lymphoma, is a form of immunotherapy through its complement- and antibody-dependent cell-mediated cytotoxicity. Graft-versus-leukemia or -lymphoma phenomenon is a crucial element of the therapeutic role of allogeneic hematopoietic cell transplantation (HCT) and, in itself, is a well-established effective form of immunotherapy.

There are certainly several features that make hematologic malignancies ideal targets for treatment with immune checkpoint inhibitors. Firstly, immune dysregulation is known to accompany these neoplasms and is recognized as an important step in their development and progression. In addition, other immunotherapies have already proven to be effective in this field as mentioned earlier. Furthermore, hematologic malignant cells are in constant contact with the immune cells in the bone marrow, peripheral circulation, and/or lymph nodes and thus are immunologically accessible. Lastly, preclinical data suggest an added benefit from combining immune checkpoint inhibitors with other established treatment modalities including other types of immunotherapy, molecularly targeted agents, radiotherapy, and HCT. All of these factors and the unmet need for more effective and safer treatments have put hematologic malignancies at the forefront of immune checkpoint inhibitors. However, there are also some important challenges. Hematologic malignancies are a diverse group of individually uncommon diseases that have different biologies and a wide array of clinical behaviors. In addition to immune checkpoint pathways, other pathways of immune dysregulation can play a role in hematologic malignancy immune escape. Lastly, there might be unique or excessive toxicities with the use of immune checkpoint inhibitors in this patient population, especially in the post-HCT setting or when combined with other treatment modalities.

Although the full potential of immune checkpoint inhibitors in hematologic malignancies is yet to be explored, there is certainly early evidence of a remarkable benefit in Hodgkin lymphoma (HL) that has fueled the enthusiasm in this field.

IMMUNE CHECKPOINT PATHWAY DYSREGULATION IN HEMATOLOGIC MALIGNANCIES

Cytotoxic T-Lymphocyte Antigen 4

Cytotoxic T-lymphocyte antigen 4 (CTLA-4) (also known as CD152) is a protein encoded on chromosome 2q33.2 and belongs to the immunoglobulin superfamily. It acts as a negative regulator of CD28-dependent T-cell responses and plays a critical role in suppressing effector T-cells, enhancing the immunosuppressive activity of regulatory T-cells, and resulting in peripheral T-cell tolerance or anergy.[1–3]

The current knowledge of the role of CTLA-4 in the regulation of T-cell immune responses in hematologic malignancies is limited. Most patients with acute and chronic myeloid leukemia and B- and T-lymphocytic leukemia express CTLA-4 on the leukemic cell surface and/or in the cytoplasm.[4] CTLA-4 expression is also upregulated in patients with peripheral and cutaneous T-cell lymphomas (TCLs).[5] Furthermore, the CTLA4-CD28 gene rearrangement has been described in patients with Sézary syndrome (SS), angioimmunoblastic TCL, peripheral TCL, not otherwise specified, extranodal natural killer (NK)/TCLs, and T-cell leukemia/lymphoma.[6–8] The fusion gene codes for the transmembrane domain of CTLA-4 and the cytoplasmic domain of CD28, which results in converting inhibitory signals into stimulatory ones for T-cell activation.[7] Although several polymorphisms within the *CTLA4* gene have been linked to an increased risk of developing autoimmune diseases, the "tolerogenic" CT60 AA genotype has been associated with high rates of relapse and lower overall survival (OS) in patients with acute myeloid leukemia (AML).[9]

Programmed Cell Death 1 and Its Ligands (PD-L1 and PD-L2)

Programmed cell death ligand-1 (PD-L1) (also known as B7–H1 or CD274) is normally expressed on the surface of B-cells, T-cells, NK cells, and macrophages while PD-L2 (also known as B7-DC or CD273) is expressed on antigen-presenting cells.[10] In various types of solid malignancies, PD-L1 is expressed on tumor cells, whereas PD-1 is upregulated in tumor-infiltrating lymphocytes (TILs).[3,10,11] PD-1 interaction with its ligands provides an escape mechanism for malignant cells and is exploited by many solid and hematologic malignancies.[10] As discussed in details throughout this chapter, both PD-L1 and PD-L2 expression have been reported on tumor cells in several hematologic malignancies. In addition, PD-1 can be upregulated in the malignant cells of certain neoplasms such as chronic lymphocytic leukemia (CLL) and some types of peripheral TCL.[12–14] Various mechanisms contribute to the upregulation of PD-1 ligand expression including induction by inflammatory cytokines, genetic alterations, viral infections, and transcriptional activation by oncogenic signaling pathways as discussed in detail later (Fig. 9.1). PD-1–positive TILs and nonmalignant stromal cells of the tumor microenvironment also play a critical role in creating a tumor-permissive microenvironment.[11] Our knowledge of this pathway is expanding rapidly and warrants a more detailed discussion for each tumor type.

HODGKIN LYMPHOMA

HL is divided into two major subgroups: classical HL (cHL) and nodular lymphocyte-predominant HL (NLPHL), based on morphologic and immunophenotypic characteristics of their cell of origin. cHL accounts for 95% of all cases and is characterized by a small number of neoplastic Reed–Sternberg (RS) cells or its variants within a dense infiltrate of inflammatory cells, including different types of lymphocytes, macrophages, eosinophils, neutrophils, and fibroblasts.[15] RS cells actively affect the composition of the cells of the microenvironment that in turn support the growth and survival of RS cells. However, despite the abundance of these immune cells in the tumor microenvironment, there is minimal effective host antitumor response highlighting the importance of immune evasion for survival of lymphoma cells.[15,16]

RS cells use several mechanisms to escape immune detection of which the PD-1 signaling pathway seems to play a key role. RS cells express PD-L1 and PD-L2 whereas PD-1 is expressed on TILs and peripheral T-cells. By engaging the PD-1 receptor on T-cells, RS cells are capable of reversibly inhibiting T-cell activation and proliferation, inducing a state of "T-cell exhaustion" to evade the antitumor immune response.[17] Macrophages and monocytes within the tumor microenvironment can also express PD-1 ligands and thus contribute to T-cell exhaustion and immune tolerance. Increased numbers of these tumor-associated macrophages expressing PD-1 ligands and of PD-1–positive TILs have been associated with poor outcomes in cHL.[18,19] Furthermore, blockade of the PD-1 signaling pathway in vitro was shown to restore the function of TILs.[17]

Mechanisms of PD-L1 and PD-L2 Overexpression in cHL

There are several mechanisms that lead to the upregulation of PD-L1 and PD-L2 in cHL. These mechanisms are not mutually exclusive and have also been described in other types of lymphoma, myeloma, and leukemia as discussed later (Fig. 9.1). *PD-L1* and *PD-L2* genes are located on chromosome 9p24.1, which has been shown to be a recurrent genetic abnormality in cHL.[20] In a series of 108 patients with newly diagnosed cHL, fluorescent in situ hybridization (FISH) assay showed that 97% of patients had alterations of the *PD-L1* and *PD-L2* loci on chromosome 9p24.1 (polysomy 5%, copy gain 56%, and amplification 36%).[21] Janus Kinase 2 (JAK2) is also located in close proximity on 9p24.1 and was coamplified with *PD-L1* and *PD-L2*.[20,21] JAK2/Signal Transducer and Activator of Transcription (STAT) pathway activation leads to PD-1 ligand induction, which further augments PD-1 ligand expression.[20] These alterations were associated with clinical outcomes, as progression-free survival (PFS) was significantly shorter for patients with 9p24.1 amplification who were also more likely to have advanced stage disease.[21] In another study of 265 patients with cHL, PD-L1 expression by immunohistochemistry (IHC) was noted on more than 5% of tumor cells in 70% of patients with cHL.[22] Alterations involving the major histocompatibility complex (MHC) class II transactivator (CIITA) (MHC2TA, a highly active promoter) have also been linked to PD-L1 and PD-L2 overexpression in cHL.[23]

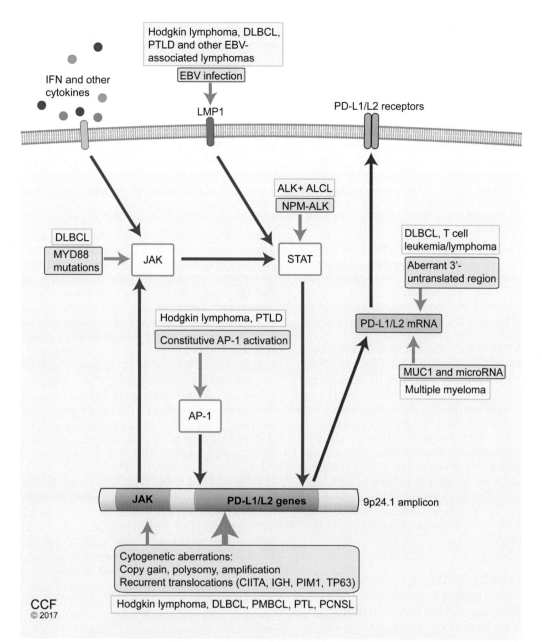

FIG. 9.1 Mechanisms of PD-L1 and PD-L2 overexpression in various hematologic malignancies. *PD-L1* and *PD-L2* genes are located on chromosome 9p24.1 and are target for recurrent cytogenetic aberrations leading to their overexpression. Such cytogenetic aberrations can also result in *JAK2* gene coamplification and, subsequently, further induction of PD-L1 expression through the JAK/STAT pathway activity on *PD-L1* promoter. Inflammatory cytokines, EBV infection, MYD88 mutations, and NPM-ALK fusion gene induce PD-L1/ L2 overexpression through the JAK/STAT pathway. AP-1 stimulates *PD-L1* enhancer. EBV infection also leads to AP-1 activation (not shown in figure). Structural variations disrupting the 3′ region of the *PD-L1* gene lead to elevated expression of abnormal *PD-L1* transcripts and increased expression of PD-L1 proteins. MUC1 oncoprotein induces PD-L1 expression by downregulating *PD-L1* specific microRNAs. *ALCL*, anaplastic large cell lymphoma; *CIITA*, class II transactivator; *DLBCL*, diffuse large B-cell lymphoma; *EBV*, Epstein–Barr virus; *IFN*, interferon; *JAK*, janus kinase; *PCNSL*, primary CNS lymphoma; *PMBCL*, primary mediastinal B-cell lymphoma; *PTL*, primary testicular lymphoma; *PTLD*, posttransplant lymphoproliferative disorders; *TCL*, T-cell lymphoma.

Infection with Epstein—Barr virus (EBV) is another alternative mechanism for PD-1 ligand overexpression in cHL tumor cells with normal 9p24.1 copy number.[24] EBV is implicated in 30%—40% of cHL cases where infected RS cells express several EBV proteins.[15] The EBV-encoded latent membrane protein-1 activates the promoter and enhancer of *PD-L1* by increasing signaling through the JAK/STAT pathway and activation of the transcription factor AP-1, respectively.[24] In this way, stimulation of PD-L1 expression in EBV-infected cells is crucial for EBV to avoid immune detection. Constitutive AP-1 signaling in RS cells is another reported mechanism for upregulation of PD-L1 expression.[24]

Based on these findings, cHL was felt to be a prime target for PD-1 blockade and has been the most heavily studied hematologic malignancy in this regards. In fact, cHL has the highest response rates to PD-1 blockade among all cancers studied so far, highlighting the pivotal role for the PD-1 pathway for tumor survival.

Nodular Lymphocyte Predominant Hodgkin Lymphoma

NLPHL is an uncommon subtype of HL characterized by the presence of TILs that form rosettes around atypical RS cells called lymphocytic and histiocytic cells. Less data are available on the PD-1 pathway expression in NLPHL given its rarity. However, PD-L1 positivity by IHC (more than 5% of tumor cells) has been reported in 54% of patients in one study and in 13% in another study, although the number of patients in each study was small.[22,25] The TILs in NPLHL have been shown to express PD-1 uniformly; a feature that can help differentiate NLPHL from other types of non-Hodgkin lymphoma (NHL).[14,22,26]

DIFFUSE LARGE B-CELL LYMPHOMA

Compared with HL, PD-L1 expression on lymphoma cells in diffuse large B-cell lymphoma (DLBCL) is in general less prevalent (11%—31%), although this depends on the study and the cutoff used to define positive expression. Notably, PD-L1 expression is mainly restricted to the more aggressive, non—germinal center B-cell—like (non-GCB) subtype.[22,25,27,28]

Mechanisms of PD-L1 Overexpression in Diffuse Large B-Cell Lymphoma

Several mechanisms have been reported for PD-L1 overexpression in DLBCL, a few of which have already been discussed in cHL (Fig. 9.1). Genetic/cytogenetic aberrations involving *PD-L1/PD-L2* locus on chromosome

9p24.1 have been described in 20% of DLBCL cases. In a study using whole-genome sequencing analysis on DLBCL samples, the *PD-L1/PD-L2* locus was found to be a recurrent translocation partner for the immunoglobulin heavy chain locus.[28] Two other translocation partners were also recognized (PIM1 and TP63). Using a FISH assay on 179 samples in the same study, the *PD-L1/PD-L2* locus was affected by gains (12%), amplifications (3%), and translocations (4%).[28] These aberrations were more commonly seen in the non-GCB subtype. Another study reported an association between PD-L1 expression on DLBCL cells and chromosome 9p24.1 gain but not structural abnormalities.[27] In contrast to other types of lymphoma,[17,29,30] these cytogenetic abnormalities correlated with increased expression of PD-L1 but not PD-L2.[28] Enhanced expression of JAK/STAT has been reported in non-GCB DLBCL and can result in PD-L1 overexpression as mentioned previously.[31] Additionally, 30% of non-GCB cases harbor MYD88 mutations that lead to constitutive expression and activation of the JAK/STAT pathway.[32] Furthermore, PD-L1 expression in DLBCL has been linked with EBV infection through mechanisms described earlier in this chapter.[27,28,33] Finally, a small subset of patients with DLBCL (and adult T-cell leukemia/lymphoma) had PD-L1 transcripts with an aberrant 3'-untranslated region, which resulted in delayed clearance of PD-L1 transcripts and therefore PD-L1 overexpression.[34]

Impact of PD-L1 Overexpression on Clinical Outcomes in Diffuse Large B-cell Lymphoma

Importantly, PD-1 and PD-L1 expression in DLBCL has been linked to clinical outcomes. In a study of 1253 untreated patients with DLBCL, PD-L1 and PAX5 double staining was performed to identify PD-L1—positive lymphoma cells and distinguish them from PD-L1—positive tumor microenvironment cells (predominantly macrophages).[27] PD-L1 expression (using a positivity cutoff $\geq$30% for malignant cells and $\geq$20% for nonmalignant cells) was positive in 11% of lymphoma cells and 15% of tumor microenvironment cells. PD-L1 expression on lymphoma cells was significantly associated with the presence of B symptoms, elevated soluble interleukin-2 receptor levels, international prognostic index high-risk group, non-GCB subtype, and inferior OS. The prognostic effect of PD-L1 expression on OS was maintained in multivariable analysis. The number of PD-1—positive TILs was significantly lower in patients with adverse clinical features (presence of B symptoms, extranodal involvement, and bulky disease) and in those with positive PD-L1 expression on lymphoma or tumor microenvironment cells whereas it was higher in patients with a GCB subtype. Combining the median number of PD-1—positive TILs with positive or negative PD-L1 expression on lymphoma or tumor microenvironment cells, patients with positive PD-L1 expression and a low number of TILs had worse outcomes than those with negative PD-L1 expression and a low number of TILs.[27] High levels of soluble PD-L1 (sPD-L1) were also found to be associated with poor outcomes in DLBCL.[35,36] Plasma sPD-L1 levels were retrospectively analyzed in 288 patients enrolled on a French phase III clinical trial comparing the efficacy of R-CHOP (rituximab plus cyclophosphamide, doxorubicin, vincristine, and prednisone) with R-high-dose chemotherapy followed by autologous HCT. Compared with healthy subjects, sPD-L1 levels were elevated (at a defined level of 1.52 ng/mL) in 30% of DLBCL patients at diagnosis. Patients with high sPD-L1 had a significantly inferior 3-year OS compared with those with low sPD-L1 levels (76% vs. 89%), which remained significant on multivariable analysis.[35] A US study of an independent cohort of patients with newly diagnosed DLBCL treated with R-CHOP or R-CHOP—like regimens confirmed the association between elevated sPD-L1 levels and inferior OS.[36] Notably, these two studies showed no association between sPD-L1 levels and PD-L1 expression on lymphoma or nonmalignant cells, and sPD-L1 levels normalized in patients who achieved complete remission (CR). This indicates the existence of a complex system for sPD-L1 production, and that sPD-L1 levels reflect the extent of the host antitumor immune response, more than the mere presence of tumor cells.[36] Taken together, these studies demonstrate that upregulation of PD-L1 is associated with worse clinical outcomes in patients with DLBCL. The predictive role of PD-1 and PD-L1 expression in patients with DLBCL treated with immune checkpoint inhibitors is yet to be elucidated.

PD-L1/PD-L2 Overexpression in Variants/Subtypes of Diffuse Large B-Cell Lymphoma

PD-L1 is particularly overexpressed in the uncommon variant of DLBCL: T-cell—/histiocyte-rich large B-cell lymphoma (THRLB), with positive expression in 31%—91% of the small number of examined cases.[25,27] THRLB is characterized by the presence of rare malignant B-cells in a cytokine-rich inflammatory background of reactive T-cells and histiocytes. These lymphoma-surrounding cells also show strong PD-L1 expression indicating a potential role in providing immune escape signals.[25]

PD-L1 expression on malignant cells has also been reported in several other related types of lymphoma including primary CNS (central nervous system) lymphoma (PCNSL) (10% of cases), primary testicular large B-cell lymphoma (PTL) (54%), EBV-associated DLBCL of the elderly (100%), plasmablastic lymphoma (23%—44%), posttransplant lymphoproliferative disorders (59%), and HHV-8 associated primary effusion lymphoma (50%).[30,37,38] Chromosome 9p24.1 aberrations including copy number alterations and translocations have been reported in more than 50% of PTL and PCNSL cases.[25,30] It is worth mentioning here that, similar to EBV, infection with the human immunodeficiency virus (HIV) can lead to PD-1 and PD-L1 overexpression. PD-1 expression is upregulated in HIV-specific CD8+ T-cells and correlates with higher viral load and impaired cytokine production and cellular proliferation, indicating that the PD-1/PD-L1 axis is used by HIV for host immune evasion.[39]

Primary mediastinal large B-cell lymphoma (PMBCL) is a subtype of DLBCL with unique epidemiologic, clinical, and pathologic features. Gene expression analysis shows that it is distinct from typical DLBCL and shares many parts of its molecular signature with cHL.[40] Similarly, PD-1 ligands are expressed in PMBCL in 36%—100% of the cases with a strong association between PD-L1 and PD-L2 overexpression and genetic alteration involving chromosome 9p24.1 (Fig. 9.1).[20,29] These genetic alterations include locus amplification in 63% of cases with results similar to those mentioned previously in cHL and DLBCL and chromosomal rearrangements in 20% of cases resulting in the juxtaposition of CIITA adjacent to PD-1 ligand locus leading to overexpression of both PD-L1 and PD-L2.[20,41,42] CIITA rearrangements also lead to decreased expression of MHC class II molecules on the cell surface, which further enhances the immunosuppressive tumor microenvironment in PMBCL.[42]

Chromosome 9p24.1 locus aberrations have so far been reported in cHL, PMBCL, PTL, and PCNSL,[20,21,29,30] which lead to overexpression of both PD-L1 and PD-L2. Because both ligands, PD-L1 and PD-L2, are overexpressed concurrently, treatment of these lymphomas with agents targeting PD-1 is expected to have more therapeutic benefit than targeting either ligand alone. However, early results of a phase I trial using an anti—PD-L1 antibody in cHL have shown results comparable with those obtained with PD-1 inhibitors.[43] Although more data are needed, this might indicate that PD-1/PD-L1 interactions have a more dominant role in evading antitumor host immune responses than those of PD-1/PD-L2.[43]

FOLLICULAR LYMPHOMA

In contrast to HL and DLBCL, PD-L1 and PD-L2 expression have not been reported on tumor cells in follicular lymphoma (FL).[22,44–46] Nonetheless, the FL tumor microenvironment is rich with PD-L1−positive histiocytes and PD-1−positive TILs and follicular helper T-cells (TFH).[44,46] The reduced cytokine responsiveness of these PD-1−positive TILs implies that they receive suppressive signals from the surrounding PD-L1−positive histiocytes.[46] This again highlights the fundamental role for the tumor microenvironment in facilitating immune evasion in lymphoma and points to the potential therapeutic role of PD-1 inhibition in FL.

Studies regarding the prognostic significance of PD-1−positive TILs on clinical outcomes in FL have had conflicting results. This might be related to the presence of various subtypes of PD-1−positive TILs (TFH, regulatory T-cells, exhausted T-cells) that have distinct functions and localization patterns in lymph nodes (intra- vs. interfollicular areas).[46,47] One study showed that a higher number of PD-1−positive regulatory T-cells was associated with superior PFS and OS and lower risk of transformation to DLBCL,[48] wheras another study showed that a higher number of PD-1−positive TFH cells was associated with poor survival.[49] Another study identified two subpopulations of cells depending on PD-1 expression intensity (low or high); the number of exhausted CD4+PD-1^{low} T-cells was significantly associated with inferior OS whereas the number of CD4+PD-1^{high} T-cells was not.[47] Two other studies showed no effect on outcomes.[50,51] The effect of PD-1/PD-L1 blockade on these different subsets of TILs in FL is yet to be clarified.

CHRONIC LYMPHOCYTIC LEUKEMIA

PD-L1 is expressed on CLL cells, including those circulating in the blood and bone marrow, as well as on cells of the tumor microenvironment.[12,13] In contrast to most other hematologic malignancies, PD-1 is also expressed on the malignant cells in CLL, although the significance of this remains unclear.[12,13] PD-1−positive T-cells lie in close proximity to PD-L1−positive CLL cells and have reduced cytotoxic and proliferation capabilities, but they retain the ability to produce CLL growth-stimulating cytokines such as IFN-γ and TNF-α.[12,52] In a mouse model, PD-1 blockade was shown to restore T-cell cytotoxicity and prevent CLL development.[53] The prognostic significance of PD-1 and PD-L1 expression on tumor cells and TILs in patients with CLL has not been well studied and remains unclear.

OTHER B-CELL LYMPHOMAS

Data regarding the PD-1/PD-1 ligand axis in mantle cell lymphoma, lymphoplasmacytic lymphoma, marginal zone lymphoma (MZL), and Burkitt lymphoma are limited. However, from the few small available studies, none of these lymphomas seems to express PD-L1,[22,45,54] with the exception of one study reporting PD-L1 expression in 11% of cases of MZL with a high-grade component.[22]

T-CELL LYMPHOMA

Angioimmunoblastic TCL and around 20% of peripheral TCL not otherwise specified manifest a T follicular helper phenotype for which PD-1 is a common marker.[14,55] Cutaneous TCL can also have a similar phenotype, and PD-1 is expressed by the lymphoma cells in patients with mycosis fungoides, SS, and primary cutaneous CD4-positive small/medium TCL.[56,57] Furthermore, PD-L1 is overexpressed by ALK+ anaplastic large cell lymphoma (ALK+ ALCL), mycosis fungoides/SS, and NK/TCL-nasal type.[25,58,59] In ALK+ ALCL, the NPM-ALK fusion protein induces PD-L1 expression through the transcription factor STAT3 (Fig. 9.1).[58]

A study of 135 patients with adult T-cell leukemia/lymphoma reported PD-L1 expression on malignant cells in 7% of the patients.[60] Furthermore, among patients with negative PD-L1 expression on malignant cells, 59% had PD-L1 expression on nonmalignant cells of the tumor microenvironment. PD-L1 expression on malignant cells was an independent prognostic factor for inferior survival, whereas its expression on nonmalignant cells was an independent prognostic factor for superior survival.[60] The biology of the association between PD-L1 expression on tumor microenvironment cells and better clinical outcomes is not clear but has been reported in solid tumors.[61,62]

ACUTE LYMPHOCYTIC LEUKEMIA

PD-L1 expression was found to be increased in pediatric patients with relapsed B-cell acute lymphocytic leukemia (ALL) and in patients with ALL refractory to prior treatment with blinatumomab (a bispecific T-cell engaging monoclonal antibody).[63] This indicates a role for PD-1/PD-L1 axis in mediating resistance to blinatumomab and suggests a potential therapeutic benefit from combining immune checkpoint inhibitors with blinatumomab in patients with ALL.[63]

MULTIPLE MYELOMA

PD-L1 is overexpressed on plasma cells from patients with multiple myeloma (MM) but not on plasma cells from healthy donors or those with monoclonal gammopathy of undetermined significance.[64–67] In contrast, PD-L2 expression has not been reported in MM.[67,68] PD-L1 overexpression in myeloma cells can be mediated by PD-L1 gene copy number alterations in a way similar to cHL[67] or alternative mechanisms such as MUC1 oncoprotein expression and microRNA suppression (Fig. 9.1).[69] A study reported that increased PD-L1 expression was associated with higher bone marrow myeloma burden and serum lactate dehydrogenase levels and increased resistance to melphalan. Furthermore, PD-L1 expression was increased in patients with refractory or relapsed MM.[66] Likewise, higher serum levels of sPD-L1 were found to be associated with worse PFS in patients with MM.[70] PD-L1 expression is also present on the tumor microenvironment cells including plasmacytoid dendritic cells. These cells are increased in the bone marrow of MM patients and contribute to the immune dysfunctional state through interacting with the surrounding PD-1–positive T-cells and NK cells.[68] Murine models show that these PD-1–positive T-cells are present in large numbers at sites of myeloma cells but have an exhausted phenotype with impaired cytotoxic capabilities and that PD-L1 blockade improves survival in the myeloma-bearing mice.[71]

Lenalidomide is a very effective immunomodulatory agent commonly used in the treatment of newly diagnosed and relapsed MM. Lenalidomide exerts part of its therapeutic effect by acting on myeloid-derived suppressor cells, plasmacytoid dendritic cells, and the other cells of the tumor microenvironment.[72,73] Lenalidomide reduces the production of proangiogenic and anti-inflammatory cytokines and downregulates PD-1 expression on helper and cytotoxic T-cells and NK cells and PD-L1 expression on MM cells, which restores the cytotoxic functions of NK and T-cells.[67,73,74] Importantly, in vitro studies show that the combination of lenalidomide and immune checkpoint inhibitors might have a synergistic effect on MM tumor growth inhibition.[67] Based on these findings, multiple clinical trials are currently evaluating the safety and efficacy of combining lenalidomide, or its related drug pomalidomide, with immune checkpoint inhibitors, as discussed later.

Daratumumab is another drug that has an immunomodulatory effect in MM and can potentially augment the therapeutic benefit of immune checkpoint inhibitors. In addition to its known activity against CD38-expressing myeloma cells, daratumumab has recently been shown to be effective in targeting CD38-expressing immunosuppressive regulatory T- and B-cells and myeloid-derived suppressor cells and increasing the numbers of helper and cytotoxic T-cells in patients with MM.[75]

MYELOID MALIGNANCIES

Our current understanding of the PD-1 axis among the myeloid malignancies is most established in AML. In mice injected with AML cells, PD-L1 expression on leukemia cells was upregulated in vivo compared with baseline levels.[76] In addition, the number of CD8+ T-cells expressing PD-1 increased significantly at major sites of leukemic cell dissemination. In addition, PD-1 knock-out mice had enhanced number and functionality of CD8+ T-cells and slower AML progression compared with PD-1 wild-type mice. Similar antitumor results were seen after injecting PD-1 wild-type mice with PD-L1 blocking antibodies.[76] These observations demonstrate how AML cells engage the PD-1 axis for immune evasion.

Clinical studies confirmed these findings and showed expression of PD-1 and its ligands in hematopoietic cells of patients with AML, myelodysplastic syndrome (MDS), and chronic myelomonocytic leukemia (CMML).[77] A study of 124 patients with myeloid malignancies (69 with MDS, 46 with CMML, and 9 with AML) at different stages of treatment showed that PD-L1 mRNA expression level was upregulated by ≥twofold in 36%, 32%, and 25% of CD34+ cells in MDS, CMML, and AML, respectively, compared with CD34+ normal control cells.[77] PD-L2 and PD-1 were also upregulated but in smaller proportions. Similarly, PD-L1, PD-L2, and PD-1 expression were upregulated in peripheral blood mononuclear cells, with higher levels for PD-L2 and PD-1 than in CD34+ cells. By IHC of bone marrow biopsies, 20% of the leukemic blasts were positive for PD-L1, and PD-1 expression in stroma cells was also detected. Interestingly, PD-L1, PD-L2, PD-1, and CTLA-4 gene expression were upregulated ≥twofold in >50% of patients treated with hypomethylating agents, with a trend toward increased expression in resistant patients compared with sensitive patients. Furthermore, upregulation of PD-L1 and PD-L2 was associated with inferior OS, which was statistically significant for PD-L2. This indicates that the PD-1 pathway might be involved in developing resistance to treatment with hypomethylating agents and that adjunctive therapy with immune checkpoint inhibitors might potentiate the therapeutic benefits of hypomethylating agents.[77] Another study of 154 patients with AML showed that although PD-L1 was not overexpressed in AML patients compared with healthy donors, simulation with IFN-γ significantly increased PD-L1 expression on AML blasts and not in normal controls. Notably, the increase in PD-L1 expression on myeloid blasts was more pronounced in samples from patients in CR or at relapse than in those with newly diagnosed AML.[78] This pattern of inducible PD-L1 expression suggests that chronic inflammatory conditions and the accompanying cytokine milieu might play a key role in inducing expression of immune-inhibitory signals on myeloid blasts that lead to immune evasion.[78] There is also evidence showing that the leukemic blasts use the PD-1 axis to induce alloreactive T-lymphocyte dysfunction in the setting of disease relapse after allogeneic HCT.[79,80]

Data regarding the PD-1 axis in other myeloid malignancies are limited. Patients with chronic myeloid leukemia (CML) have been shown to have impaired immune responses at diagnosis, as demonstrated by the increased number of myeloid-derived suppressor cells, regulatory T-cells, and exhausted cytotoxic T-cells and NK cells.[81,82] The PD-1 axis plays an important role in mediating this immunosuppressive tumor environment. CML cells express PD-L1, and PD-1−expressing T-cells are dysfunctional in patients with CML.[81−83] In murine models, PD-L1 is expressed on CML stem and progenitor cells, and is upregulated by IFN-γ secreted by cytotoxic T-cells.[83] A recent study showed recovery of the immune function and reduction in PD-1 expression on cytotoxic T-cells in patients who achieved deep molecular remissions after treatment with tyrosine kinase inhibitors (TKIs).[82] This demonstrates that the state of antitumor immune dysfunction that accompanies CML can be reversed and suggests a potential therapeutic benefit from immune checkpoint inhibitors in combination with TKIs in CML.[82]

TREATMENT WITH IMMUNE CHECKPOINT INHIBITORS

Hodgkin Lymphoma

Ipilimumab, a fully human IgG1 anti−CTLA-4 antibody, was the first immune checkpoint inhibitor tested in a phase I trial of a single infusion at doses between 0.1 and 3.0 mg/kg in 14 patients with relapsed or refractory cHL after allogeneic HCT. Two patients achieved CR, and importantly, there were no cases of significant graft-versus-host disease (GVHD).[84]

Based on the success of anti−PD-1 therapy in solid tumors, a phase I study of nivolumab (CheckMate 039) was initiated in patients with relapsed or refractory cHL, NHL and MM (Table 9.1). The cHL cohort consisted of 23 heavily treated patients, most of whom had received three or more prior treatments, including 18 patients who had received prior autologous HCT followed by brentuximab vedotin (BV). Despite this, nivolumab showed an impressive objective response rate (ORR) of 87% (CR = 17%).[85] A subsequent phase II study (CheckMate 205) confirmed nivolumab's activity in patients with relapsed or refractory cHL after autologous HCT.[86,87] CheckMate 205 enrolled patients into one of three cohorts. Cohort A consisted of patients with no prior exposure to BV; cohort B included patients who received BV only after autologous HCT; and cohort C included patients who received BV before and/or after autologous HCT. Nivolumab was given at a dose of 3 mg/kg every 2 weeks until disease progression or unacceptable toxicity. In cohort C, patients with CR for 1 year were required to discontinue treatment with nivolumab with an option to resume it at relapse. Early results of cohort B in 2016, after a median follow-up of 15 months, showed an ORR of 68% (CR = 8%). Even though the rate of CR was low, responses lasted a median duration of 13 months, and median PFS was 15 months while median OS was not reached.[86,87] Based on these results, nivolumab was granted accelerated approval by the U.S. Food and Drug Administration (FDA) for the treatment of patients with cHL following failure of autologous HCT and posttransplantation BV (May 2016). A recent update of the CheckMate 205 trial reported the outcomes of 243 treated patients: 63 BV-naïve patients (cohort A), 80 patients treated with BV after autologous HCT (cohort B), and 100 patients treated with BV before and/or after autologous HCT (cohort C; 33 had BV before, 58 after, and 9 before and after autologous HCT). Median duration of follow-up was 19, 23, and 16 months for cohorts A, B, and C, respectively. For cohort A, ORR was 65% (CR = 29%) and median duration of response and PFS were 20 and 18 months, respectively. For cohort B, ORR was 68% (CR = 13%) and median duration of response and PFS were 16 and 15 months, respectively. For cohort C, ORR was 73% (CR = 12%) and median duration of response and PFS were 15 and 12 months, respectively. Median OS for the 243 patients was not reached.[88]

Similarly, a phase Ib study (KEYNOTE-013) of another anti−PD-1 monoclonal antibody, pembrolizumab, included an independent cohort of 31 patients with cHL. Patients had failed prior treatment with BV, and 22 patients had also failed prior autologous HCT. Pembrolizumab showed similar encouraging results with an ORR of 58% (CR = 19%). The

TABLE 9.1
Selected Trials of Immune Checkpoint Inhibitors in Relapsed/Refractory Hodgkin Lymphoma

Trial Name[References]	Phase	Drug	No. of Pts[a]	Description	OUTCOMES					Median Follow-Up (m)	Safety (G3/4/5 DRAE)
					ORR (%)	CR (%)	PFS (m)	OS (m)	DOR (m)		
CheckMate 039[85]	I	Nivolumab	23	18 pts had prior auto HCT and BV	87	17	NR	83% at 18m	NR	10	G3: 22% (one pneumonitis and one colitis). No G4/5
CheckMate 205[86–88]	II	Nivolumab	243	Cohort A (n = 63): BV-naïve	65	29	18	NR	20	19	Infusion reactions 2% Pneumonitis 1%
				Cohort B (n = 80): BV after auto HCT	68	13	15	NR	16	23	
				Cohort C (n = 100): BV before and/or after auto HCT	73	12	12	NR	15	16	
KEYNOTE-013[89,90]	I	Pembrolizumab	31	Failed BV (22 failed auto HCT)	58	19	11	NR	NR	25	G3: 16% (one colitis) No G4/5
KEYNOTE-087[91]	II	Pembrolizumab	210	Three treatment cohorts:	69	22	72% at 6 m	NR	NR	10	G3: 7% (one colitis) No G4/5
				Cohort 1 (n = 69): after auto HCT and BV	74	22	–	–	–	–	
				Cohort 2 (n = 81): ineligible for auto HCT, after BV	64	25	–	–	–	–	
				Cohort 3 (n = 60): after auto HCT, no BV	70	20	–	–	–	–	
ECOG-ACRIN (E4412)[93]	I	Nivolumab + BV	17	Eight pts had prior auto HCT and four had prior BV	89	50	91% at 6 m	NR	–	6	Two pneumonitis (one G3 + one G5)
NCT02572167[94]	I/II	Nivolumab + BV	55	45% of pts with primary refractory disease	85	64	–	–	–	–	G 3/4: 33% One G4 pneumonitis
JAVELIN Hodgkin[43]	I	Avelumab	31	Failed prior auto or allo HCT or HCT-ineligible.	55	7	–	–	–	–	G 3/4: 37% Two G3 liver GVHD

Allo, allogeneic; *Auto HCT*, autologous hematopoietic cell transplantation; *BV*, brentuximab vedotin; *CR*, complete response; *DOR*, duration of response; *DRAE*, drug-related adverse events; *G*, grade; *GVHD*, graft versus host disease; *m*, month; *No.*, number; *NR*, not reached; *ORR*, overall response rate; *OS*, overall survival; *PFS*, progression-free survival; *Pts*, patients.
[a]Number of patients evaluable for response.

median duration of response was not reached after a median follow-up of 25 months.[89,90] In the phase II KEYNOTE-087 study of 210 patients with relapsed or refractory cHL, pembrolizumab was evaluated in three cohorts of patients defined by history of exposure to BV and autologous HCT.[91] Cohort 1 consisted of patients with relapsed or refractory disease after autologous HCT and subsequent BV; cohort 2 included patients with no response to salvage chemotherapy and were therefore ineligible for autologous HCT and whose disease subsequently progressed on BV; and cohort 3 included patients with relapsed or refractory disease after autologous HCT but who had not received posttransplant treatment with BV. With a median duration of follow-up of 10 months, the ORR was 69% (CR = 22%) across all cohorts (74% in cohort 1; 64% in cohort 2; and 70% in cohort 3). ORR was 80% (CR = 25%) in patients with primary refractory disease and 64% (CR = 23%) in transplant-ineligible patients secondary to failure of salvage therapy and BV. ORRs were similar between patients who received <three prior lines of therapy versus those who received ≥three lines.[91] These remarkable results granted pembrolizumab an accelerated FDA approval for the treatment of patients with refractory cHL or those who have relapsed after ≥three prior lines of therapy (March 2017). Safety analysis in all four trials did not show any new safety concerns, and toxicities of anti–PD-1 monotherapy in cHL were similar to those reported in solid tumors. Grade 3 or higher drug-related adverse events occurred in around 20% of the patients. The incidence of any grade pneumonitis was comparable with what is seen in solid tumors (less than 5%),[92] despite the prior exposure to pneumotoxic agents such as bleomycin, carmustine, radiotherapy, and/or BV in most of these patients.

Correlative studies in these trials confirmed the earlier genetic studies, with all of the examined tumor samples showing copy number gain at 9p24.1 and associated overexpression of PD-L1 and PD-L2, in addition to the activation of JAK-STAT signaling pathway in RS cells.[86] PD-1 blockade was also shown to expand T-cell and NK cell populations and upregulate IFN-γ–activated pathways.[89] Patients with chromosome 9p24.1 amplification and high PD-L1 expression on RS cells, previously reported to have worse clinical outcomes when treated with chemotherapy,[21] had higher response rates with PD-L1 blockade.[86] In contrast, PD-L1 expression on infiltrating nonmalignant cells was not associated with improved response.[86]

As discussed earlier, RS overexpress both PD-L1 and PD-L2; therefore, the use of blocking either of these two ligands and leaving the other unopposed has been questioned. However, the phase I JAVELIN Hodgkin trial (NCT02603419) of the anti–PD-L1 monoclonal antibody, avelumab, suggests that PD-L1 blockade alone can result in significant therapeutic responses in cHL.[43] This study evaluated avelumab in patients with cHL whose disease progressed following either autologous or allogeneic HCT or in those ineligible for HCT. Patients received one of five dosing intensities (70, 350 or 500 mg every 2 weeks, 500 mg every 3 weeks, or 10 mg/kg every 2 weeks). Five patients had disease progression after autologous HCT; eight, after allogeneic HCT, and the remaining patients were ineligible for transplant. The ORR in the 31 evaluable patients was 55% (CR = 7%). Responses were observed in all dosing groups (ORR range 14%–83%). ORR was 20% in the five postautologous HCT patients (1 partial remission (PR)), and 75% in the eight postallogeneic HCT patients (1 CR and 5 PR). In the 30 patients analyzed for safety, the most common treatment-related adverse events of any grade were infusion-related reaction (27%), nausea (20%), rash (20%), and fatigue (13%). Two patients discontinued treatment owing to infusion-related reactions. Grade ≥3 treatment-related adverse events occurred in 11 patients (37%) with no treatment-related deaths.[43]

Combining PD-1 blockade with other active agents in Hodgkin lymphoma

The great clinical efficacy and favorable safety profile of PD-1 monotherapy in cHL encouraged investigators to combine it with other active agents. To date, two studies have tested the combination of nivolumab with BV in patients with relapsed or refractory cHL (Table 9.1). Preliminary data from these two trials show promising results with deeper responses than with either agent alone.[93,94] Nonetheless, further follow-up is needed to update efficacy and safety data. In the phase I ECOG-ACRIN (E4412) trial, patients received nivolumab 3 mg/kg plus BV 1.2 or 1.8 mg/kg every 21 days for 16 cycles.[93] Nivolumab was allowed to be continued for an additional year. Patients were heavily treated, with a median of three prior therapies; eight patients had received prior autologous HCT, and four patients had prior treatment with BV. For the 17 evaluable patients, the ORR was highly impressive at 89% (CR = 50%). With a median follow-up of 6 months, the 6 month PFS was 91% and median OS was not reached. Of the 19 patients evaluable for safety, two patients developed pneumonitis—one was grade 5 and the other one was grade 3 from which the patient fully recovered. Rash, pruritis, and neutropenia were the other grade 3 toxicities, and there were no other grade 4 or 5 toxicities. Only one grade 1–2 infusion reaction was reported.[93] The other study (NCT02572167) was a similar phase I/II study in patients with relapsed or refractory disease, with around half of the patients with primary refractory disease.[94] Patients were treated with nivolumab 3 mg/kg plus BV 1.8 mg/kg in 21-day cycles for up to four cycles. For the 55 evaluable patients, the ORR was 85% (CR = 64%), and 29 patients proceeded to autologous HCT. Of the 98% patients who had treatment-related adverse events, 28% and 5% were grade 3 and 4, respectively. Two patients developed pneumonitis—one grade 4 and one grade 2. Infusion-related reactions occurred in 41% of the patients, most frequently during cycle 2 of treatment. Even though most of these reactions were grade 1–2 (grade 3 in <5%), dose interruptions were required in 25%.[94]

Future directions

Taken together, these studies have shown striking responses for treatment with immune checkpoint inhibitors in patients with relapsed or refractory cHL. In addition, these results have validated the genetically determined dependence of cHL on the PD-1 pathway for survival. Responses were durable but longer follow-up is needed and confirmation of improvement in OS is awaited. Treatment with PD-1 monotherapy was overall well tolerated with no new or unexpected adverse events reported; however, further data are needed regarding the use of immune checkpoint inhibitors in combination with other therapeutic agents or following HCT.

The success of PD-1 antibody therapy in the relapsed or refractory setting has encouraged investigators to use these agents earlier in the treatment course of cHL to increase the cure rates of patients with high-risk disease and to reduce treatment toxicity in lower risk patients. A phase III trial was initiated to compare pembrolizumab versus BV in patients with relapsed or refractory cHL (NCT02684292). A phase II clinical trial is currently evaluating the safety and efficacy of the combination of nivolumab with doxorubicin, vinblastine, and dacarbazine (AVD) in patients with newly diagnosed cHL. Another study is evaluating nivolumab plus BV in elderly patients or those who cannot tolerate conventional chemotherapy. Other studies are testing PD-1 blockade in combination with ipilimumab with (NCT01896999) or without BV (NCT02304458 and NCT01592370) or with ibrutinib (NCT02940301) in the relapsed or refractory setting.

Diffuse Large B-Cell Lymphoma, Primary Mediastinal Large B-Cell Lymphoma, and Other Large Cell Lymphomas

Ipilimumab was the first immune checkpoint inhibitor evaluated in DLBCL despite the lack of a clear role for the CTLA-4 pathway in this disease. The phase I trial of ipilimumab enrolled 18 patients with relapsed or refractory B-cell NHL. Overall, the ORR was low (11%); however, of the three patients with DLBCL, two responded with one patient achieving CR that lasted for more than 2.5 years.[95]

Pidilizumab, a humanized IgG-1 κ monoclonal antibody, was the first PD-1 inhibitor tested in hematologic malignancies in a phase I study that enrolled 17 patients with various hematologic malignancies. The study showed a favorable safety profile for pidilizumab, but there were no objective responses in the two patients with DLBCL.[96] Subsequently, a phase II trial of pidilizumab was conducted in patients with recurrent DLBCL, PMBCL, or transformed indolent lymphoma undergoing autologous HCT (Table 9.2).[97] Pidilizumab was given at a dose of 1.5 mg/kg every 42 days for three cycles from 1 to 3 months after autologous HCT. This setting was selected, as the posttransplant period is characterized by minimal residual disease and immune system remodeling, and PD-1 blockade can potentially inhibit a tumor-driven, PD-1–dependent state of immune tolerance.[97] The overall PFS for the 66 evaluable patients was 72% at 16 months, which exceeded the study's prespecified 16-month PFS of 69%. The 16-month OS was 85%. Among the 35 patients with residual disease on CT imaging posttransplant, the ORR was 51% (CR = 34%). The ORR dropped to 33% for the nine patients with residual disease after transplant and a positive PET scan. No significant autoimmune toxicity, infusion reactions, or treatment-related mortality was reported. Pidilizumab resulted in a significant increase in the number of PD-L1–positive activated helper T-cells within 24 h of drug infusion, which lasted for at least 16 weeks. The exact mechanism for this anti–PD-1–induced increase in circulating PD-L1–expressing cells is still unclear, but it might be related to inhibition of PD-1–mediated lymphocyte apoptosis and increase in mobilization of lymphocytes from their reservoirs.[97]

Nivolumab was evaluated in a phase I trial of patients with various relapsed or refractory hematologic malignancies. Eleven patients had DLBCL of whom four patients responded to treatment (ORR = 36%, 2 CR and 2 PR) and three patients had stable disease. Median PFS was 7 weeks. The two patients who had PMBCL did not respond to treatment but had stable disease without evidence of progression at 24 weeks.[98]

TABLE 9.2
Selected Trials of Immune Checkpoint Inhibitors in Relapsed/Refractory Non-Hodgkin Lymphoma, T-cell Lymphoma, and Multiple Myeloma

| Trial[References] | Phase | Drug | Disease | No of Pts[a] | Description/ Comments | OUTCOMES | | | | Median Follow-Up (m) | Safety (G3/4/5) DRAE |
						ORR (%)	CR (%)	PFS (m)	DOR (m)		
NCT00532259[97]	II	Pidilizumab	DLBCL, PMBCL, transformed iNHL	66	Pidilizumab was given for three cycles from 1 to 3 months post auto HCT	51[b]	34	72% at 16m	—	—	G 3/4: 4% No immune-related toxicities
NCT01592370[98]	I	Nivolumab	DLBCL	11	91% received ≥2 prior tx	36	18	2	—	6	G ≥3: 22% One G5 pneumonitis
			FL	10	70% received ≥2 prior tx	40	10	NR	—	23	
			TCL	23	87% received ≥2 prior tx	17	0	3	—	—	
			MM	27	56% received prior auto HCT, 89% double refractory	4	4	3	—	16	
NCT02220842[99]	I	Atezolizumab, obinutuzumab	DLBCL	23	87% refractory to last tx	16	—	—	2	—	G 3/4: pain (8%), anemia (6%), neutropenia (6%)
			FL	26	52% refractory to last tx	57	—	—	6	—	
KEYNOTE-013[100]	I	Pembrolizumab	PMBCL	20	67% transplant-ineligible owing to refractory disease	50	25	—	NR	14	G 3/4: 25%. One G4 veno-occlusive liver disease after allo HCT

Trial	Phase	Agent(s)	Disease	No. pts	Prior therapy						DRAE
KEYNOTE-170[101]	II	Pembrolizumab	PMBCL	23	70% transplant-ineligible owing to refractory disease	35	13	—	—	2.5	G 3/4: 30%. One G4 neutropenia
NCT00904722[103]	II	Pidilizumab, rituximab	FL	29	1–4 prior tx, rituximab-sensitive	66	52	19	20	15	No G3/4 immune-related toxicities
NCT02446457[106]	II	Pembrolizumab, rituximab	FL	15	Received ≥ 1 prior tx, rituximab-sensitive	80	60	NR	NR	7	No G3/4 immune-related toxicities
KEYNOTE-023[110]	I	Pembrolizumab, lenalidomide, dexamethasone	MM	40	Median of 4 prior tx. 75% refractory to lenalidomide and 53% double refractory	50	2.5	—	—	—	One G5 hepatic failure and one G5 ischemic stroke
NCT02289222[111]	II	Pembrolizumab, pomalidomide, dexamethasone	MM	48	70% had prior auto HCT. 73% double refractory	60	8	17	15	16	One G3 pneumonitis

Allo, allogeneic; Auto HCT, autologous hematopoietic cell transplantation; CR, complete response; DLBCL, diffuse large B-cell lymphoma; DOR, duration of response; DRAE, drug-related adverse events; FL, follicular lymphoma; G, grade; GVHD, graft versus host disease; IMiDs, immunomodulators; iNHL, indolent non-Hodgkin lymphoma; m, month; MM, multiple myeloma; No., number; NR, not reached; ORR, overall response rate; PFS, progression-free survival; PIs, proteasome inhibitors; PMBCL, primary mediastinal B-cell lymphoma; Pts, patients; TCL, T-cell lymphoma; tx, therapy.

[a]Number of patients evaluable for response.

[b]35 pts had measurable disease posttransplant and before receiving pidilizumab.

PD-L1 blockade has also been explored in DLBCL. Atezolizumab (a humanized IgG1 monoclonal anti—PD-L1 antibody), in combination with obinutuzumab (a humanized anti-CD20 monoclonal antibody), was evaluated in a phase I study in patients with relapsed or refractory DLBCL. Treatment with the combination had a favorable safety profile, but the ORR was low (16%).[99] As discussed earlier, PD-L1 upregulation is more common in the more aggressive non-GCB subtype of DLBCL; however, none of the DLBCL trials mentioned so far has compared the responses of immune checkpoint inhibitors in GCB versus non-GCB subtypes.

In contrast to the limited success in DLBCL, early results with anti—PD-1 monotherapy seem to be more encouraging in PMBCL and possibly PCNS and PTL (Table 9.2); however, larger trials and longer follow-up are needed.[100–102] An independent cohort of the phase Ib trial of pembrolizumab (KEYNOTE-013) enrolled patients with relapsed or refractory PMBCL.[100] The ORR was 50% (CR = 25%) in the 20 evaluable patients. Median duration of response was not reached after a median follow-up of 14 months. Duration of response in patients with CR ranged from 1 to 27 months. Based on these results, an international phase II trial (KEYNOTE-170) of pembrolizumab in patients with relapsed or refractory PMBCL was launched. Preliminary results showed an ORR of 35% (CR = 13%) in the 23 evaluable patients. Of note, more than two-thirds of the patients enrolled in these two trials had primary refractory disease and were therefore ineligible for autologous HCT.[100,101] A pilot series of five patients with relapsed or refractory PCNS and PTL treated with nivolumab showed radiographic responses in all patients, including four complete responses and one partial response. Three patients remained with no evidence of disease progression for more than a year.[102] A phase II study of nivolumab in patients with relapsed or refractory PCNS and PTL is currently recruiting (CheckMate 647, NCT02857426).

Follicular Lymphoma

In the aforementioned phase I trial of nivolumab in relapsed or refractory hematologic malignancies, 4 of the 10 patients with FL responded to treatment (ORR = 40%, CR = 10%)[98] (Table 9.2). Of note, none of the other patients with B-cell NHL responded (mantle cell [n = 4], small lymphocytic [n = 2], MZL [n = 1], and B-cell NHL not otherwise specified [n = 1]).[98]

A phase II trial of patients with relapsed, rituximab-sensitive, grade 1—2 FL evaluated the use of pidilizumab

in combination with rituximab.[103] Pidilizumab was given at a dose of 3 mg/kg every 4 weeks while rituximab was given at a standard dose every week, each for four infusions. Responders and those with stable disease were given eight optional pidilizumab infusions every 4 weeks. The ORR was 66% (CR = 52%) in the 29 evaluable patients. The median time to response was 88 days (range 53—392 days), and six patients had delayed initial responses occurring more than 4 months after the first pidilizumab infusion. With a median follow-up duration of 15 months, PFS was 19 months for all patients and not reached for responders; the median duration of response was 20 months. Understanding the limitations of comparing different studies, these results compare favorably with historical data of patients with relapsed FL treated with rituximab monotherapy (ORR = 40—49%, CR = 11—14%).[104,105] No grade 3 or 4 treatment-related adverse events were detected. The baseline expression of PD-L1, but not PD-1 or PD-L2, was significantly higher in peripheral blood CD4+ cells, CD8+ cells, and CD14+ cells of responders than that of nonresponders; however, this was not associated with PFS.[103] The lack of autoimmune toxicity with pidilizumab in the DLBCL and FL trials so far is worth mentioning, which might be attributed to the lower dose and less frequent administration of pidilizumab compared with the other anti—PD-1 antibodies.[97,103]

An ongoing phase II trial is evaluating the use of pembrolizumab in combination with rituximab in patients with relapsed, rituximab-sensitive, grade 1—3a FL. Rituximab is given weekly for 4 weeks while pembrolizumab is given every 3 weeks for up to 16 cycles. Preliminary results showed an ORR of 80% (CR = 60%) in the 15 evaluable patients. With a median follow-up of 7 months, median duration of response, PFS, and OS was not reached. For the 27 treated patients, grade 3 adverse events included aseptic meningitis and pneumonia, in one patient each. Immune-related adverse events included grade 2 diarrhea in two patients and grade 2 pneumonitis and skin rash in one patient each.[106]

Chronic Lymphocytic Leukemia

A phase II study of pembrolizumab in patients with transformed CLL with Richter transformation or relapsed CLL showed an ORR of 44% in the 9 patients with Richter transformation, while none of the 16 patients with relapsed disease responded.[107] Notably, all responses were observed in patients with Richter transformation who had disease progression after prior therapy with ibrutinib. With a median follow-up duration of 11 months, the median OS for patients with Richter transformation was 11 months but was not reached in patients previously treated with ibrutinib. No new or excessive toxicities were reported. Responders had increased expression of PD-L1 on cells of the tumor microenvironment on pretreatment samples.[107]

In addition to inhibiting Bruton tyrosine kinase that is vital for the survival of malignant B-lymphocytes, ibrutinib also inhibits interleukin-2—inducible kinase (ITK) that has an essential role in the activation of regulatory T-cells.[108] By inhibiting ITK, ibrutinib can potentially shift the balance toward an antitumor immune response.[108] Based on this reasoning, combining ibrutinib with PD-1 blockade was attempted in vitro and in mice and showed significant therapeutic efficacy.[109] Ongoing trials are exploring the combination of immune checkpoint inhibitors with ibrutinib in CLL.

T-Cell Lymphoma

Data regarding the use of immune checkpoint inhibitors in patients with TCL are limited to 23 patients (including 5 with peripheral TCL and 13 with mycosis fungoides) treated on a phase I trial with nivolumab (Table 9.2). The ORR was 17% (all PR, two patients with mycosis fungoides and two with peripheral TCL). With a median follow-up of 10 months, responses were ongoing for three patients.[98]

Multiple Myeloma

Twenty-seven patients with MM were included in the phase Ib trial of nivolumab in hematologic malignancies mentioned previously[98] (Table 9.2). Almost all patients received two or more prior treatments; more than half of them had received autologous HCT, and 24 patients had disease progression after prior therapy with an immunomodulatory drug and a proteasome inhibitor. Despite the lack of objective responses to treatment after a median follow-up of 9 weeks, 63% of the patients achieved stable disease that lasted for a median of 11 weeks.[98]

As discussed previously, there is preclinical rationale for combining immune checkpoint inhibitors with other agents active in MM such as lenalidomide and/or daratumumab for a synergistic therapeutic effect. The phase I trial KEYNOTE-023 (NCT02036502) included patients with relapsed or refractory MM treated with two or more prior therapies.[110] Patients received pembrolizumab 200 mg every 2 weeks, lenalidomide 25 mg daily on day 1–21, and dexamethasone

40 mg weekly, each on a 28-day cycle. Patients were heavily treated with a median of four prior therapies; 75% were refractory to lenalidomide, and 53% were refractory to both proteasome inhibitors and immunomodulatory agents. Preliminary results for the 40 evaluable patients showed an ORR of 50% (1 stringent CR, 5 very good PR, 14 PR). ORR for lenalidomide refractory patients was 38%. Neutropenia (33%), thrombocytopenia (18%), and anemia (12%) were the most common serious treatment-related adverse events. Two patients had grade 5 treatment-related adverse events (liver failure and ischemic stroke). Immune-related adverse events occurred in 10% of the patients, but no cases of pneumonitis were reported. Flow cytometry analysis of bone marrow biopsies at time of diagnosis showed that all CD38+ CD138+ cells expressed PD-L1, while PD-L2 expression was variable. Treatment with lenalidomide and pembrolizumab increased the frequency of circulating HLA-DR+ and memory T-cells in peripheral blood.[110] Similarly, a single-institution phase II trial of pembrolizumab, pomalidomide, and dexamethasone in patients with relapsed or refractory MM was conducted.[111] Patients received pembrolizumab 200 mg every 2 weeks, pomalidomide 4 mg daily for 21 days, and dexamethasone 40 mg weekly in a 28-day cycle. Forty-eight patients were enrolled with a median of three prior therapies; 70% had prior autologous HCT, and 73% were refractory to both proteasome inhibitors and immunomodulatory agents. The ORR was 60% (stringent CR/CR = 8%, very good PR = 9%, and PR = 33%). With a median follow-up duration of 16 months, the median duration of response and PFS were 15 and 17 months, respectively, and OS was not reached. Grade 3 or higher treatment-related adverse events occurred in 42% of patients with hematologic toxicities being the most common. Six patients developed pneumonitis—grade 3 in one patient and grades 1–2 in the rest. IHC of pretreatment bone marrow biopsies showed a trend toward increased PD-L1 expression in responding patients (54% vs. 20%, $P = .06$) but with no correlation between PD-L1 staining and PFS. There was also a trend for longer PFS with increased number of TILs, irrespective of PD-1 expression.[111] Bearing in mind the caveats of indirect comparisons of clinical trial data, the response rates in these two trials were remarkably higher than those seen in other lenalidomide or pomalidomide studies, and responses were more durable. For example, in the NIMBUS and STRATUS studies of heavily treated MM patients (median number of prior therapies = 5), patients who received pomalidomide and low-dose dexamethasone had an ORR of 33%

and median PFS of 4—5 months.[112,113] Nonetheless, larger multicenter trials and longer follow-up are needed to confirm these results. Furthermore, although adding pembrolizumab to lenalidomide or pomalidomide did not seem to cause new or unexpected toxicities in these two trials; enrollment of new patients on two phase III clinical trials evaluating pembrolizumab in combination with lenalidomide and dexamethasone in newly diagnosed (KEYNOTE-185; NCT02579863) or relapsed/refractory (KEYNOTE-183; NCT02576977) MM patients was put on hold on June 12, 2017, given concerns of unexpected deaths in the cohorts receiving pembrolizumab.[114]

A phase I trial (CheckMate 039; NCT01592370) is testing nivolumab in combination with daratumumab, with or without pomalidomide and dexamethasone, for relapsed or refractory MM. Other trials are evaluating PD-L1 blockade in MM with durvalumab (an anti—PD-L1 monoclonal antibody) and atezolizumab. Durvalumab is being evaluated in combination with lenalidomide in newly diagnosed MM (NCT02685826), alone and in combination with pomalidomide for relapsed or refractory MM (NCT02616640) and in combination with pomalidomide, dexamethasone, and daratumumab for refractory MM (NCT02807454). Atezolizumab is being studied in combination with an immunomodulatory drug (lenalidomide or pomalidomide) and/or daratumumab in patients with refractory MM (NCT02431208) and as monotherapy in patients with asymptomatic MM to assess its biological and clinical effects (NCT02784483).

Regarding the use of CTLA-4 inhibitors in MM, none of the six patients with MM enrolled in a previously mentioned phase I clinical trial of ipilimumab in relapsed hematologic malignancies after allogeneic HCT had objective responses.[84] There are ongoing trials looking at the combination of ipilimumab and nivolumab in patients with MM or lymphoma at high risk for recurrence after autologous HCT (CPIT001, NCT02681302) or the combination of tremelimumab (a fully human IgG2 anti—CTLA-4 monoclonal antibody) and durvalumab (NCT02716805) in patients with MM who are at high risk for relapse postautologous HCT.

Myeloid Malignancies

In a phase I study of ipilimumab in 28 patients with various hematologic malignancies relapsed after allogeneic HCT, 12 patients had AML (including 3 with leukemia cutis and 1 with a myeloid sarcoma), 2 had MDS, and 1 had a myeloproliferative neoplasm.[115] No responses were seen in patients treated with ipilimumab

at 3 mg/kg dose. Among the 22 patients treated with the 10 mg/kg dose, seven patients (32%) achieved an objective response, including CR in five patients: all three patients with leukemia cutis, one with myeloid sarcoma, and one with smoldering MDS developing into AML.[115] Another phase I study of ipilimumab in 11 patients with high-risk MDS who had failed hypomethylating agents did not show any objective responses. Three patients underwent allogeneic HCT after treatment with ipilimumab without any additional toxicities.[116] In a phase I trial of pidilizumab that included eight patients with AML, one patient achieved reduction in the number of peripheral blasts from 50% to 5% but the seven other patients did not respond.[96]

Preliminary results of a single-institution phase I/II study of nivolumab in combination with azacitidine in 53 patients with relapsed AML showed encouraging results.[117,118] Patients received azacitidine 75 mg/m^2 on days 1—7 and nivolumab 3 mg/kg on day 1 and 14, every 4—5 weeks indefinitely. The ORR was 35% (CR = 21%, hematologic improvement = 14%), and 26% had more than 50% bone marrow blast reduction. Responses were durable with 82% of the patients in CR alive at 1 year. OS was superior to historical controls treated with salvage azacitidine at the same institution. Grade 3—4 immune-mediated toxicities were detected in 14% of patients. One patient died from grade 4 pneumonitis/epiglottitis. One of four patients who had prior allogeneic HCT developed grade 3 flare of skin and gastrointestinal GVHD. Flow cytometry analysis and bone marrow aspirates of responders had higher baseline number of CD3+ and CD8+ cells and showed progressive increase in CD4+ and CD8+ TILs with therapy. Interestingly, all evaluable patients showed increased number of CTLA4+ CD8+ cells while on therapy, indicating a possible role for the CTLA-4 pathway in mediating resistance to PD-1 blockade in AML.[117,118]

A phase II study was designed to test different combinations of ipilimumab, nivolumab, and azacitidine in patients previously treated or untreated MDS.[119] Preliminary results showed an ORR of 22% with ipilimumab monotherapy in the nine previously treated MDS patients, while no patients responded to nivolumab monotherapy. In treatment-naïve patients, the combination of nivolumab and azacitidine had on ORR of 69% (9/13).[119] The cohort of patients with MDS who had failed treatment with a hypomethylating in KEYNOTE-013 also showed disappointing results with pembrolizumab monotherapy as the ORR was 4% (1 PR).[120]

Ongoing trials are currently evaluating the role of anti−PD-1 monotherapy in patients with relapsed or refractory AML (NCT02768792) or those in remission (NCT02708641, NCT02275533 and NCT02532231) or in combination with chemotherapy for newly diagnosed AML patients (NCT02464657). Other trials are studying the combination of durvalumab with oral azacitidine (NCT02281084) or with subcutaneous azacitidine and/or tremelimumab (NCT02117219) in patients with MDS or AML.

THE USE OF IMMUNE CHECKPOINT INHIBITORS IN THE PERI-HCT SETTING

As discussed earlier in this chapter, the post-HCT period is characterized by low disease burden and immune remodeling that make it an ideal setting for checkpoint inhibition.[121] Results of the use of pidilizumab after autologous HCT in patients with DLBCL were discussed earlier and appear to be promising.[97] However, in the setting of allogeneic HCT, the effect of checkpoint inhibition on graft-versus-tumor effect and the incidence and severity of GVHD are still unclear. Two previously mentioned phase I trials of ipilimumab were conducted in patients with relapsed hematologic malignancies after allogeneic HCT.[84,115] In the first trial, single infusions of ipilimumab were given at doses ranging from 0.1 to 3.0 mg/kg, at a median of 366 days (range, 125 to 2368) after transplant. No cases of GVHD were reported in the 29 treated patients.[84] In the second study, ipilimumab was given at a dose of 3 or 10 mg/kg, at a median of 675 days (range, 198−1830) after transplantation. Four cases of GVHD (three chronic and one acute) that precluded further administration of ipilimumab were detected in the 28 treated patients.[115] Of note, patients were excluded from these studies if they had a prior history of grade 3 or 4 acute GVHD. In the previously discussed phase I trial of pidilizumab in 17 patients with various hematologic malignancies, one of the four patients who had received allogeneic HCT developed grade 4 GVHD of the gastrointestinal tract and died of persistent AML and GVHD.[96] Of the eight patients with cHL who had received prior allogeneic HCT and were then treated with avelumab, two had grade 3 liver GVHD that completely resolved after immunosuppressive therapy and discontinuation of avelumab.[43] A recent multicenter retrospective study looked at the outcomes and toxicities of anti−PD-1 therapy after allogeneic HCT in 31 patients with relapsed lymphoma (30 patients had cHL).[122] Although 61% of the patients had a history of GVHD, it was inactive in the majority of patients, and most of

them (74%) were off immunosuppressive therapy at the time of anti−PD-1 treatment initiation. Anti−PD-1 therapy consisted of nivolumab in 28 patients and pembrolizumab in 3 patients, with a median time from transplantation to starting treatment of about 2 years. The ORR was remarkable at 77% (CR = 50%), and median PFS was about 20 months. However, this was associated with significant toxicity, as 17 patients (55%) developed GVHD after anti−PD-1 treatment (six acute, seven chronic and four overlap), five of whom (29%) had no prior history of GVHD. GVHD occurred after one or two doses in 16 of these patients, with a median onset time of 2−3 weeks. Skin and liver were the most common sites of involvement. GVHD attributed to PD-1 therapy (four acute and four chronic) resulted in eight deaths (26%).[122]

These concerns also extend to the use of immune checkpoint inhibitors in the preallogeneic HCT setting, as their immunomodulatory effects can last after transplantation. A retrospective study of 39 patients with lymphoma treated on several clinical trials with a PD-1 inhibitor before allogeneic HCT showed a higher than expected rate of early severe posttransplant complications.[123] The median time from last dose of PD-1 therapy to transplantation was 62 days (range, 7−260), and almost all patients received reduced-intensity conditioning regimens. Although the 1-year incidences of acute and chronic GVHD were within the expected range, the incidence of grade 4 acute GVHD (13%) was higher than seen in prior studies (3%−4%).[124,125] All four patients treated with a combination of anti−PD-1 with ipilimumab developed acute GVHD, including one grade 4. Three patients died from acute GVHD that occurred within 2 weeks of transplantation.[123] This urged the FDA to issue a warning for use of allogeneic HCT after prior exposure to anti−PD-1 therapy.

CONCLUSIONS AND FUTURE DIRECTIONS

Early evidence shows that the excitement surrounding the use of immune checkpoint inhibitors in the treatment of hematologic malignancies is justified but needs further exploration. Although monotherapy with immune checkpoint inhibitors is effective in HL and possibly PMBCL, it has been of limited benefit so far in other diseases such as MM, NHL, and MDS. On the other hand, combining immune checkpoint inhibitors with other active agents seems to be more promising. So far, the use of ICI in this field has been limited to heavily treated patients, and their therapeutic effect might be more substantial in patients with a less compromised immune system. Toxicities with immune checkpoint inhibitors monotherapy seem to be similar to what is seen in solid tumors, whereas those with treatment combinations or in the peri-allogeneic HCT period warrant careful attention and further evaluation. The need for larger trials and longer follow-up to validate efficacy results and assess toxicities cannot be overstated. There is also a need to identify biomarkers that can help select patients who would respond to treatment.

As our knowledge expands in understanding the biology of different hematologic malignancies and the role the PD-1 axis plays in mediating antitumor immune evasion in each disease, newer promising treatment combinations might emerge. Few examples have already been discussed through this chapter including the combination with immunomodulators such as lenalidomide and pomalidomide, monoclonal antibodies such as daratumumab, and ibrutinib. The use of chimeric antigen receptor-modified T-cells in the treatment of several hematologic malignancies is a rapidly evolving field, and there is a rationale for added benefit if combined with immune checkpoint inhibitors.[126] Combinations with various types of conventional chemotherapy, vaccines, radiotherapy, and HCT are also being explored. Determining the optimal timing and sequencing of these different treatments will be of utmost importance to achieve higher therapeutic efficacy and acceptable toxicity.

DISCLOSURE STATEMENT

Yazeed Sawalha: none.

Anjali Advani: Amgen (research funding) and Regeneron (research funding).

REFERENCES

1. Brunet JF, Denizot F, Luciani MF, et al. A new member of the immunoglobulin superfamily—CTLA-4. *Nature*. 1987; 328(6127):267–270.
2. Teft WA, Kirchhof MG, Madrenas J. A molecular perspective of CTLA-4 function. *Annu Rev Immunol*. 2006;24:65–97.
3. Topalian SL, Drake CG, Pardoll DM. Immune checkpoint blockade: a common denominator approach to cancer therapy. *Cancer Cell*. 2015;27(4):450–461.
4. Pistillo MP, Tazzari PL, Palmisano GL, et al. CTLA-4 is not restricted to the lymphoid cell lineage and can function as a target molecule for apoptosis induction of leukemic cells. *Blood*. 2003;101(1):202–209.
5. Wong HK, Wilson AJ, Gibson HM, et al. Increased expression of CTLA-4 in malignant T cells from patients with mycosis fungoides — cutaneous T-cell lymphoma. *J Investig Dermatol*. 2006;126(1):212–219.
6. Sekulic A, Liang WS, Tembe W, et al. Personalized treatment of Sezary syndrome by targeting a novel CTLA4: CD28 fusion. *Mol Genet Genomic Med*. 2015;3(2): 130–136.
7. Yoo HY, Kim P, Kim WS, et al. Frequent CTLA4-CD28 gene fusion in diverse types of T-cell lymphoma. *Haematologica*. 2016;101(6):757–763.
8. Kataoka K, Nagata Y, Kitanaka A, et al. Integrated molecular analysis of adult T cell leukemia/lymphoma. *Nat Genet*. 2015;47(11):1304–1315.
9. Perez-Garcia A, Brunet S, Berlanga JJ, et al. CTLA-4 genotype and relapse incidence in patients with acute myeloid leukemia in first complete remission after induction chemotherapy. *Leukemia*. 2008;23(3):486–491.
10. Keir ME, Butte MJ, Freeman GJ, Sharpe AH. PD-1 and its ligands in tolerance and immunity. *Annu Rev Immunol*. 2008;26:677–704.
11. Ahmadzadeh M, Johnson LA, Heemskerk B, et al. Tumor antigen–specific CD8 T cells infiltrating the tumor express high levels of PD-1 and are functionally impaired. *Blood*. 2009;114(8):1537–1544.
12. Brusa D, Serra S, Coscia M, et al. The PD-1/PD-L1 axis contributes to T-cell dysfunction in chronic lymphocytic leukemia. *Haematologica*. 2013;98(6):953–963.
13. Grzywnowicz M, Karczmarczyk A, Skorka K, et al. Expression of programmed death 1 ligand in different compartments of chronic lymphocytic leukemia. *Acta Haematol*. 2015;134(4):255–262.
14. Dorfman DM, Brown JA, Shahsafaei A, Freeman GJ. Programmed death-1 (PD-1) is a marker of germinal center-associated T cells and angioimmunoblastic T-cell lymphoma. *Am J Surg Pathol*. 2006;30(7):802–810.
15. Mathas S, Hartmann S, Kuppers R. Hodgkin lymphoma: pathology and biology. *Semin Hematol*. 2016;53(3): 139–147.
16. Aldinucci D, Gloghini A, Pinto A, De Filippi R, Carbone A. The classical Hodgkin's lymphoma microenvironment and its role in promoting tumour growth and immune escape. *J Pathol*. 2010;221(3):248–263.
17. Yamamoto R, Nishikori M, Kitawaki T, et al. PD-1-PD-1 ligand interaction contributes to immunosuppressive microenvironment of Hodgkin lymphoma. *Blood*. 2008; 111(6):3220–3224.
18. Steidl C, Lee T, Shah SP, et al. Tumor-associated macrophages and survival in classic Hodgkin's lymphoma. *N Engl J Med*. 2010;362(10):875–885.
19. Muenst S, Hoeller S, Dirnhofer S, Tzankov A. Increased programmed death-1+ tumor-infiltrating lymphocytes in classical Hodgkin lymphoma substantiate reduced overall survival. *Hum Pathol*. 2009;40(12): 1715–1722.
20. Green MR, Monti S, Rodig SJ, et al. Integrative analysis reveals selective 9p24.1 amplification, increased PD-1 ligand expression, and further induction via JAK2 in nodular sclerosing Hodgkin lymphoma and primary mediastinal large B-cell lymphoma. *Blood*. 2010; 116(17):3268–3277.

21. Roemer MG, Advani RH, Ligon AH, et al. PD-L1 and PD-L2 genetic alterations define classical Hodgkin lymphoma and predict outcome. *J Clin Oncol.* 2016;34(23):2690−2697.
22. Menter T, Bodmer-Haecki A, Dirnhofer S, Tzankov A. Evaluation of the diagnostic and prognostic value of PDL1 expression in Hodgkin and B-cell lymphomas. *Hum Pathol.* 2016;54:17−24.
23. Steidl C, Shah SP, Woolcock BW, et al. MHC class II trans-activator CIITA is a recurrent gene fusion partner in lymphoid cancers. *Nature.* 2011;471(7338):377−381.
24. Green MR, Rodig S, Juszczynski P, et al. Constitutive AP-1 activity and EBV infection induce PD-L1 in Hodgkin lymphomas and posttransplant lymphoproliferative disorders: implications for targeted therapy. *Clin Cancer Res.* 2012;18(6):1611−1618.
25. Chen BJ, Chapuy B, Ouyang J, et al. PD-L1 expression is characteristic of a subset of aggressive B-cell lymphomas and virus-associated malignancies. *Clin Cancer Res.* 2013;19(13):3462−3473.
26. Nam-Cha SH, Roncador G, Sanchez-Verde L, et al. PD-1, a follicular T-cell marker useful for recognizing nodular lymphocyte-predominant Hodgkin lymphoma. *Am J Surg Pathol.* 2008;32(8):1252−1257.
27. Kiyasu J, Miyoshi H, Hirata A, et al. Expression of programmed cell death ligand 1 is associated with poor overall survival in patients with diffuse large B-cell lymphoma. *Blood.* 2015;126(19):2193−2201.
28. Georgiou K, Chen L, Berglund M, et al. Genetic basis of PD-L1 overexpression in diffuse large B-cell lymphomas. *Blood.* 2016;127(24):3026−3034.
29. Shi M, Roemer MG, Chapuy B, et al. Expression of programmed cell death 1 ligand 2 (PD-L2) is a distinguishing feature of primary mediastinal (thymic) large B-cell lymphoma and associated with PDCD1LG2 copy gain. *Am J Surg Pathol.* 2014;38(12):1715−1723.
30. Chapuy B, Roemer MG, Stewart C, et al. Targetable genetic features of primary testicular and primary central nervous system lymphomas. *Blood.* 2016;127(7):869−881.
31. Ok CY, Chen J, Xu-Monette ZY, et al. Clinical implications of phosphorylated STAT3 expression in de novo diffuse large B-cell lymphoma. *Clin Cancer Res.* 2014;20(19):5113−5123.
32. Ngo VN, Young RM, Schmitz R, et al. Oncogenically active MYD88 mutations in human lymphoma. *Nature.* 2011;470(7332):115−119.
33. Kwon D, Kim S, Kim PJ, et al. Clinicopathological analysis of programmed cell death 1 and programmed cell death ligand 1 expression in the tumour microenviroments of diffuse large B cell lymphomas. *Histopathology.* 2016;68(7):1079−1089.
34. Kataoka K, Shiraishi Y, Takeda Y, et al. Aberrant PD-L1 expression through 3′-UTR disruption in multiple cancers. *Nature.* 2016;534(7607):402−406.
35. Rossille D, Gressier M, Damotte D, et al. High level of soluble programmed cell death ligand 1 in blood impacts overall survival in aggressive diffuse large B-cell lymphoma: results from a French multicenter clinical trial. *Leukemia.* 2014;28(12):2367−2375.
36. Rossille D, Azzaoui I, Feldman AL, et al. Soluble programmed death-ligand 1 as a prognostic biomarker for overall survival in patients with diffuse large B-cell lymphoma: a replication study and combined analysis of 508 patients. *Leukemia.* 2017;31(4):988−991.
37. Berghoff AS, Ricken G, Widhalm G, et al. PD1 (CD279) and PD-L1 (CD274, B7H1) expression in primary central nervous system lymphomas (PCNSL). *Clin Neuropathol.* 2014;33(1):42−49.
38. Laurent C, Fabiani B, Do C, et al. Immune-checkpoint expression in Epstein-Barr virus positive and negative plasmablastic lymphoma: a clinical and pathological study in 82 patients. *Haematologica.* 2016;101(8):976−984.
39. Trautmann L, Janbazian L, Chomont N, et al. Upregulation of PD-1 expression on HIV-specific CD8+ T cells leads to reversible immune dysfunction. *Nat Med.* 2006;12(10):1198−1202.
40. Savage KJ, Monti S, Kutok JL, et al. The molecular signature of mediastinal large B-cell lymphoma differs from that of other diffuse large B-cell lymphomas and shares features with classical Hodgkin lymphoma. *Blood.* 2003;102(12):3871−3879.
41. Twa DD, Chan FC, Ben-Neriah S, et al. Genomic rearrangements involving programmed death ligands are recurrent in primary mediastinal large B-cell lymphoma. *Blood.* 2014;123(13):2062−2065.
42. Steidl C, Gascoyne RD. The molecular pathogenesis of primary mediastinal large B-cell lymphoma. *Blood.* 2011;118(10):2659−2669.
43. Chen R, Gibb AL, Collins GP, et al. Blockade of the PD-1 checkpoint with anti−PD-L1 antibody avelumab is sufficient for clinical activity in relapsed/refractory classical Hodgkin lymphoma (CHL). *Hematol Oncol.* 2017;35:67.
44. Laurent C, Charmpi K, Gravelle P, et al. Several immune escape patterns in non-Hodgkin's lymphomas. *Oncoimmunology.* 2015;4(8):e1026530.
45. Andorsky DJ, Yamada RE, Said J, Pinkus GS, Betting DJ, Timmerman JM. Programmed death ligand 1 is expressed by non-Hodgkin lymphomas and inhibits the activity of tumor-associated T cells. *Clin Cancer Res.* 2011;17(13):4232−4244.
46. Myklebust JH, Irish JM, Brody J, et al. High PD-1 expression and suppressed cytokine signaling distinguish T cells infiltrating follicular lymphoma tumors from peripheral T cells. *Blood.* 2013;121(8):1367−1376.
47. Yang ZZ, Grote DM, Ziesmer SC, Xiu B, Novak AJ, Ansell SM. PD-1 expression defines two distinct T-cell sub-populations in follicular lymphoma that differentially impact patient survival. *Blood Cancer J.* 2015;5:e281.
48. Carreras J, Lopez-Guillermo A, Roncador G, et al. High numbers of tumor-infiltrating programmed cell death 1-positive regulatory lymphocytes are associated with improved overall survival in follicular lymphoma. *J Clin Oncol.* 2009;27(9):1470−1476.

49. Richendollar BG, Pohlman B, Elson P, Hsi ED. Follicular programmed death 1-positive lymphocytes in the tumor microenvironment are an independent prognostic factor in follicular lymphoma. *Hum Pathol.* 2011;42(4): 552–557.

50. Takahashi H, Tomita N, Sakata S, et al. Prognostic significance of programmed cell death-1-positive cells in follicular lymphoma patients may alter in the rituximab era. *Eur J Haematol.* 2013;90(4):286–290.

51. Koch K, Hoster E, Unterhalt M, et al. The composition of the microenvironment in follicular lymphoma is associated with the stage of the disease. *Hum Pathol.* 2012; 43(12):2274–2281.

52. Riches JC, Davies JK, McClanahan F, et al. T cells from CLL patients exhibit features of T-cell exhaustion but retain capacity for cytokine production. *Blood.* 2013; 121(9):1612–1621.

53. McClanahan F, Hanna B, Miller S, et al. PD-L1 checkpoint blockade prevents immune dysfunction and leukemia development in a mouse model of chronic lymphocytic leukemia. *Blood.* 2015;126(2):203–211.

54. Xerri L, Chetaille B, Serriari N, et al. Programmed death 1 is a marker of angioimmunoblastic T-cell lymphoma and B-cell small lymphocytic lymphoma/chronic lymphocytic leukemia. *Hum Pathol.* 2008;39(7): 1050–1058.

55. de Leval L, Rickman DS, Thielen C, et al. The gene expression profile of nodal peripheral T-cell lymphoma demonstrates a molecular link between angioimmunoblastic T-cell lymphoma (AITL) and follicular helper T (TFH) cells. *Blood.* 2007;109(11):4952–4963.

56. Cetinozman F, Jansen PM, Vermeer MH, Willemze R. Differential expression of programmed death-1 (PD-1) in Sezary syndrome and mycosis fungoides. *Arch Dermatol.* 2012;148(12):1379–1385.

57. Cetinozman F, Jansen PM, Willemze R. Expression of programmed death-1 in primary cutaneous CD4-positive small/medium-sized pleomorphic T-cell lymphoma, cutaneous pseudo-T-cell lymphoma, and other types of cutaneous T-cell lymphoma. *Am J Surg Pathol.* 2012; 36(1):109–116.

58. Marzec M, Zhang Q, Goradia A, et al. Oncogenic kinase NPM/ALK induces through STAT3 expression of immunosuppressive protein CD274 (PD-L1, B7-H1). *Proc Natl Acad Sci USA.* 2008;105(52):20852–20857.

59. Wilcox RA, Feldman AL, Wada DA, et al. B7-H1 (PD-L1, CD274) suppresses host immunity in T-cell lymphoproliferative disorders. *Blood.* 2009;114(10): 2149–2158.

60. Miyoshi H, Kiyasu J, Kato T, et al. PD-L1 expression on neoplastic or stromal cells is respectively a poor or good prognostic factor for adult T-cell leukemia/lymphoma. *Blood.* 2016;128(10):1374–1381.

61. Droeser RA, Hirt C, Viehl CT, et al. Clinical impact of programmed cell death ligand 1 expression in colorectal cancer. *Eur J Cancer (Oxf, Engl 1990).* 2013;49(9): 2233–2242.

62. Taube JM, Anders RA, Young GD, et al. Colocalization of inflammatory response with B7-H1 expression in human melanocytic lesions supports an adaptive resistance mechanism of immune escape. *Sci Transl Med.* 2012; 4(127):127ra137.

63. Feucht J, Kayser S, Gorodezki D, et al. T-cell responses against CD19+ pediatric acute lymphoblastic leukemia mediated by bispecific T-cell engager (BiTE) are regulated contrarily by PD-L1 and CD80/CD86 on leukemic blasts. *Oncotarget.* 2016;7(47):76902–76919.

64. Liu J, Hamrouni A, Wolowiec D, et al. Plasma cells from multiple myeloma patients express B7-H1 (PD-L1) and increase expression after stimulation with IFN-γ and TLR ligands via a MyD88-, TRAF6-, and MEK-dependent pathway. *Blood.* 2007;110(1):296–304.

65. Yousef S, Marvin J, Steinbach M, et al. Immunomodulatory molecule PD-L1 is expressed on malignant plasma cells and myeloma-propagating pre-plasma cells in the bone marrow of multiple myeloma patients. *Blood Cancer J.* 2015;5:e285.

66. Tamura H, Ishibashi M, Yamashita T, et al. Marrow stromal cells induce B7-H1 expression on myeloma cells, generating aggressive characteristics in multiple myeloma. *Leukemia.* 2013;27(2):464–472.

67. Gorgun G, Samur MK, Cowens KB, et al. Lenalidomide enhances immune checkpoint blockade-induced immune response in multiple myeloma. *Clin Cancer Res.* 2015;21(20):4607–4618.

68. Ray A, Das DS, Song Y, et al. Targeting PD1-PDL1 immune checkpoint in plasmacytoid dendritic cell interactions with T cells, natural killer cells and multiple myeloma cells. *Leukemia.* 2015;29(6):1441–1444.

69. Rajabi H, Coll MD, Rosenblatt J, et al. Mucin-1 (MUC1) oncoprotein in multiple myeloma cells inhibits the Th1 responses by down regulating the expression of mir-200c and up-regulating the PDL1 expression. *Blood.* 2014;124(21):2072.

70. Wang L, Wang H, Chen H, et al. Serum levels of soluble programmed death ligand 1 predict treatment response and progression free survival in multiple myeloma. *Oncotarget.* 2015;6(38):41228–41236.

71. Hallett WH, Jing W, Drobyski WR, Johnson BD. Immunosuppressive effects of multiple myeloma are overcome by PD-L1 blockade. *Biol Blood Marrow Transplant.* 2011; 17(8):1133–1145.

72. Busch A, Zeh D, Janzen V, et al. Treatment with lenalidomide induces immunoactivating and counter-regulatory immunosuppressive changes in myeloma patients. *Clin Exp Immunol.* 2014;177(2):439–453.

73. Luptakova K, Rosenblatt J, Glotzbecker B, et al. Lenalidomide enhances anti-myeloma cellular immunity. *Cancer Immunol Immunother.* 2013;62(1):39−49.

74. Benson Jr DM, Bakan CE, Mishra A, et al. The PD-1/PD-L1 axis modulates the natural killer cell versus multiple myeloma effect: a therapeutic target for CT-011, a novel monoclonal anti-PD-1 antibody. *Blood.* 2010;116(13): 2286−2294.

75. Krejcik J, Casneuf T, Nijhof IS, et al. Daratumumab depletes CD38+ immune regulatory cells, promotes T-cell expansion, and skews T-cell repertoire in multiple myeloma. *Blood.* 2016;128(3):384−394.

76. Zhang L, Gajewski TF, Kline J. PD-1/PD-L1 interactions inhibit antitumor immune responses in a murine acute myeloid leukemia model. *Blood.* 2009;114(8): 1545−1552.

77. Yang H, Bueso-Ramos C, DiNardo C, et al. Expression of PD-L1, PD-L2, PD-1 and CTLA4 in myelodysplastic syndromes is enhanced by treatment with hypomethylating agents. *Leukemia.* 2014;28(6):1280−1288.

78. Kronig H, Kremmler L, Haller B, et al. Interferon-induced programmed death-ligand 1 (PD-L1/B7-H1) expression increases on human acute myeloid leukemia blast cells during treatment. *Eur J Haematol.* 2014;92(3): 195−203.

79. Norde WJ, Maas F, Hobo W, et al. PD-1/PD-L1 interactions contribute to functional T-cell impairment in patients who relapse with cancer after allogeneic stem cell transplantation. *Cancer Res.* 2011;71(15):5111−5122.

80. Kong Y, Zhang J, Claxton DF, et al. PD-1(hi)TIM-3(+) T cells associate with and predict leukemia relapse in AML patients post allogeneic stem cell transplantation. *Blood Cancer J.* 2015;5:e330.

81. Mumprecht S, Schurch C, Schwaller J, Solenthaler M, Ochsenbein AF. Programmed death 1 signaling on chronic myeloid leukemia-specific T cells results in T-cell exhaustion and disease progression. *Blood.* 2009; 114(8):1528−1536.

82. Hughes A, Clarson J, Tang C, et al. CML patients with deep molecular responses to TKI have restored immune effectors and decreased PD-1 and immune suppressors. *Blood.* 2017;129(9):1166−1176.

83. Riether C, Gschwend T, Huguenin AL, Schurch CM, Ochsenbein AF. Blocking programmed cell death 1 in combination with adoptive cytotoxic T-cell transfer eradicates chronic myelogenous leukemia stem cells. *Leukemia.* 2015;29(8):1781−1785.

84. Bashey A, Medina B, Corringham S, et al. CTLA4 blockade with ipilimumab to treat relapse of malignancy after allogeneic hematopoietic cell transplantation. *Blood.* 2009; 113(7):1581−1588.

85. Ansell SM, Lesokhin AM, Borrello I, et al. PD-1 blockade with nivolumab in relapsed or refractory Hodgkin's lymphoma. *N Engl J Med.* 2015;372(4):311−319.

86. Younes A, Santoro A, Shipp M, et al. Nivolumab for classical Hodgkin's lymphoma after failure of both autologous stem-cell transplantation and brentuximab vedotin: a multicentre, multicohort, single-arm phase 2 trial. *Lancet Oncol.* 2016;17(9):1283−1294.

87. Timmerman JM, Engert A, Younes A, et al. Checkmate 205 update with minimum 12-month follow up: a phase 2 study of nivolumab in patients with relapsed/refractory classical Hodgkin lymphoma. *Blood.* 2016;128(22):1110.

88. Fanale M, Engert A, Younes A, et al. Nivolumab for relapsed/refractory classical Hodgkin lymphoma after autologous transplant: full results after extended follow-up of the phase 2 checkmate 205 trial. *Hematol Oncol.* 2017;35:135−136.

89. Armand P, Shipp MA, Ribrag V, et al. Programmed death-1 blockade with pembrolizumab in patients with classical Hodgkin lymphoma after brentuximab vedotin failure. *J Clin Oncol.* 2016;34.

90. Armand P, Shipp MA, Ribrag V, et al. Pembrolizumab in patients with classical Hodgkin lymphoma after brentuximab vedotin failure: long-term efficacy from the phase 1b Keynote-013 study. *Blood.* 2016;128(22):1108.

91. Chen R, Zinzani PL, Fanale MA, et al. Phase II study of the efficacy and safety of pembrolizumab for relapsed/refractory classic Hodgkin lymphoma. *J Clin Oncol.* 2016;0(0): JCO.2016.2072.1316.

92. Naidoo J, Wang X, Woo KM, et al. Pneumonitis in patients treated with anti−programmed death-1/programmed death ligand 1 therapy. *J Clin Oncol.* 2017;35(7):709−717.

93. Diefenbach CS, Hong F, David K, et al. Safety and efficacy of combination of brentuximab vedotin and nivolumab in relapsed/refractory Hodgkin lymphoma: a trial of the ECOG-ACRIN Cancer Research Group (E4412). *Hematol Oncol.* 2017;35:84−85.

94. Herrera AF, Moskowitz AJ, Bartlett NL, et al. Interim results from a phase 1/2 study of brentuximab vedotin in combination with nivolumab in patients with relapsed or refractory Hodgkin lymphoma. *Hematol Oncol.* 2017; 35:85−86.

95. Ansell SM, Hurvitz SA, Koenig PA, et al. Phase I study of ipilimumab, an anti-CTLA-4 monoclonal antibody, in patients with relapsed and refractory B-cell non-Hodgkin lymphoma. *Clin Cancer Res.* 2009;15(20):6446−6453.

96. Berger R, Rotem-Yehudar R, Slama G, et al. Phase I safety and pharmacokinetic study of CT-011, a humanized antibody interacting with PD-1, in patients with advanced hematologic malignancies. *Clin Cancer Res.* 2008;14(10):3044−3051.

97. Armand P, Nagler A, Weller EA, et al. Disabling immune tolerance by programmed death-1 blockade with pidilizumab after autologous hematopoietic stem-cell transplantation for diffuse large B-cell lymphoma: results of an international phase II trial. *J Clin Oncol.* 2013; 31(33):4199−4206.

98. Lesokhin AM, Ansell SM, Armand P, et al. Nivolumab in patients with relapsed or refractory hematologic malignancy: preliminary results of a phase Ib study. *J Clin Oncol.* 2016;34(23):2698–2704.

99. Palomba ML, Till BG, Park SI, et al. A phase IB study evaluating the safety and clinical activity of atezolizumab combined with obinutuzumab in patients with relapsed or refractory non-Hodgkin lymphoma (NHL). *Hematol Oncol.* 2017;35:137–138.

100. Zinzani P, Ribrag V, Moskowitz CH, et al. Phase 1B study of pembrolizumab in patients with relapsed/refractory primary mediastinal large B-cell lymphoma (RRPMBCL): updated results from the KEYNOTE-013 trial. *Hematol Oncol.* 2017;35:189–190.

101. Zinzani P, Thieblemont C, Melnichenko V, et al. Efficacy and safety of pembrolizumab in relapsed/refractory primary mediastinal large B-cell lymphoma (rrPMBCL): interim analysis of the KEYNOTE-170 phase 2 trial. *Hematol Oncol.* 2017;35:62–63.

102. Nayak L, Iwamoto FM, LaCasce A, et al. PD-1 blockade with nivolumab in relapsed/refractory primary central nervous system and testicular lymphoma. *Blood.* 2017; 129(23):3071–3073.

103. Westin JR, Chu F, Zhang M, et al. Safety and activity of PD1 blockade by pidilizumab in combination with rituximab in patients with relapsed follicular lymphoma: a single group, open-label, phase 2 trial. *Lancet Oncol.* 2014;15(1):69–77.

104. Coiffier B, Osmanov EA, Hong X, et al. Bortezomib plus rituximab versus rituximab alone in patients with relapsed, rituximab-naive or rituximab-sensitive, follicular lymphoma: a randomised phase 3 trial. *Lancet Oncol.* 2011;12(8):773–784.

105. Davis TA, Grillo-Lopez AJ, White CA, et al. Rituximab anti-CD20 monoclonal antibody therapy in non-Hodgkin's lymphoma: safety and efficacy of re-treatment. *J Clin Oncol.* 2000;18(17):3135–3143.

106. Nastoupil LJ, Westin JR, Fowler NH, et al. Response rates with pembrolizumab in combination with rituximab in patients with relapsed follicular lymphoma: interim results of an on open-label, phase II study. *J Clin Oncol.* 2017;35(suppl 15):7519.

107. Ding W, LaPlant BR, Call TG, et al. Pembrolizumab in patients with chronic lymphocytic leukemia with Richter's transformation and relapsed CLL. *Blood.* 2017;129.

108. Dubovsky JA, Beckwith KA, Natarajan G, et al. Ibrutinib is an irreversible molecular inhibitor of ITK driving a Th1-selective pressure in T lymphocytes. *Blood.* 2013; 122(15):2539–2549.

109. Sagiv-Barfi I, Kohrt HE, Czerwinski DK, Ng PP, Chang BY, Levy R. Therapeutic antitumor immunity by checkpoint blockade is enhanced by ibrutinib, an inhibitor of both BTK and ITK. *Proc Natl Acad Sci USA.* 2015;112(9): E966–E972.

110. Ocio EM, Mateos M-V, Orlowski RZ, et al. Pembrolizumab (Pembro) plus lenalidomide (Len) and low-dose dexamethasone (Dex) for relapsed/refractory multiple myeloma (RRMM): efficacy and biomarker analyses. *J Clin Oncol.* 2017;35(suppl 15):8015.

111. Badros A, Hyjek E, Ma N, et al. Pembrolizumab, pomalidomide and low dose dexamethasone for relapsed/refractory multiple myeloma. *Blood.* 2017;130.

112. San Miguel J, Weisel K, Moreau P, et al. Pomalidomide plus low-dose dexamethasone versus high-dose dexamethasone alone for patients with relapsed and refractory multiple myeloma (MM-003): a randomised, open-label, phase 3 trial. *Lancet Oncol.* 2013;14(11): 1055–1066.

113. Dimopoulos MA, Palumbo A, Corradini P, et al. Safety and efficacy of pomalidomide plus low-dose dexamethasone in STRATUS (MM-010): a phase 3b study in refractory multiple myeloma. *Blood.* 2016;128(4):497–503.

114. Merck. *Update on Multiple Myeloma Studies KEYNOTE-183 and 185 of KEYTRUDA® (pembrolizumab) in Combination with Other Therapies;* 2017. http://investors.merck.com/news/press-release-details/2017/Merck-Provides-Update-on-Multiple-Myeloma-Studies-KEYNOTE-183-and-185-of-KEYTRUDA-pembrolizumab-in-Combination-with-Other-Therapies/default.aspx.

115. Davids MS, Kim HT, Bachireddy P, et al. Ipilimumab for patients with relapse after allogeneic transplantation. *N Engl J Med.* 2016;375(2):143–153.

116. Zeidan AM, Zeidner JF, Duffield A, et al. Stabilization of myelodysplastic syndromes (MDS) following hypomethylating agent (HMAs) failure using the immune checkpoint inhibitor ipilimumab: a phase I trial. *Blood.* 2015; 126(23):1666.

117. Daver N, Basu S, Garcia-Manero G, et al. Phase IB/II study of nivolumab in combination with azacytidine (AZA) in patients (pts) with relapsed acute myeloid leukemia (AML). *Blood.* 2016;128(22):763.

118. Daver NG, Basu S, Garcia-Manero G, et al. Phase IB/II study of nivolumab with azacytidine (AZA) in patients (pts) with relapsed AML. *J Clin Oncol.* 2017;35(suppl 15):7026.

119. Garcia-Manero G, Daver NG, Montalban-Bravo G, et al. A phase II study evaluating the combination of nivolumab (Nivo) or ipilimumab (Ipi) with azacitidine in pts with previously treated or untreated myelodysplastic syndromes (MDS). *Blood.* 2016;128(22):344.

120. Garcia-Manero G, Tallman MS, Martinelli G, et al. Pembrolizumab, a PD-1 inhibitor, in patients with myelodysplastic syndrome (MDS) after failure of hypomethylating agent treatment. *Blood.* 2016;128(22):345.

121. Guillaume T, Rubinstein DB, Symann M. Immune reconstitution and immunotherapy after autologous hematopoietic stem cell transplantation. *Blood.* 1998;92(5): 1471–1490.

122. Haverkos BM, Abbott D, Hamadani M, et al. PD-1 blockade for relapsed lymphoma post allogeneic hematopoietic cell transplant: high response rate but frequent GVHD. *Blood*. 2017;130.
123. Merryman RW, Kim HT, Zinzani PL, et al. Safety and efficacy of allogeneic hematopoietic stem cell transplant after PD-1 blockade in relapsed/refractory lymphoma. *Blood*. 2017;129(10):1380−1388.
124. Sureda A, Robinson S, Canals C, et al. Reduced-intensity conditioning compared with conventional allogeneic stem-cell transplantation in relapsed or refractory Hodgkin's lymphoma: an analysis from the Lymphoma Working Party of the European Group for Blood and Marrow Transplantation. *J Clin Oncol*. 2008;26(3):455−462.
125. Robinson SP, Sureda A, Canals C, et al. Reduced intensity conditioning allogeneic stem cell transplantation for Hodgkin's lymphoma: identification of prognostic factors predicting outcome. *Haematologica*. 2009;94(2):230−238.
126. Brudno JN, Somerville RP, Shi V, et al. Allogeneic T cells that express an anti-CD19 chimeric antigen receptor induce remissions of B-cell malignancies that progress after allogeneic hematopoietic stem-cell transplantation without causing graft-versus-host disease. *J Clin Oncol*. 2016;34(10):1112−1121.

CHAPTER 10

Pediatric Malignancies

ERIC K. RING, MD • G. YANCEY GILLESPIE, PHD • GREGORY K. FRIEDMAN, MD

INTRODUCTION

Over 15,000 children are diagnosed with cancer each year in the United States. With advances in treatment and supportive care, the overall 5-year survival rate is approximately 80%, but cancer remains the leading cause of death due to disease in children.[1,2] Acute lymphocytic leukemia (ALL) is the most common pediatric cancer followed by central nervous system (CNS) tumors and extracranial solid tumors. CNS tumors, which are the most common solid tumors in children, account for 20%−25% of childhood malignancies. Cancer is approximately 30 times less common in children than in adults, and while most adult tumors tend to be carcinomas derived from epithelial tissue, most pediatric tumors are embryonic, derived from nonectodermal embryonal tissue. In contrast to adult malignancies, pediatric cancers rarely arise in the setting of risk factors, and the spectrum of mutations seen in pediatric malignancies are strikingly different than that of adults, even in tumors with the same histopathology.[3] Adults with leukemia, for example, have a higher frequency of genomic subgroups resistant to standard therapy such as Philadelphia chromosome-positive ALL, whereas favorable genetic subgroups, such as hyperdiploid ALL or ALL with the *ETV6-RUNX1* fusion gene, commonly seen in pediatrics, are rarely seen in adult patients.[4,5]

Standard therapy for children with cancer includes various combinations of surgery, cytotoxic chemotherapy, and radiation, which contribute to acute and chronic morbidity and mortality for young patients. Although survival rates have improved for children with cancer, outcomes are extremely poor for patients with recurrent, high-grade, refractory, or metastatic disease. Novel therapies, such as checkpoint inhibitors, are opportunities to improve outcomes and lessen toxicities for children with a variety of malignancies, and several Food and Drug Administration (FDA)−approved checkpoint inhibitors have shown significant benefit in human adult cancer studies.[6−12] However, differences between pediatric and adult malignancies illustrate potential barriers to successful adaptation of immune checkpoint blockade in children. For example, tumor mutational burden (TMB), which is directly associated with response to PD-1 (programmed death protein-1) and PD-L1 (programmed death ligand-1) blockade due to the revelation of novel epitopes, is significantly different between pediatric and adult cancers, with adults showing a more than twofold increase in TMB compared with their pediatric counterparts.[13] Although there is limited research evaluating the role of immune checkpoint molecules in pediatric malignancy, evidence is rapidly emerging for the use of checkpoint blockade in children with cancer.[14] In this chapter, we examine preclinical studies of immune checkpoint proteins and clinical applications of checkpoint blockade in pediatric cancer.

PD-1/PD-L1

PD-L1 (B7-H1) is a member of the B7 family of costimulatory molecules used in the regulation of humoral and cellular immune responses as well as peripheral tolerance and autoimmunity.[15] PD-L1 exists as a 40-kDa type 1 transmembrane cell surface glycoprotein on various hematopoietic and parenchymal cells and exerts its effects through interaction with the PD-1 receptor on activated T- and B-cells.[16] Binding of PD-1 with PD-L1 dramatically downregulates T-cell−mediated proliferation and production of interleukin-2 (IL-2) and interferon gamma (IFN-γ).

Cancer cells that express surface PD-L1 can suppress the antitumor immune response leading to tumor growth and immune escape.[15] Studies evaluating PD-L1 expression in patient soft tissue sarcoma tumor samples demonstrate a correlation between PD-L1 expression and shorter overall survival (OS).[17] Several studies have demonstrated PD-L1 expression in various pediatric malignancies (see Table 10.1 for summary of checkpoint protein expression by pediatric

TABLE 10.1
Summary of Checkpoint Protein Expression by Pediatric Malignancy

Cancer Type	CTLA-4	PD-1/PD-L1	CD200	IDO	References
ALL	NA	High	Med/High	NA	40,65,66
Burkitt lymphoma	NA	High	NA	NA	23
Hodgkin lymphoma	NA	NA	NA	High	78
Non-Hodgkin's lymphoma	NA	High	NA	NA	19
Ewing sarcoma	NA	Low/Med/High	NA	NA	17–19,22,29
DSRCT	NA	Low/High	NA	NA	24
Alveolar RMS	NA	Med/High	NA	NA	17,18
Embryonal RMS	High	Med	NA	NA	53,18
Synovial sarcoma	NA	Med/High	NA	NA	17,23
Epithelioid sarcoma	NA	Med	NA	NA	17
Mesenchymal chondrosarcoma	NA	NA	NA	NA	17
Osteosarcoma	High	Med/Hi	NA	High	53,18,34,22,23,77
Neuroblastoma	High	Neg/Low/Med/High	High	High	53,18,19,21,27, 67,22,23,71
Retinoblastoma	NA	High	NA	NA	26
Nasopharyngeal carcinoma	NA	NA	NA	High	76
Wilms, favorable	NA	Neg/Low	NA	NA	20–22
Wilms, anaplastic	NA	Med	NA	NA	20
Clear cell sarcoma of kidney	NA	Neg	NA	NA	21
Hepatoblastoma	NA	Neg	NA	NA	21
Yolk sac tumor	NA	Neg	NA	NA	21
Teratoma	NA	Neg	NA	NA	21
INTRACRANIAL SOLID TUMORS					
Ependymoma	NA	Low/Med	High	NA	23,68,79
Germinoma	NA	Neg/High	NA	NA	21
Glioblastoma	NA	Med	NA	NA	19,23
Medulloblastoma	NA	Neg/High	NA	NA	19,21,80
ATRT	NA	Neg/Low	NA	NA	21,23
Supratentorial Peripheral Neuroectodermal Tumor	NA	Med	NA	NA	23

Checkpoint protein expression was graded as follows: *ALL*, acute lymphocytic leukemia; *ATRA*, atypical teratoid/rhabdoid tumor; *ATRT*, atypical teratoid/rhabdoid tumor; *CTLA*, Cytotoxic T-lymphocyte antigen-4; *DSRCT*, desmoplastic small round cell tumor; *High*, 60%–100% of tumors tested; *IDO*, indoleamine 2,3-dioxygenase; *Low*, 1%–19% of tumors tested; *Med*, 20%–59% of tumors tested; *NA*, no data available; *Neg*, no expression; *PD-L1*, programmed death ligand-1; *RMS*, rhabdomyosarcoma.

malignancy).[17–24] Results vary widely likely owing to different methods for immunohistochemical staining procedures and scoring and PD-L1 antibodies that differ in their targeted epitope, isotype, source, and binding affinity.[25] Despite these limitations, moderate to high PD-L1 expression was seen in clinically aggressive pediatric malignancies such as sarcomas, neuroblastoma, Burkitt and non-Hodgkin lymphoma, and anaplastic Wilms tumor.[17,18,20,21] PD-L1 expression in Wilms tumors with "favorable histology" was associated with an increased risk of recurrence compared with PD-L1–negative favorable histology tumors.

Pediatric cancers with the highest proportion of PD-L1 positivity showed the poorest survival.[17,18,23,24]

In preclinical studies, PD-L1 surface expression was upregulated in response to immunogenic stimuli such as IFNγ in pediatric leukemia (acute myelogenous leukemia [AML]), extracranial solid tumors (Ewing sarcoma, neuroblastoma, rhabdomyosarcoma, retino-blastoma), and brain tumors (atypical teratoid/rhabdoid tumor [ATRT], and glioblastoma).[26–29] PD-L1–blocking antibody treatment enhances T-cell activation and proliferation further supporting PD-L1 as a negative regulator of the antitumor immune response. In murine AML models, targeting the PD-1/PD-L1 interaction with an anti-PD-L1 monoclonal antibody increased the function and proliferation of cytotoxic T-cells at tumor sites and reduced AML tumor burden with significantly prolonged survival compared with untreated controls.[30,31] This antileukemia effect was enhanced when combined with T-regulatory cell (Treg) depletion before PD-L1 blockade. Similar findings were reported by Mao et al. and Rigo et al. in murine neuroblastoma models using PD-L1–blocking antibodies with a selective colony stimulating factor-1 receptor inhibitor (BLZ945) that blocks induction of suppressive myeloid-derived suppressor cells (MDSCs) and anti-CD4 monoclonal antibody, respectively.[32,33] Significant tumor responses were seen using these combinations; however, PD-L1 blockade alone was insufficient to control tumor growth. These findings suggest that combining immunotherapy approaches may be necessary in some diseases.

PD-L1 expression and tumor response to PD-L1 blockade varies between primary versus metastatic tumors and within different subtypes of the same tumor.[34,35] In contrast to human primary osteosarcoma, human metastatic osteosarcoma cells had greater surface expression of PD-L1 and had PD-1 expression on CD8+ metastasis-infiltrating lymphocytes.[34] An anti-PD-L1 antibody significantly increased survival and improved function of infiltrating lymphocytes in a metastatic murine osteosarcoma model suggesting that PD-L1+ tumors are able to tolerize infiltrating T-cells leading to tumor escape. Group 3 murine medulloblastomas with a higher proportion of CD8+/PD-1+ T-cells were more sensitive to blockade with PD-1 antibodies than sonic hedgehog (Shh) murine tumors.[35] Immunologic differences within tumor microenvironments likely exist and may be exploited for therapeutic benefit.

With promising adult data rapidly emerging, off-trial use of checkpoint inhibition in pediatric patients with relapsed or refractory disease is a becoming more common practice; however, results have been mixed. Significant responses to nivolumab (anti-PD-1) in two young siblings with recurrent multifocal glioblastoma and biallelic mismatch repair deficiency have been reported, supporting the evidence that high TMB predicts a clinical response to PD-1/PD-L1 blockade.[13,36] Another report describes a 19-year-old male with recurrent heavily pretreated metastatic Ewing sarcoma who achieved a clinical and radiological remission after three doses of pembrolizumab (anti-PD-1).[37] In contrast, five children with recurrent primary CNS tumors treated with pembrolizumab all had progressive disease while receiving treatment without any signs of clinical or radiographic response to treatment.[38] Foran et al. reported the first pediatric patient with primary refractory Hodgkin lymphoma with a partial response to nivolumab and sustained benefit for 11 months until radiographic disease progression.[39] This patient experienced severe cytokine release syndrome requiring inotropic support and corticosteroids following the first infusion of nivolumab but tolerated subsequent infusions with steroids and antihistamines as premedications. Combination of blinatumomab, an anti-CD19 bispecific T-cell engager that enables a patient's T-cells to recognize malignant B-cells, and pembrolizumab induced a morphologic remission in a 12-year-old girl with refractory ALL and was well tolerated with expected fever and transient increase in laboratory inflammatory markers.[40]

Although the development of immune-related side effects is associated with an increased likelihood of treatment response, the potential severity of immune-mediated toxicities requires great caution when considering these treatments for children with cancer. This is best exemplified by the report of a 10-year-old girl with glioblastoma treated with nivolumab who died from immune-mediated inflammation and tumor necrosis that resulted in cerebral edema and uncal herniation.[38,41] Controlled clinical trials are vital to explore and describe the safest and most effective age- and disease-specific treatment regimens.

Phase I and II clinical trials using PD-1/PD-L1 blockade for pediatric malignancies are currently recruiting patients (see Table 10.2 for summary of pediatric checkpoint inhibitor trials). These studies are testing nivolumab alone or in combination with conventional chemotherapy such as cyclophosphamide for relapsed pediatric solid tumors (NCT02901145) or ifosfamide, carboplatin, and etoposide (ICE) for relapsed/refractory Hodgkin lymphoma (NCT03016871). The primary outcomes include event-free survival (EFS), OS, adverse events, and safety. Secondary outcome measures include

TABLE 10.2
Clinical trials using checkpoint inhibition for pediatric cancers

Protein	Drug	Disease	Phase	Age (years)	Status	NCT Identifier
CTLA-4	Ipilimumab	Stage III or IV melanoma	2	12–17	Terminated owing to slow accrual	NCT01696045
	Ipilimumab	Recurrent/refractory solid tumors	1	3–21	Completed	NCT01445379
	Ipilimumab	Advanced synovial sarcoma	2	≥13	Terminated owing to poor accrual	NCT00140855
	Ipilimumab	Metastatic renal cell carcinoma	2	≥16	Completed	NCT00057889
	Ipilimumab + imatinib	Advanced cancers	1	≥15	Recruiting	NCT01738139
	Ipilimumab + paclitaxel	Metastatic melanoma	2	12–70	Active, not recruiting	NCT01827111
	Ipilimumab or interferon α-2b	Recurrent or stage III/IV melanoma	3	>12	Active, not recruiting	NCT01274338
	Ipilimumab + CD19-CAR T-cells	B-cell Non-Hodgkin lymphoma, ALL, CLL	1	Any	Active, not recruiting	NCT00586391
	Ipilimumab + gene-modified T-cells and dendritic cell vaccine	Locally advanced or metastatic cancers	1	≥16	Recruiting	NCT02070406
PD-1	Nivolumab	Refractory or recurrent hypermutated malignancies in biallelic mismatch repair deficiency	1, 2	1–18	Recruiting	NCT02992964
	Nivolumab	Glioblastoma	2	≥1	Completed	NCT02550249
	Nivolumab + cyclophosphamide	Relapsed solid tumors	1, 2	1–21	Not yet recruiting	NCT02901145
	Nivolumab + anti-GD2 antibody	Relapsed or refractory Neuroblastoma	1	1–18	Not yet recruiting	NCT02914405
	Nivolumab + brentuximab vedotin	Refractory Hodgkin lymphoma	2	5–30	Recruiting	NCT02927769
	Nivolumab + brentuximab vedotin	Relapsed/refractory Non-Hodgkin lymphoma	1, 2	≥15	Recruiting	NCT02581631
	Nivolumab + Epstein-Barr Virus (EBV)-specific T-cells	Relapsed/refractory EBV + lymphoma	1	All	Recruiting	NCT02973113
	Nivolumab ± stereotactic radiosurgery	Recurrent, advanced or metastatic chordoma	1	≥15	Recruiting	NCT02989636
	Nivolumab + ICE	Relapsed/refractory Hodgkin lymphoma	2	≥15	Recruiting	NCT03016871
	Nivolumab + gene-modified T-cells and NY-ESO-1 vaccine	Stage IV or locally advanced solid tumors expressing NY-ESO-1	1	≥16	Recruiting	NCT02775292

	Agent	Condition	Phase	Age	Status	Identifier
	Nivolumab + Cyclophosphamide ± radiotherapy	Relapsed/refractory cancers	1, 2	≤18	Recruiting	NCT02813135
	Pembrolizumab	Recurrent, progressive or refractory high-grade gliomas, DIPG or hypermutated tumors	1	1–29	Recruiting	NCT02359565
	Pembrolizumab	Advanced melanoma or advanced, relapsed/refractory PD-L1+ solid tumors or lymphoma	1, 2	0.5–17	Recruiting	NCT02332668
	Pembrolizumab	Advanced sarcomas	2	≥12	Recruiting	NCT02301039
	Pembrolizumab	Natural killer/T-cell lymphoma	2	≥15	Recruiting	NCT03107962
	Pembrolizumab + IL2	Stage III or IV melanoma	2	≥15	Recruiting	NCT02748564
	Pembrolizumab + cyclophosphamide, fludarabine, IL2 and tumor-infiltrating lymphocyte infusion	Metastatic melanoma	2	16–70	Recruiting	NCT02621021
	Pembrolizumab + axitinib	Alveolar soft part sarcomas and other soft tissue sarcomas	2	≥16	Recruiting	NCT02636725
	Pembrolizumab + third-generation GD-2 CAR T-cell	Relapsed/refractory Neuroblastoma	1	Any	Active, not recruiting	NCT01822652
	Pembrolizumab + GSK3359609	Advanced solid tumors	1	≤18	Recruiting	NCT02723955
	Pidilizumab	DIPG	1, 2	3–21	Active, not recruiting	NCT01952769
	Anti-PD-1 antibody + decitabine	Relapsed/refractory malignancies	1, 2	12–80	Recruiting	NCT02961101
PD-L1	Atezolizumab	Refractory solid tumors	1, 2	≤30	Active, not recruiting	NCT02541604
	Avelumab	Recurrent or progressive osteosarcoma	2	12–49	Recruiting	NCT03008848
	Durvalumab	Relapsed/Refractory solid tumors, lymphoma or CNS tumors	1	1–17	Recruiting	NCT02793466
PD-1 + CTLA-4	Nivolumab ± ipilimumab	Relapsed/refractory solid tumors	1, 2	1–30	Recruiting	NCT02304458
	Nivolumab + ipilimumab	Untreated, unresected or metastatic melanoma	3	≥15	Active, not recruiting	NCT02905266
	Nivolumab + ipilimumab	Resected stage III/IV melanoma	2	≥16	Active, not recruiting	NCT02970981
	Nivolumab + blinatumomab ± ipilimumab	Poor risk relapsed/refractory CD19+ B-cell ALL	1	≥16	Recruiting	NCT02879695

Continued

TABLE 10.2
Clinical trials using checkpoint inhibition for pediatric cancers—cont'd

Protein	Drug	Disease	Phase	Age (years)	Status	NCT Identifier
	Nivolumab + NY-ESO-1 vaccine ± ipilimumab	Resected stage III/IV melanoma	1	≥16	Active, not recruiting	NCT01176474
	Durvalumab + tremelimumab	Advanced rare tumors	2	≥16	Recruiting	NCT02879162
	Durvalumab + tremelimumab	Recurrent stage IV lung cancer	2	≥3	Recruiting	NCT03373760
B7-H3	Enoblituzumab	B7-H3+ relapsed/refractory solid tumors	1	1–30	Recruiting	NCT02982941
	^{131}I-8H9	DSRCT and other solid tumors involving the peritoneum	1	≥1	Recruiting	NCT01099644
	^{131}I-8H9	Relapsed/refractory or advanced CNS or leptomeningeal cancer	1	Any	Recruiting	NCT00089245
	^{131}I-8H9	Nonprogressive DIPG previously treated with external beam radiation	1	3–21	Recruiting	NCT01502917
IDO	Indoximod + temozolomide	Progressive primary malignant brain tumors	1	3–21	Recruiting	NCT02502708

ALL, acute lymphocytic leukemia; CLL, chronic lymphocytic leukemia; CNS, central nervous system; CTLA, cytotoxic T-lymphocyte antigen-4; DSRCT, desmoplastic small round cell tumor; DIPG, diffuse intrinsic pontine glioma; ICE, ifosfamide, carboplatin, and etoposide; TMB, tumor mutational burden.

antitumor response and the role of PD-L1/L2 on tumor specimens and T-cell, B-cell, and NK-cell subsets in the peripheral blood. Other active phase I and II clinical trials of PD-1/PD-L1 inhibitors for pediatric malignancies are using PD-1/PD-L1 blockade combined with a disease-specific targeted therapy. A phase I trial in children with relapsed or refractory neuroblastoma is studying the safety, tolerability, and antitumor response to nivolumab plus anti-GD2 antibody (ch14.18/CHO). Two phase II clinical trials using nivolumab plus brentuximab vedotin, an antibody–drug conjugate that selectively targets the CD30 antigen commonly found on various forms of lymphoma, for patients with relapsed or refractory Hodgkin lymphoma or non-Hodgkin lymphoma are currently recruiting adult and pediatric patients.

CYTOTOXIC T-LYMPHOCYTE ANTIGEN-4

Cytotoxic T-lymphocyte antigen-4 (CTLA-4) is a cell surface glycoprotein that shares 30% homology with CD28 and binds the B7 family of proteins with very high affinity. It is predominantly found within the intracellular compartment of CD4+, CD8+ T-cells and Tregs and can be transported to be expressed on the cell surface in response to T-cell activation.[42,43] On the cell surface, CTLA-4 competes with CD28 by interacting with CD80 (B7-1)/CD86 (B7-2), leading to decreased activation and expansion of T-cells and accelerating the death of activated T-cells.[44]

Patients with germline mutations in the *CTLA-4* gene have severe immune dysregulation, and *CTLA-4* knockout mice develop uncontrolled lymphoproliferation.[45,46] Anti-CTLA-4 antibodies inhibit Tregs while expanding CD8+ T-cells at tumor sites.[47] The full therapeutic effects of anti-CTLA-4 antibodies likely result from the combination of enhanced cytotoxic T-cell function and inhibition of Treg activity.[48] Normal expression of CTLA-4 may be critical for circulating immunomodulatory cells to maintain physiologic self-tolerance and homeostasis.

There are few preclinical studies examining CTLA-4 expression and response to anti-CTLA-4 antibodies in pediatric malignancies.[49–51] Increased expression of peripheral blood CTLA-4+ T-cells in pediatric patients with newly diagnosed or relapsed osteosarcoma and Ewing sarcoma and tumor cytoplasmic and surface expression of CTLA-4 in pediatric neuroblastoma, rhabdomyosarcoma, and osteosarcoma cell lines has been reported (Table 10.1).[52,53] The significance of CTLA-4 cell surface expression in pediatric malignancies is not fully known; however, in vitro treatment of

human CTLA-4-expressing osteosarcoma cell lines with CTLA-4-ligands induced tumor cell apoptosis. This suggests that tumor surface CTLA-4 may be targetable by checkpoint inhibitors. In murine models of neuroblastoma, treatment with systemic anti-CTLA-4 antibodies in combination with PD-L1 inhibition, radiation, and IL-2–linked tumor-specific antibody (hu14.18) or Prussian blue nanoparticle-based photothermal therapy improved tumor response and animal survival compared with any of the respective treatments alone.[54–56]

Volejnikova et al. reported a 5-year-old boy with congenital melanocytic nevi and metastatic melanoma who had rapid disease progression while being treated with ipilimumab, an anti-CTLA-4 monoclonal antibody.[57] The first clinical study using checkpoint inhibition in pediatric cancer was a phase I trial of ipilimumab in pediatric patients with recurrent or refractory solid tumors (Table 10.2).[58] Ipilimumab was given intravenously every 3 weeks to 33 patients with melanoma (n = 12), sarcoma (n = 17), renal or bladder carcinoma (n = 3), or neuroblastoma (n = 1). Responses were assessed at 6 and 12 weeks and then every 3 months. There were no partial or complete responses, but stable disease was seen in six patients for 4–10 cycles. Interestingly, presence of immune-related toxicities was associated with increased OS. Overall, half of patients developed any grade immune-related adverse event (irAE) with a similar spectrum of symptoms as described in adults. Grade 3 or 4 irAEs were seen in 27% of patients, including pancreatitis, pneumonitis, colitis, endocrinopathies, and transaminitis. No fatalities occurred, but one patient developed hypophysitis and subsequent panhypopituitarism. One patient developed colitis that responded to steroids but resulted in colonic perforation.

Phase I and II studies examining ipilimumab for pediatric solid tumors with conventional chemotherapies such as imatinib (NCT00057889) or paclitaxel (NCT01827111) or immune stimulators such as interferon α-2 (NCT01274338) have primary outcome measures of maximum tolerated dose of ipilimumab, rate of adverse events, and progression-free survival. A phase I study for patients with non-Hodgkin lymphoma, ALL, and chronic lymphocytic leukemia (CLL) using ipilimumab combined with CD19-CAR T-cells is currently recruiting patients ≥16 years of age. Primary outcomes measured include treatment-related adverse events and safety of the combination therapy. Secondary outcomes will examine the survival and function of CD19-CAR T-cells with ipilimumab as well as tumor response.

CD200

CD200 is a transmembrane protein related to the B7 family of costimulatory receptors involved in T-cell signaling and likely plays a role in physiologic immune tolerance. It is normally expressed on lymphoid and neuronal tissue, and its receptor, CD200R, is expressed on antigen-presenting cells and T-cells. [59] Binding of CD200 with its receptor leads to expansion of Tregs, downregulation of T-cell–mediated immune response, and decreased production of IL-2 and IFN-γ by monocytes and macrophages. [60–63] CD200 can be expressed on the surface of malignant cells and results in tumor immune escape. [62,64]

Few preclinical studies in pediatric cancers exist. There are two reports of pediatric precursor B-cell ALL expressing surface CD200 and two neuroblastoma samples expressing surface CD200 (Table 10.1). [65–67] Further evaluation of the neuroblastoma cells revealed that IL-2 and IFN-γ, cytokines necessary for efficient T-cell function, were decreased when neuroblastoma cells expressing CD200 were added to mixed lymphocyte reactions. Addition of an anti-CD200 antibody restored IL-2 and IFN-γ responses suggesting that CD200 suppresses antitumor T-cell responses. Compared with normal brain tissue, pediatric ependymoma, medulloblastoma, and diffuse intrinsic pontine glioma had greater CD200 expression by western blot. [68] Supratentorial ependymoma showed increased CD200 mRNA compared with posterior fossa ependymoma. Similarly, CD200 mRNA was increased in group 4 medulloblastoma compared with Shh or group 3 medulloblastoma. In a murine glioma model, mice treated with a CD200 antagonist had extended survival and enhanced production of tumor necrosis factor-α and IFN-γ compared with untreated mice. [68] Further research and randomized clinical trials are needed to clarify immunologic differences between tumor types and within tumor subtypes and evaluate the safety and efficacy of CD200 blockade in pediatric cancer patients. There are currently no active adult or pediatric cancer clinical trials examining or targeting CD200.

INDOLEAMINE 2,3-DIOXYGENASE

Indoleamine 2,3-dioxygenase (IDO) is an intracellular enzyme that catalyzes the initial and rate-limiting step in the kynurenine pathway, the major pathway of L-tryptophan catabolism in mammals. [69] This pathway produces the active metabolites L-kynurenine, kynurenic acid (KYNA), quinolinic acid (QUIN), 3-hydroxykynurenine (3-HK), and picolinic acid (PIC). QUIN is a potent NMDA receptor agonist; QUIN, L-kynurenine, and PIC inhibit T- and NK-cell proliferation; and 3-HK has immunomodulatory properties indirectly by the production of free radicals. [70] In the setting of inflammation and IFN-γ, IDO is upregulated in monocytes and tumors cells leading to the depletion of tryptophan that T-cells and NK cells need for efficient activation. IDO likely plays a crucial role in the physiologic termination of the inflammatory cascade and control of peripheral tolerance. [71–73]

Increased IDO expression has been shown to correlate with aggressive tumor growth and resistance to therapies that use cytotoxic killing by T-cells owing to the recruitment and activation of MDSCs through a Treg-dependent mechanism. [74,75] Murine mastocytoma tumor cells expressing IDO had decreased T-cell accumulation at the tumor site compared with tumor cells with low or absent IDO expression, and tumor progression was significantly slowed when treated with 1-methyl-tryptophan (1MT), an IDO inhibitor. [75]

Similar to other checkpoint molecules, there are few studies examining IDO in pediatric malignancy. Patients with nasopharyngeal carcinoma with high IDO expression and low tumor T-cell infiltration were found to have significantly lower survival rates (Table 10.1). [76] Pediatric osteosarcoma patients with high IDO expression had significantly lower metastasis-free survival (53% vs. 81%) and 5-year OS (60% vs. 92%) compared with patients with lower IDO expression. This suggests that the immune tolerance mediated by IDO may play an important role in the metastatic potential of osteosarcoma. [77]

A phase I clinical trial for pediatric patients with progressive primary brain tumors using indoximod (1-methyl-tryptophan), an orally available IDO inhibitor, in combination with temozolomide is currently recruiting patients (NCT02502708). Indoximod will be administered orally to patients in escalating doses, beginning at 12.8 mg/kg/dose twice daily and increasing to 22.4 mg/kg/dose twice daily along with temozolomide 200 mg/m^2 daily for 5 days. Patients will also be eligible to receive up-front indoximod plus radiation followed by 12 cycles of indoximod plus temozolomide. The study will evaluate incidence of regimen-limiting toxicities and objective response rate as primary outcome measures, and indoximod pharmacokinetics, progression-free survival, OS, and feasibility of indoximod combined with conformal radiation as secondary outcomes.

CONCLUSIONS

Checkpoint inhibition is an emerging and exciting avenue of therapy that has shown efficacy in adult cancer and is being explored in pediatric cancer. In contrast to the preclinical evidence in adult malignancies, preclinical studies of checkpoint expression and activity in pediatric malignancies are limited. Because of the stark differences in adult and pediatric cancer genetics, biology, and treatment, reliable preclinical models for testing new forms of immunotherapy such as checkpoint inhibitors are critical. Young children with naïve immune systems, adolescents with developing immune systems, and young adults with relatively mature immune systems present complex challenges of adapting immunotherapy in children and young adults. Serious immune-related adverse events associated with checkpoint inhibition pose a particularly difficult challenge in this diverse and fragile population. Clinical trials using checkpoint inhibition for pediatric cancer are ongoing and few have been completed. Preclinical data and clinical treatment trials will be vital to accurately define the ideal patients and to match the most effective checkpoint inhibition therapy for each patient.

FINANCIAL SUPPORT

St. Baldrick's Foundation, the Rally Foundation for Childhood Cancer Research, The Truth 365, Department of Defense (W81XWH-15-1-0108), Kaul Pediatric Research Institute to GKF, and the National Institutes of Health (P20CA151129 to GYG and P01CA071933 to GYG).

REFERENCES

1. Ward E, DeSantis C, Robbins A, Kohler B, Jemal A. Childhood and adolescent cancer statistics. *CA Cancer J Clin*. 2014;64(2):83−103.
2. Murphy SL, Xu J, Kochanek KD. Deaths: final data for 2010. *Natl Vital Stat Rep*. 2013;61(4):1−117.
3. Downing JR, Wilson RK, Zhang J, et al. The pediatric cancer genome project. *Nat Genet*. 2012;44(6):619−622.
4. Pui CH, Robison LL, Look AT. Acute lymphoblastic leukaemia. *Lancet*. 2008;371(9617):1030−1043.
5. Loh ML, Zhang J, Harvey RC, et al. Tyrosine kinome sequencing of pediatric acute lymphoblastic leukemia: a report from the Children's Oncology Group TARGET Project. *Blood*. 2013;121(3):485−488.
6. Ribas A, Kefford R, Marshall MA, et al. Phase III randomized clinical trial comparing tremelimumab with standard-of-care chemotherapy in patients with advanced melanoma. *J Clin Oncol*. 2013;31(5):616−622.
7. Eggermont AM, Chiarion-Sileni V, Grob JJ, et al. Adjuvant ipilimumab versus placebo after complete resection of high-risk stage III melanoma (EORTC 18071): a randomised, double-blind, phase 3 trial. *Lancet Oncol*. 2015; 16(5):522−530.
8. Robert C, Schachter J, Long GV, et al. Pembrolizumab versus ipilimumab in advanced melanoma. *N Engl J Med*. 2015;372(26):2521−2532.
9. Larkin J, Chiarion-Sileni V, Gonzalez R, et al. Combined nivolumab and ipilimumab or monotherapy in untreated melanoma. *N Engl J Med*. 2015;373(1):23−34.
10. Motzer RJ, Escudier B, McDermott DF, et al. Nivolumab versus everolimus in advanced renal-cell carcinoma. *N Engl J Med*. 2015;373(19):1803−1813.
11. Rosenberg JE, Hoffman-Censits J, Powles T, et al. Atezolizumab in patients with locally advanced and metastatic urothelial carcinoma who have progressed following treatment with platinum-based chemotherapy: a single-arm, multicentre, phase 2 trial. *Lancet*. 2016;387(10031):1909−1920.
12. Brahmer J, Reckamp KL, Baas P, et al. Nivolumab versus docetaxel in advanced squamous-cell non-small-cell lung cancer. *N Engl J Med*. 2015;373(2):123−135.
13. Chalmers ZR, Connelly CF, Fabrizio D, et al. Analysis of 100,000 human cancer genomes reveals the landscape of tumor mutational burden. *Genome Med*. 2017;9(1):34.
14. Ring EK, Markert JM, Gillespie GY, Friedman GK. Checkpoint proteins in pediatric brain and extracranial solid tumors: opportunities for immunotherapy. *Clin Cancer Res*. 2017;23(2):342−350.
15. Dong H, Strome SE, Salomao DR, et al. Tumor-associated B7-H1 promotes T-cell apoptosis: a potential mechanism of immune evasion. *Nat Med*. 2002;8(8):793−800.
16. Keir ME, Liang SC, Guleria I, et al. Tissue expression of PD-L1 mediates peripheral T cell tolerance. *J Exp Med*. 2006;203(4):883−895.
17. Kim C, Kim EK, Jung H, et al. Prognostic implications of PD-L1 expression in patients with soft tissue sarcoma. *BMC Cancer*. 2016;16:434.
18. Chowdhury F, Dunn S, Mitchell S, Mellows T, Ashton-Key M, Gray JC. PD-L1 and CD8+PD1+ lymphocytes exist as targets in the pediatric tumor microenvironment for immunomodulatory therapy. *Oncoimmunology*. 2015; 4(10):e1029701.
19. Majzner RG, Simon JS, Grosso JF, et al. Assessment of PD-L1 expression and tumor-associated lymphocytes in pediatric cancer tissues. *Cancer Res*. 2015;75(suppl 15):249.
20. Routh JC, Ashley RA, Sebo TJ, et al. B7-H1 expression in Wilms tumor: correlation with tumor biology and disease recurrence. *J Urol*. 2008;179(5):1954−1959; discussion 1959−1960.
21. Aoki T, Hino M, Koh K, et al. Low frequency of programmed death ligand 1 expression in pediatric cancers. *Pediatr Blood Cancer*. 2016;63(8):1461−1464.
22. Pinto N, Park JR, Murphy E, et al. Patterns of PD-1, PD-L1, and PD-L2 expression in pediatric solid tumors. *Pediatr Blood Cancer*. 2017;64(11). https://doi.org/10.1002/pbc. 26613. Epub 2017 May 10.

23. Majzner RG, Simon JS, Grosso JF, et al. Assessment of programmed death-ligand 1 expression and tumor-associated immune cells in pediatric cancer tissues. *Cancer*. 2017;123(19):3807−3815. https://doi.org/10.1002/cncr.30724. Epub 2017 Jun 13.

24. van Erp AEM, Versleijen-Jonkers YMH, Hillebrandt-Roeffen MHS, et al. Expression and clinical association of programmed cell death-1, programmed death-ligand-1 and CD8+ lymphocytes in primary sarcomas is subtype dependent. *Oncotarget*. 2017;8(41):71371−71384. https://doi.org/10.18632/oncotarget.19071. eCollection 2017 Sep 19.

25. Bhaijee F, Anders RA. PD-L1 expression as a predictive biomarker: is absence of proof the same as proof of absence? *JAMA Oncol*. 2016;2(1):54−55.

26. Usui Y, Okunuki Y, Hattori T, et al. Expression of costimulatory molecules on human retinoblastoma cells Y-79: functional expression of CD40 and B7H1. *Invest Ophthalmol Vis Sci*. 2006;47(10):4607−4613.

27. Boes M, Meyer-Wentrup F. TLR3 triggering regulates PD-L1 (CD274) expression in human neuroblastoma cells. *Cancer Lett*. 2015;361(1):49−56.

28. Aquino-Lopez A, Senyukov VV, Vlasic Z, Kleinerman ES, Lee DA. Interferon gamma induces changes in natural killer (NK) cell ligand expression and alters NK cell-mediated lysis of pediatric cancer cell lines. *Front Immunol*. 2017;8:391.

29. Spurny C, Kailayangiri S, Jamitzky S, et al. Programmed cell death ligand 1 (PD-L1) expression is not a predominant feature in Ewing sarcomas. *Pediatr Blood Cancer*. 2018;65(1).

30. Zhou Q, Munger ME, Highfill SL, et al. Program death-1 signaling and regulatory T cells collaborate to resist the function of adoptively transferred cytotoxic T lymphocytes in advanced acute myeloid leukemia. *Blood*. 2010;116(14):2484−2493.

31. Zhang L, Gajewski TF, Kline J. PD-1/PD-L1 interactions inhibit antitumor immune responses in a murine acute myeloid leukemia model. *Blood*. 2009;114(8):1545−1552.

32. Mao Y, Eissler N, Blanc KL, Johnsen JI, Kogner P, Kiessling R. Targeting suppressive myeloid cells potentiates checkpoint inhibitors to control spontaneous neuroblastoma. *Clin Cancer Res*. Aug 1 2016;22(15):3849−3859. https://doi.org/10.1158/1078-0432.CCR-15-1912. Epub 2016 Mar 8.

33. Rigo V, Emionite L, Daga A, et al. Combined immunotherapy with anti-PDL-1/PD-1 and anti-CD4 antibodies cures syngeneic disseminated neuroblastoma. *Sci Rep*. 2017;7(1):14049.

34. Lussier DM, O'Neill L, Nieves LM, et al. Enhanced T-cell immunity to osteosarcoma through antibody blockade of PD-1/PD-L1 interactions. *J Immunother*. 2015;38(3):96−106.

35. Pham CD, Flores C, Yang C, et al. Differential immune microenvironments and response to immune checkpoint blockade among molecular subtypes of murine medulloblastoma. *Clin Cancer Res*. 2016;22(3):582−595.

36. Bouffet E, Larouche V, Campbell BB, et al. Immune checkpoint inhibition for hypermutant glioblastoma multiforme resulting from germline biallelic mismatch repair deficiency. *J Clin Oncol*. 2016;34(19):2206−2211.

37. McCaughan GJ, Fulham MJ, Mahar A, et al. Programmed cell death-1 blockade in recurrent disseminated Ewing sarcoma. *J Hematol Oncol*. 2016;9(1):48.

38. Blumenthal DT, Yalon M, Vainer GW, et al. Pembrolizumab: first experience with recurrent primary central nervous system (CNS) tumors. *J Neurooncol*. 2016;129(3):453−460.

39. Foran AE, Nadel HR, Lee AF, Savage KJ, Deyell RJ. Nivolumab in the treatment of refractory pediatric hodgkin lymphoma. *J Pediatr Hematol Oncol*. 2017;39(5):e263−e266.

40. Feucht J, Kayser S, Gorodezki D, et al. T-cell responses against CD19+ pediatric acute lymphoblastic leukemia mediated by bispecific T-cell engager (BiTE) are regulated contrarily by PD-L1 and CD80/CD86 on leukemic blasts. *Oncotarget*. 2016;7(47):76902−76919.

41. Zhu X, McDowell MM, Newman WC, Mason GE, Greene S, Tamber MS. Severe cerebral edema following nivolumab treatment for pediatric glioblastoma: case report. *J Neurosurg Pediatr*. 2017;19(2):249−253.

42. Alegre ML, Noel PJ, Eisfelder BJ, et al. Regulation of surface and intracellular expression of CTLA4 on mouse T cells. *J Immunol*. 1996;157(11):4762−4770.

43. Linsley PS, Bradshaw J, Greene J, Peach R, Bennett KL, Mittler RS. Intracellular trafficking of CTLA-4 and focal localization towards sites of TCR engagement. *Immunity*. 1996;4(6):535−543.

44. Noel PJ, Boise LH, Green JM, Thompson CB. CD28 costimulation prevents cell death during primary T cell activation. *J Immunol*. 1996;157(2):636−642.

45. Kuehn HS, Ouyang W, Lo B, et al. Immune dysregulation in human subjects with heterozygous germline mutations in CTLA4. *Science*. 2014;345(6204):1623−1627.

46. Waterhouse P, Penninger JM, Timms E, et al. Lymphoproliferative disorders with early lethality in mice deficient in Ctla-4. *Science*. 1995;270(5238):985−988.

47. Selby MJ, Engelhardt JJ, Quigley M, et al. Anti-CTLA-4 antibodies of IgG2a isotype enhance antitumor activity through induction of intratumoral regulatory T cells. *Cancer Immunol Res*. 2013;1(1):32−42.

48. Peggs KS, Quezada SA, Chambers CA, Korman AJ, Allison JP. Blockade of CTLA-4 on both effector and regulatory T cell compartments contributes to the antitumor activity of anti-CTLA-4 antibodies. *J Exp Med*. 2009;206(8):1717−1725.

49. Hurwitz AA, Yu TF, Leach DR, Allison JP. CTLA-4 blockade synergizes with tumor-derived granulocyte-macrophage colony-stimulating factor for treatment of an experimental mammary carcinoma. *Proc Natl Acad Sci U S A*. 1998;95(17):10067−10071.

50. Kwon ED, Hurwitz AA, Foster BA, et al. Manipulation of T cell costimulatory and inhibitory signals for immunotherapy of prostate cancer. *Proc Natl Acad Sci U S A*. 1997;94(15):8099−8103.

51. Leach DR, Krummel MF, Allison JP. Enhancement of anti-tumor immunity by CTLA-4 blockade. *Science*. 1996; 271(5256):1734−1736.

52. Hingorani P, Maas ML, Gustafson MP, et al. Increased CTLA-4(+) T cells and an increased ratio of monocytes with loss of class II (CD14(+) HLA-DR(lo/neg)) found in aggressive pediatric sarcoma patients. *J Immunother Cancer*. 2015;3:35.

53. Contardi E, Palmisano GL, Tazzari PL, et al. CTLA-4 is constitutively expressed on tumor cells and can trigger apoptosis upon ligand interaction. *Int J Cancer*. 2005; 117(4):538−550.

54. Morris ZS, Guy EI, Francis DM, et al. In situ tumor vaccination by combining local radiation and tumor-specific antibody or immunocytokine treatments. *Cancer Res*. 2016; 76(13):3929−3941.

55. Cano-Mejia J, Burga RA, Sweeney EE, et al. Prussian blue nanoparticle-based photothermal therapy combined with checkpoint inhibition for photothermal immunotherapy of neuroblastoma. *Nanomedicine*. 2017;13(2): 771−781.

56. Srinivasan P, Wu X, Basu M, Rossi C, Sandler AD. PD-L1 checkpoint inhibition and anti-CTLA-4 whole tumor cell vaccination counter adaptive immune resistance: a mouse neuroblastoma model that mimics human disease. *PLoS Med*. 2018;15(1):e1002497.

57. Volejnikova J, Bajciova V, Sulovska L, et al. Bone marrow metastasis of malignant melanoma in childhood arising within a congenital melanocytic nevus. *Biomed Pap Med Fac Univ Palacky Olomouc Czech Repub*. 2016;160(3): 456−460.

58. Merchant MS, Wright M, Baird K, et al. Phase I clinical trial of ipilimumab in pediatric patients with advanced solid tumors. *Clin Cancer Res*. 2016;22(6):1364−1370.

59. Wright GJ, Jones M, Puklavec MJ, Brown MH, Barclay AN. The unusual distribution of the neuronal/lymphoid cell surface CD200 (OX2) glycoprotein is conserved in humans. *Immunology*. 2001;102(2):173−179.

60. Hoek RM, Ruuls SR, Murphy CA, et al. Down-regulation of the macrophage lineage through interaction with OX2 (CD200). *Science*. 2000;290(5497):1768−1771.

61. Jenmalm MC, Cherwinski H, Bowman EP, Phillips JH, Sedgwick JD. Regulation of myeloid cell function through the CD200 receptor. *J Immunol*. 2006;176(1): 191−199.

62. McWhirter JR, Kretz-Rommel A, Saven A, et al. Antibodies selected from combinatorial libraries block a tumor antigen that plays a key role in immunomodulation. *Proc Natl Acad Sci U S A*. 2006;103(4):1041−1046.

63. Gorczynski RM, Lee L, Boudakov I. Augmented Induction of CD4+CD25+ Treg using monoclonal antibodies to CD200R. *Transplantation*. 2005;79(9):1180−1183.

64. Kretz-Rommel A, Qin F, Dakappagari N, et al. CD200 expression on tumor cells suppresses antitumor immunity: new approaches to cancer immunotherapy. *J Immunol*. 2007;178(9):5595−5605.

65. Tembhare PR, Ghogale S, Ghatwai N, et al. Evaluation of new markers for minimal residual disease monitoring in B-cell precursor acute lymphoblastic leukemia: CD73 and CD86 are the most relevant new markers to increase the efficacy of MRD 2016; 00B: 000−000. *Cytometry B Clin Cytom*. 2018;94(1):100−111. https://doi.org/ 10.1002/cyto.b.21486. Epub 2016 Oct 27.

66. Adnan Awad S, Kamel MM, Ayoub MA, Kamel AM, Elnoshokaty EH, El Hifnawi N. Immunophenotypic characterization of cytogenetic subgroups in egyptian pediatric patients with B-cell acute lymphoblastic leukemia. *Clin Lymphoma Myeloma Leuk*. 2016;16(suppl):S19−S24.e11.

67. Siva A, Xin H, Qin F, Oltean D, Bowdish KS, Kretz-Rommel A. Immune modulation by melanoma and ovarian tumor cells through expression of the immunosuppressive molecule CD200. *Cancer Immunol Immunother*. 2008;57(7):987−996.

68. Moertel CL, Xia J, LaRue R, et al. CD200 in CNS tumor-induced immunosuppression: the role for CD200 pathway blockade in targeted immunotherapy. *J Immunother Cancer*. 2014;2(1):46.

69. Takikawa O. Biochemical and medical aspects of the indoleamine 2,3-dioxygenase-initiated L-tryptophan metabolism. *Biochem Biophys Res Commun*. 2005;338(1):12−19.

70. Frumento G, Rotondo R, Tonetti M, Damonte G, Benatti U, Ferrara GB. Tryptophan-derived catabolites are responsible for inhibition of T and natural killer cell proliferation induced by indoleamine 2,3-dioxygenase. *J Exp Med*. 2002;196(4):459−468.

71. Werner-Felmayer G, Werner ER, Fuchs D, Hausen A, Reibnegger G, Wachter H. Characteristics of interferon induced tryptophan metabolism in human cells in vitro. *Biochim Biophys Acta*. 1989;1012(2):140−147.

72. Guillemin GJ, Smythe G, Takikawa O, Brew BJ. Expression of indoleamine 2,3-dioxygenase and production of quinolinic acid by human microglia, astrocytes, and neurons. *Glia*. 2005;49(1):15−23.

73. Dai X, Zhu BT. Indoleamine 2,3-dioxygenase tissue distribution and cellular localization in mice: implications for its biological functions. *J Histochem Cytochem*. 2010; 58(1):17−28.

74. Holmgaard RB, Zamarin D, Li Y, et al. Tumor-expressed IDO recruits and activates MDSCs in a treg-dependent manner. *Cell Rep*. 2015;13(2):412−424.

75. Uyttenhove C, Pilotte L, Theate I, et al. Evidence for a tumoral immune resistance mechanism based on tryptophan degradation by indoleamine 2,3-dioxygenase. *Nat Med*. 2003;9(10):1269−1274.

76. Ben-Haj-Ayed A, Moussa A, Ghedira R, et al. Prognostic value of indoleamine 2,3-dioxygenase activity and expression in nasopharyngeal carcinoma. *Immunol Lett*. 2016; 169:23−32.

77. Urakawa H, Nishida Y, Nakashima H, Shimoyama Y, Nakamura S, Ishiguro N. Prognostic value of indoleamine 2,3-dioxygenase expression in high grade osteosarcoma. *Clin Exp Metastasis*. 2009;26(8):1005−1012.

78. Shahlaee A, Al-Quran S, Hou W, Schwartz C, Munn D. Aberrant indoleamine 2, 3 dioxygenase (IDO) expression is present in pediatric patients with Hodgkin's lymphoma. *Paper Presented at: ASCO Annual Meeting Proceedings.* 2007.

79. Witt DA, Donson AM, Amani V, et al. Specific expression of PD-L1 in RELA-fusion supratentorial ependymoma: implications for PD-1-targeted therapy. *Pediatr Blood Cancer.* 2018;65(5):e26960.

80. Vermeulen JF, Van Hecke W, Adriaansen EJM, et al. Prognostic relevance of tumor-infiltrating lymphocytes and immune checkpoints in pediatric medulloblastoma. *Oncoimmunology.* 2018;7(3):e1398877.

CHAPTER 11

Toxicities in Immune Checkpoint Inhibitors

SUNYOUNG S. LEE, MD, PhD • MATTHEW LOECHER, MD •
IGOR PUZANOV, MD, MSCI, FACP

INTRODUCTION

Immune checkpoint inhibitors (ICIs) have extended the scope of cancer treatment in patients with metastatic disease refractory to systemic chemotherapy or those with disease relapse after surgery, radiation, or systemic treatment. ICIs have been used for the treatment of many solid and hematologic malignancies. Currently, there are multiple clinical trials evaluating monotherapy ICIs, combination ICIs, and regimens including an ICI plus chemotherapy, radiation therapy, or molecular targeted therapy.

Several immune checkpoint molecules have been identified, including programmed death protein 1 (PD-1), programmed death-ligand 1 (PD-L1), cytotoxic T-lymphocyte–associated protein 4 (CTLA-4), lymphocyte-activation gene 3, T-cell membrane protein 3, V-domain Ig suppressor of T-cell activation, B- and T-cell lymphocyte attenuator, and killer cell immunoglobulin-like receptors.[1–3] PD-1 and CTLA-4 are the two main immune checkpoint molecules that therapies have targeted. Immune cells including T- and B-cells express PD-1; and complementary molecules, PD-L1, and PD-L2 bind to PD-1. This specific pathway exhausts immune system surveillance and enables regulatory T-cell (Treg) upregulation.[4] CTLA-4 is responsible for muting the immune response. Increased activation of T-cell receptors results in increased CTLA-4 expression and subsequent immune system downregulation.[5] By inhibiting PD-1/PD-L1 and CTLA-4, immune cell antitumor activity can be restored.

Many ICIs have been developed, seven of which have been extensively investigated: nivolumab and pembrolizumab are antibodies against PD-1; atezolizumab, avelumab, and durvalumab are PD-L1 inhibitors; and ipilimumab and tremelimumab are antibodies against CTLA-4. Several of these have been approved by the US Food and Drug Administration (FDA) for metastatic cancer, with their use now expanded into the neoadjuvant or first-line setting as monotherapy or with other treatment modalities.

One factor contributing to the diverse use of ICIs is their mild side effect profile. However, ICIs have been reported to cause immune-related adverse events (irAEs) similar to autoimmune diseases. These adverse events (AEs) are expected side effects, given ICI's mechanism of action—reactivating the immune system to chronic antigens, both malignant and benign. These side effects are distinct from those observed in cytotoxic chemotherapy or molecular targeted therapy.

With the advent of ICIs not too long ago, many new irAEs are still being first reported in the literature. Therefore, the strategic algorithm to manage ICI-induced irAEs has not been well established. This chapter will extensively review the toxicities associated with ICIs including organ system–based side effect profiles and the use of ICIs in challenging populations.

DIAGNOSIS AND CLINICAL MANIFESTATION OF IMMUNE-RELATED ADVERSE EVENTS

The diagnosis of irAEs is clinically made. Although circulating autoimmune antibodies are suspected in irAEs, no specific antibodies have been recognized to confirm the diagnosis of ICI-induced AEs.[6,7] Therefore, antibody recognition assays are not used to support the clinical diagnosis.

Immune-related side effects often follow a characteristic pattern of timing after the administration of an ICI. For example, patients with metastatic melanoma receiving ipilimumab developed skin-related irAEs during weeks 3–11, hepatotoxicity at 6–14 weeks, colitis at 5–11 weeks, and hypophysitis after 6–7 weeks of treatment.[8,9]

The grade, frequency, and involved organ systems of ICI-induced irAEs vary between malignancies and ICIs. For example, in a retrospective analysis of 576 patients with advanced melanoma who received nivolumab 3 mg/kg every 2 weeks,[10] 71% experienced any-grade treatment-related AEs. The most common AE was fatigue (25%). The organ systems associated with irAEs were skin (33%), gastrointestinal (14%), endocrine (8%), hepatic (4%), pulmonary (2%), and renal (2%) systems. The median times to onset were 5 (0.1–57), 7.3 (0.1–37.6), 10.4 (3.6–46.9), 7.7 (2.0–38.9), 8.9 (3.6–22.1), and 15.1 (3.9–26.4) weeks, respectively in these organ systems. The objective response rate was significantly better in patients who experienced treatment-related AEs of any grade, compared with those who did not. More importantly, 114 patients who received systemic immunosuppressants to manage irAEs did not have a significant difference in the objective response rate, compared with 462 patients who did not receive systemic immunosuppressants.

A different retrospective study analyzed patients with advanced melanoma who received ipilimumab 3 mg/kg every 2 weeks.[11] Of 298 patients, 254 (85%) experienced an irAE of any grade. Grade 3, 4, and 5 AEs were observed in 91 (31%) patients, 20 (7%) patients, and 1 patient, respectively. The organ systems associated with irAEs were hepatic (66%), skin (41%), gastrointestinal (29%), pituitary gland (6%), eyes (3%), and others (5%). Corticosteroids were given to 103 patients (35%), and anti-tumor necrosis factor-alpha (TNF-α) agents were given in 29 cases (10%), in which irAEs did not respond to systemic corticosteroids. No difference in overall survival (OS) or time to treatment failure (TTF) was detected in patients who had irAEs or those who did not. There was no difference in OS or TTF when patients were stratified by the administration of corticosteroids to treat irAEs.

ORGAN-SPECIFIC TOXICITIES
Grades of each AE are summarized in Table 11.1. Table 11.2 shows management of each grade of AEs.

DERMATOLOGIC AND MUCOSAL TOXICITY
Dermatologic side effects are very common immune-related events in patients on ICIs. These tend to occur 3 weeks or more after the patient's first infusion.[12] In particular, dermatologic toxicity is most frequently reported in patients with melanoma. This is likely due to common antigens between melanoma and benign

skin tissues.[13,14] Histopathology of most skin lesions reveals lymphocytic infiltration. Most commonly noticed dermatologic events are pruritus, rash, and vitiligo, but a wide variety of skin changes are seen including pustules, maculopapular rash, urticarial dermatitis, Sweet syndrome, lichenoid dermatitis, bullous pemphigoid, Stevens Johnson syndrome, and toxic epidermal necrolysis.[15–18] Nivolumab caused dermatologic irAEs in 34% of patients with advanced melanoma,[18] and up to 39% of patients with advanced melanoma had skin manifestations on pembrolizumab.[19,20] Ipilimumab caused skin AEs in up to 43.5% of melanoma patients.[21,22] The degree of skin manifestations is usually mild, but high-grade toxicities have been reported, resulting in the discontinuation of ICIs. For example, 1.5% of patients who received ipilimumab for advanced melanoma developed grade 3 dermatologic irAEs.[23] Another study comparing pembrolizumab with ipilimumab in advanced melanoma[20] shows that 13.4% and 14.1% of patients who received pembrolizumab developed rashes and pruritus, respectively, and 14.5% and 25.4% of those who received ipilimumab developed rashes and pruritus, respectively. Of note, no grade 3–5 toxicities were reported in pembrolizumab, but 1.2% of patients developed grade 3–5 toxicities with ipilimumab. CTLA-4 inhibitors, ipilimumab and tremelimumab caused more dermatologic toxicities, both mild and severe, than anti-PD-1 antibodies (see Table 11.3).

Mucosal toxicities are less common than skin AEs. For example, 0.7% and 0.4% of melanoma patients who received pembrolizumab compared with ipilimumab developed mucositis, respectively.[20] Another study of nivolumab shows that 6.5% of melanoma patients developed mucositis.[24]

Table 11.1 has grades of skin and mucosal AEs. Dermatologic and mucosal abnormalities are usually reversible, and therefore, those developing dermatologic lesions require early dermatologic evaluation. A topical corticosteroid cream is the first-line treatment. Oral antihistamine medications including diphenhydramine or hydroxyzine are also widely used. Moderate to severe rashes or pruritus (grade 2 and 3 toxicity) that do not resolve by these means should be treated by oral corticosteroids. ICIs are withheld until symptoms improve to grade 1. For grade 4 toxicities including full-thickness dermal ulceration, bullous lesions, necrosis, Stevens Johnson syndrome, or toxic epidermal necrolysis, ICIs should be discontinued permanently. ICIs also need to be permanently discontinued in abnormalities for which corticosteroid cannot be tapered

TABLE 11.1

Grades of Adverse Events (Based on National Cancer Institute Common Terminology Criteria for Adverse Events)

Adverse Event	Grade 1	Grade 2	Grade 3	Grade 4	Grade 5
General term	Mild; asymptomatic or mild symptoms; clinical or diagnostic observations only; intervention not indicated	Moderate; minimal, local, or noninvasive intervention indicated; limiting age-appropriate instrumental ADL	Severe or medically significant but not immediately life-threatening; hospitalization or prolongation of hospitalization indicated; disabling; limiting self-care ADL	Life-threatening consequences; urgent intervention indicated	Death
Maculopapular rash	Macules/papules covering <10% BSA with or without symptoms (e.g., pruritus, burning, tightness)	Macules/papules covering 10%–30% BSA with or without symptoms (e.g., pruritus, burning, tightness); limiting instrumental ADL	Macules/papules covering >30% BSA with or without associated symptoms; limiting self-care ADL	N/A	N/A
Papulopustular rash	Papules and/or pustules covering < 10% BSA, which may or may not be associated with symptoms	Papules and/or pustules covering 10%–30% BSA, which may or may not be associated with symptoms of pruritus or tenderness; associated with psychosocial impact; limiting instrumental ADL	Papules and/or pustules covering >30% BSA, which may or may not be associated with symptoms of pruritus or tenderness; limiting self-care ADL; associated with local superinfection with oral antibiotics indicated	Papules and/or pustules covering any % BSA, which may or may not be associated with symptoms of pruritus or tenderness and are associated with extensive superinfection with IV antibiotics indicated; life-threatening consequences	Death
Diarrhea	Increase of <4 stools per day over baseline; mild increase in ostomy output compared with baseline	Increase of 4–6 stools per day over baseline; moderate increase in ostomy output compared with baseline	Increase of >=7 stools per day over baseline; incontinence; hospitalization indicated; severe increase in ostomy output compared with baseline; limiting self-care ADL	Life-threatening consequences; urgent intervention indicated	Death
Enterocolitis	Asymptomatic; clinical or diagnostic observations only; intervention not indicated	Abdominal pain; mucus or blood in stool	Severe or persistent abdominal pain; fever; ileus; peritoneal signs	Life-threatening consequences; urgent intervention indicated	Death
Hepatitis	Bilirubin > ULN to 1.5×; ALT/AST > ULN to 2.5×; Albumin < LLN to 3 g/dL	Bilirubin >1.5–3.0×; ALT/AST > 2.5–5.0×; Albumin 3–2 g/dL	Bilirubin >3.0–10.0×; ALT/AST > 5.0–20.0×; Albumin <2 g/dL	Bilirubin >10.0×; ALT/AST > 20.0×	Death

Continued

TABLE 11.1
Grades of Adverse Events (Based on National Cancer Institute Common Terminology Criteria for Adverse Events)—cont'd

Adverse Event	Grade 1	Grade 2	Grade 3	Grade 4	Grade 5
Hypothyroidism	Asymptomatic; clinical or diagnostic observations only; intervention not indicated	Symptomatic; thyroid replacement indicated; limiting instrumental ADL	Severe symptoms; limiting self-care ADL; hospitalization indicated	Life-threatening consequences; urgent intervention indicated	Death
Hyperthyroidism	Asymptomatic; clinical or diagnostic observations only; intervention not indicated	Symptomatic; thyroid suppression indicated; limiting instrumental ADL	Severe symptoms; limiting self-care ADL; hospitalization indicated	Life-threatening consequences; urgent intervention indicated	Death
Adrenal insufficiency	Asymptomatic; clinical or diagnostic observations only; intervention not indicated	Moderate symptoms; medical intervention indicated	Severe symptoms; hospitalization indicated	Life-threatening consequences; urgent intervention indicated	Death
Type 1 diabetes mellitus	Asymptomatic; intervention not indicated	Symptomatic; dietary modification or oral agent indicated	Symptoms interfering with ADL; insulin indicated	Life-threatening consequences (e.g., ketoacidosis, hyperosmolar nonketotic coma)	Death
Pneumonitis	Asymptomatic; radiographic findings only	Symptomatic, not interfering with ADL	Symptomatic; interfering with ADL; O₂ indicated	Life-threatening; ventilatory support indicated	Death
Nephritis Acute kidney injury	Creatinine level increase of >0.3 mg/dL; creatinine 1.5–2.0× above baseline	Creatinine 2–3× above baseline	Creatinine >3× baseline or >4.0 mg/dL; hospitalization indicated	Life-threatening consequences; dialysis indicated	Death
Pancreatitis	N/A	Enzyme elevation or radiologic findings only	Severe pain; vomiting; medical intervention indicated (e.g., analgesia or nutritional support)	Life-threatening consequences; urgent intervention indicated	Death
Neurologic toxicity	Mild symptoms	Moderate symptoms; limiting instrumental ADL	Severe symptoms; limiting self-care ADL	Life-threatening consequences; urgent intervention indicated	Death
Uveitis	Asymptomatic; clinical or diagnostic observations only	Anterior uveitis; medical intervention indicated	Posterior uveitis or panuveitis	Blindness (20/200 or worse) in the affected eye	N/A
Heart failure Myocarditis	Asymptomatic with laboratory (BNP) or cardiac imaging abnormalities	Symptoms with mild to moderate activity or exertion	Severe with symptoms at rest or with minimal activity or exertion; intervention indicated	Life-threatening consequences; urgent intervention indicated (continuous IV therapy or mechanical hemodynamic support)	Death

Anemia	Hemoglobin (Hgb) < 10.0 g/dL	Hgb < 10.0–8.0 g/dL	Hgb < 8.0 g/dL	Life-threatening consequences; urgent intervention indicated	Death
Blood disorders	Asymptomatic or mild symptoms; clinical or diagnostic observations only; intervention not indicated	Moderate; minimal, local, or noninvasive intervention indicated; limiting age-appropriate instrumental ADL	Severe or medically significant but not immediately life-threatening; hospitalization or prolongation of existing hospitalization indicated; disabling; limiting self care ADL	Life-threatening consequences; urgent intervention indicated	Death
Arthritis	Mild pain with inflammation, erythema, or joint swelling, but not interfering with function	Moderate pain with inflammation, erythema, or joint swelling interfering with function, but not interfering with ADL	Severe pain with inflammation, erythema, or joint swelling and interfering with ADL	Disabling	Death
Fatigue	Fatigue relieved by rest	Fatigue not relieved by rest; limiting instrumental ADL	Fatigue not relieved by rest, limiting self-care ADL	N/A	N/A
Pyrexia	100.4–102.2°F	102.3–104.0°F	>104.0°F for ≤24 h	>104.0°F for >24 h	Death
Infusion reaction	Mild transient reaction; infusion interruption not indicated; intervention not indicated	Therapy or infusion interruption indicated but responds promptly to symptomatic treatment (e.g., antihistamines, NSAIDs, narcotics, IV fluids); prophylactic medications indicated for ≤24 h	Prolonged (e.g., not rapidly responsive to symptomatic medication and/or brief interruption of infusion); recurrence of symptoms following initial improvement; hospitalization indicated for clinical sequelae	Life-threatening consequences; urgent intervention indicated	Death

ADL, activities of daily living; *ALT*, alanine transaminase; *AST*, aspartate transaminase; *BNP*, brain natriuretic peptide; *BSA*, body surface area; *IV*, intravenous; *LLN*, lower limit of normal; *N/A*, not applicable; *NSAIDs*, nonsteroidal anti-inflammatory drugs; *ULN*, upper limit of normal.

TABLE 11.2
Treatment for Each Grade of Immune-Related Adverse Events

Adverse Event	Grade 1	Grade 2	Grade 3	Grade 4	Grade 5
Treatment	Supportive care; steroid or immunosuppressants not recommended; continue ICIs	Topical steroids or systemic steroids prednisone 0.5–1 mg/kg/day (or equivalent); no other immunosuppressants recommended; ICIs temporarily suspended	Hospitalization; systemic steroids methylprednisolone 1–2 mg/kg/day (or equivalent) for 3 days then reduce to 1 mg/kg/day; other immunosuppressants considered for unresolved symptoms after a 3–5-day steroid course; ICI discontinued (discuss resumption based on risk/benefit with patients)	Hospitalization or intensive care support; systemic steroids methylprednisolone 1–2 mg/kg/day (or equivalent) for 3 days then reduce to 1 mg/kg/day; other immunosuppressants considered for unresolved symptoms after a 3–5-day steroid course; ICI permanently discontinued	Death

ICI, immune checkpoint inhibitor.

down by 7.5 mg of prednisone or equivalent per day.[25] Skin lesions that do not resolve require biopsy and close monitoring with hospitalization to prevent and manage high-grade toxicities. An oral corticosteroid rinse is used to manage mucosal AEs.[26]

COLITIS AND DIARRHEA

Although dermatologic toxicities are the most common side effects of ICIs in melanoma patients, diarrhea and colitis appear to be one of the most common side effects of ICIs for all malignancies. In some articles, the terms, diarrhea and colitis are used interchangeably, but colitis designates diarrhea accompanied by abdominal pain and/or blood/mucus in stool, as well as diarrhea with evidence of colonic inflammation, mesenteric engorgement, and bowel wall thickening on imaging studies.[27,28] ICI-induced colitis shows a distinct histopathologic pattern from inflammatory bowel disease, featured by dysregulation of gastrointestinal mucosal immunity manifested as immune cell infiltration into the gastrointestinal mucosa, increased calprotectin indicating the migration of neutrophils, and deranged antibody titers in enteric flora.[29]

Diarrhea of any grade was seen in 10% of patients with non–small cell lung cancer (NSCLC)[30,31] and 11% of patients with melanoma, both of which were treated with nivolumab.[32] Pembrolizumab caused diarrhea in 13%–20% of patients with melanoma[33] and in

24% of those with metastatic carcinoma.[34] Another PD-1 antibody, pidilizumab, caused diarrhea in 17% of patients with lymphoma.[35] Combination of PD-1/PD-L1 antibody with CTLA-4 inhibitors appears to cause more diarrhea than monotherapy. The combination of nivolumab and ipilimumab caused diarrhea in 9%–44% of patients with melanoma and in 35% of those with glioblastoma multiforme.[36] When durvalumab, an anti-PD-L1 antibody, and tremelimumab, a CTLA-4 inhibitor, were given to patients with NSCLC, 27% of patients developed diarrhea.[37] The prevalence of diarrhea and colitis is summarized in Table 11.3.

Table 11.1 shows different grades of diarrhea. Diarrhea and colitis are usually manageable but can be fatal if not managed early. At the same time, cancer patients receiving ICIs are more vulnerable to gastrointestinal infections including *Clostridium difficile* or other bacterial, fungal, or viral enterocolitis. Therefore, infection should be ruled out before immunosuppressants are provided to alleviate ICI-induced inflammation. Stool cultures and *Clostridium difficile* study need to be sent. Diarrhea and colitis can cause electrolyte derangements and severe dehydration, and therefore, oral or intravenous (IV) hydration and electrolyte repletion should be maintained. For grade 1 symptoms, the focus of management is symptom control including hydration and antimotility medications. Grade 2 diarrhea or colitis requires temporary discontinuation of ICIs and supportive measures. However, patients with persistent

TABLE 11.3

Incidence of Adverse Events From Immune-Related Adverse Events

	PD-1/PD-L1 Inhibitors	CTLA-4 Inhibitors	PD-1(PD-L1)/CTLA-4 Combination
Dermatologic toxicity (pruritus or rash)	Nivolumab: 34%[50] Pembrolizumab: 11%–39%[2,4] Durvalumab: 8%–9%[31,32] Atezolizumab: 11%[33] BMS-936559: 9%[60]	Ipilimumab: 25%–44%[22,23] Tremelimumab: 59%–62%[43,44]	Nivolumab plus ipilimumab: 33%–55%[34,36] Pembrolizumab plus ipilimumab: 17%[37]
Colitis or diarrhea	Nivolumab: 8%–11%[1,3] Pembrolizumab: 3%–24%[2,10] Pidilizumab: 17%[30] Durvalumab: 7%[32] BMS-936559: 9%[60]	Ipilimumab: 9%–29%[23,45] Tremelimumab: 31%[43,44]	Nivolumab plus ipilimumab: 9%–44%[34,36] Durvalumab plus tremelimumab: 27%[38]
Hepatitis	Nivolumab: 1%–19%[8,22] Pembrolizumab: 1%–2%[2,27] Durvalumab: 4%[31] Atezolizumab: 4%[33]	Ipilimumab: 2%–18%[22,45] Tremelimumab: 6%–10%[43,44]	Nivolumab plus ipilimumab: 15%–25%[23,36] Durvalumab plus tremelimumab: 10%[38]
Hypophysitis	Pembrolizumab: 1%–2%[2,28]	Ipilimumab: 2%–16%[22,23]	Nivolumab plus ipilimumab: 12%[35]
Hypothyroidism	Nivolumab: 2%–12%[5,22] Pembrolizumab: 4%–9%[2,28] Durvalumab: 2%[31] BMS-936559: 3%[60]	Ipilimumab: 2%–3%[23,57]	Nivolumab plus ipilimumab: 15%–16%[35,36] Durvalumab plus tremelimumab: 6%[38]
Hyperthyroidism	Pembrolizumab: 5%[2] Durvalumab: 4%[32]		Nivolumab plus ipilimumab: 10%[58]
Adrenal insufficiency	BMS-936559: 2%[60]	Ipilimumab: 2%[23]	Pembrolizumab plus ipilimumab: 6%[37]
Type 1 diabetes mellitus	Pembrolizumab: 1%[2]		Nivolumab plus ipilimumab: 5%[23]
Pneumonitis	Nivolumab: 9%[24,66] Pembrolizumab: 4%[13] Durvalumab: 1%[31,32]	Ipilimumab: 2%–5%[32,45,57]	Nivolumab plus ipilimumab: 2%–10%[35,43,44] Pembrolizumab plus ipilimumab: 6%[37] Durvalumab plus tremelimumab: 5%[38]
Nephritis Acute kidney injury	Nivolumab: 1%[3] Pembrolizumab: 1%[27]		Nivolumab plus ipilimumab: 8%[58]
Pancreatitis	Nivolumab: 1%–17%[1,8] Pembrolizumab: 15%[10]	Ipilimumab: 1%[57] Tremelimumab: 3%[43,44]	Nivolumab plus ipilimumab: 13%–25%[23,34]
Neurologic toxicity	Nivolumab: 7%[116] Pembrolizumab: 2%[116]	Ipilimumab: 1%–5%[22,45,57]	Nivolumab plus ipilimumab: 3%–14%[58,116] Pembrolizumab plus ipilimumab: 6%[37] Durvalumab plus tremelimumab: 1%[38]
Ocular toxicity	Nivolumab: <1%[24] Pembrolizumab: <1%[2,83] Atezolizumab: <1%[84]	Ipilimumab: <1%[85]	Pembrolizumab plus ipilimumab: 6%[37]

Continued

TABLE 11.3
Incidence of Adverse Events From Immune-Related Adverse Events—cont'd

	PD-1/PD-L1 Inhibitors	CTLA-4 Inhibitors	PD-1(PD-L1)/CTLA-4 Combination
Heart failure or myocarditis	Case reports with no prevalence	Ipilimumab: 2%[57]	Pembrolizumab plus ipilimumab: 6%[37]
Blood disorders	Nivolumab: anemia 1%–2%,[1,8] thrombocytopenia 17%[7] Pembrolizumab: anemia 17[10] Pidilizumab: neutropenia 26%, thrombocytopenia 14%[30] Atezolizumab: thrombocytopenia 3%[6]	Ipilimumab: anemia 2%–12%,[23,57] neutropenia 1%,[57] thrombocytopenia 1%[57] Tremelimumab: neutropenia 3%[43,44]	Nivolumab plus ipilimumab: anemia 8%[58]
Arthritis or myositis	Nivolumab: 1%[5]	Ipilimumab: 2%[57] Tremelimumab: 14%[43,44]	Durvalumab plus tremelimumab: 1%[38]
Fatigue	Nivolumab: 13%–33%[31,74] Pembrolizumab: 19%–35%[19,98] Pidilizumab: 25%[30] Durvalumab: 13%–18%[31,32] Atezolizumab: 12%–24%[6,33] BMS-936559: 16%[60]	Ipilimumab: 10%–42%[23,57]	Nivolumab plus ipilimumab: 35%–38%[34,36] Pembrolizumab plus ipilimumab: 33%[61] Durvalumab plus tremelimumab: 26%[38]
Pyrexia	Nivolumab: 6%–13%[30,74] Atezolizumab: 12%[6]	Ipilimumab: 6%–12%[23,57] Tremelimumab: 24%–41%[43,44]	Nivolumab plus ipilimumab: 37%[48]
Infusion reaction	Nivolumab: 9%[22] Pembrolizumab: 3%[4] BMS-936559: 10%[60]	Ipilimumab: 6%[101]	Nivolumab plus ipilimumab: 3%[58]

CTLA-4, cytotoxic T-lymphocyte–associated protein 4; *PD-1*, programmed death protein 1; *PD-L1*, programmed death-ligand 1.

symptoms no longer on ICIs require steroid therapy and biopsy confirmation by rectosigmoidoscopy or colonoscopy. The focus of treatment is symptom control. Those with persistent grade 2 diarrhea should be started on a high-dose steroid (prednisolone 0.5–1 mg/kg/day), which should be continued until the symptoms are down to grade 1 or less. Steroids are not to be abruptly stopped. Instead, they are tapered off over 2–4 weeks. Patients with grade 3 and 4 diarrhea and colitis should be hospitalized for closer monitoring of fluid and electrolyte balances, and ICIs are permanently discontinued. A higher dose of steroid (prednisolone 1–2 mg/kg/day) is given. If symptoms do not improve within a few days, infliximab is added. Steroids are not discontinued until symptoms are stabilized, and it is tapered off over 4–8 weeks. Infliximab readministration can also be considered, as it can be given at 0, 2, and 6 weeks and every 8 weeks thereafter. Mycophenolate mofetil is also a consideration for colitis refractory to infliximab. For grade 3 and 4 colitis and diarrhea,

bowel perforation and peritonitis requiring surgical intervention should always be considered, and a gastroenterologist and gastrointestinal surgeon should be consulted.[25,27]

HEPATITIS

Immune-related hepatitis is a rare side effect that occurs in only 5% of patients treated with ICIs.[20] By definition, autoimmune hepatitis is an unexplained elevation in aspartate transaminase (AST), alanine transaminase (ALT), or bilirubin. Severity of hepatitis can be graded based on the degree of hepatic enzyme or bilirubin elevation. Patients are often asymptomatic with only mild elevations in liver function tests, but severe liver dysfunction can be fatal. Imaging studies, computed tomography (CT) scan or ultrasound, are considered to rule out biliary obstruction or disease progression. Infectious causes such as hepatitis A, B, or C and fulminant hepatitis E as well as medication-or alcohol-induced hepatitis should be excluded before managing ICI-induced hepatitis. Imaging appearances are nonspecific and can include hepatomegaly, periportal edema, and periportal lymphadenopathy. Pathology can confirm a clinical diagnosis with diffuse T-cell infiltrates in all lobes, prominent sinusoidal histiocytic infiltrates, and central vein damage with endothelialitis on liver biopsy.[38]

Nivolumab has been shown to cause immune-related hepatitis in 9% of patients with renal cell carcinoma, and 4% of patients developed grade 3−4 toxicity.[39] Up to 19% of patients with hepatocellular carcinoma developed grade 1−2 hepatitis, and up to 11% had grade 3−4 toxicity.[40] Pembrolizumab caused hepatitis in 1%−2% of patients.[20,33] Both durvalumab and atezolizumab caused grade 1−2 hepatitis in 4% of patients and grade 3−4 hepatitis in 2% of patients.[41−42] Ipilimumab and tremelimumab caused hepatitis up to 18% and 10%, respectively.[22,43−45] The combination of nivolumab and ipilimumab caused grade 1−2 hepatitis in up to 15%−25% of patients and grade 3−4 hepatitis in 6%−13% of patients.[36,46−48] The combination of durvalumab and tremelimumab caused hepatitis in 10% of patients.[37] The prevalence of hepatitis is summarized in Table 11.3.

Table 11.1 summarizes the grade of hepatitis. Grade 1 toxicity does not require discontinuation of ICIs, but liver function tests should be routinely monitored. For grade 2 toxicity, ICIs are withheld, and prednisone 1 mg/kg (or equivalent) should be initiated. For those having grade 3−4 liver toxicity, ICIs are permanently discontinued and IV methylprednisolone 2−4 mg/kg (or equivalent) is initiated with a long taper of at least 4−8 weeks. For refractory hepatitis not responding to corticosteroid treatment, mycophenolate mofetil or azathioprine is considered and infliximab is not given owing to potential hepatotoxicity. At this point, a hepatologist should be involved in patient care.[49,50]

ENDOCRINOPATHIES

Hypophysitis

Immune-related hypophysitis is most commonly associated with anti-CTLA-4 therapy but now has been observed to a lesser degree in anti-PD1/PD-L1 therapy. Hypophysitis is caused by inflammation of the pituitary gland, resulting in reduced secretion of pituitary hormones including adrenocorticotropic hormone (ACTH), thyroid-stimulating hormone (TSH), follicle-stimulating hormone (FSH), luteinizing hormone (LH), growth hormone, or prolactin. Central

hypothyroidism is the most commonly affected axis,[51] but dysfunction in each pituitary driven axis has been documented. Affected patients often have nonspecific symptoms resulting in under or delayed diagnoses. Most commonly patients report headache, fatigue, muscle weakness, paleness, constipation, weight loss, anorexia, and nausea. Patients with suspected hypophysitis should have each pituitary axis evaluated with serum levels of ACTH, morning cortisol, TSH, LH and FSH, estradiol in women, and testosterone in men as well as prolactin. Imaging is not necessary for diagnosis, but pituitary MRI (magnetic resonance imaging) often shows enlargement or areas of heterogeneity.

Hypophysitis is much more common with ipilimumab (2%−16%) than with anti-PD-1 antibodies (less than 2%).[23,29,52] Combination therapy with nivolumab and ipilimumab resulted in grade 1−2 hypophysitis in 12% of patients and grade 3−4 in 7% of patients.[41,48] Severe grade hypophysitis was observed in less than 1% of melanoma patients treated with pembrolizumab.[53] The prevalence of hypophysitis is summarized in Table 11.3 in detail.

Symptomatic patients and those with suspected hypophysitis with headache, visual change, or hypotension should be initiated on prednisone 1 mg/kg (or equivalent). Steroids should be tapered off over 2−4 weeks followed by hormone replacement as coordinated with an endocrinologist.[27] These patients should have pituitary imaging. Hypophysitis may resolve when it is managed at an earlier stage, or some patients may be weaned off from hormone replacement therapy. However, many patients often require lifelong therapy unlike other irAEs.[54]

Thyroid Dysfunction

Patients treated with ICIs can develop both immune-related hyperthyroidism and hypothyroidism, although the latter is more common. Patients with ICI-induced thyroid dysfunction may have nonspecific symptoms including fatigue, lack of appetite, or hair change, for which other differential diagnoses such as hypophysitis should be thoroughly explored. ICI-induced thyroiditis often mimics the presentation of Hashimoto thyroiditis. Often times, patients have a short period of subclinical hyperthyroidism preceding a hypothyroid state. Less commonly, patients develop TSH-receptor antibodies and progress to hyperthyroidism and Graves disease.[55] Patients with suspected thyroid dysfunction should be evaluated with serum TSH, T4, and T3 levels. Elevated TSH with low thyroid hormone indicates primary hypothyroidism; low TSH with low thyroid hormone level suggests hypophysitis. Anti-thyroglobulin and anti-thyroid peroxidase antibodies are not necessary for a diagnosis and are often undetectable.

Patients treated with nivolumab commonly develop grade 1−2 hypothyroidism seen in 2%−12% of patients,[39] but grades 3 and 4 AEs are rare, occurring in less than 1% of patients.[56] Pembrolizumab has reportedly caused hypothyroidism and hyperthyroidism in 9% and 5% of patients, respectively.[20] Durvalumab caused hypothyroidism and hyperthyroidism in 2% and 4% of patients, respectively.[41] Ipilimumab caused hypothyroidism in 2%−3% of patients.[23,57] Nivolumab and ipilimumab combination caused grade 1−2 hypothyroidism in 16% of patients,[47] but another report shows that this combination caused grade 3−4 hypothyroidism in up to 10% of patients.[36] This combination caused hyperthyroidism in 10% of patients.[58] The combination of durvalumab and tremelimumab caused it in 6% of patients.[37] The prevalence of hypothyroidism and hyperthyroidism is summarized in Table 11.3 in detail.

Patients who develop hypothyroidism often require lifelong hormone replacement with levothyroxine unless patients have acute inflammation of the thyroid, which can be managed with a short course of oral corticosteroids (prednisone 1 mg/kg or equivalent). Patients with acute episodes of hyperthyroidism may require symptom-specific treatment managed in a similar way as in those with primary hyperthyroidism. Patients with tachycardia and tremor can be treated with beta-blockers. Patients with severe symptoms may require steroid therapy and input from an endocrinologist. ICIs are most often continued, and hormone replacement is usually sufficient.[27]

Adrenal Insufficiency

Adrenal insufficiency is not a common side effect of ICIs, but it was noticed in a few reports. This may be in the setting of hypophysitis resulting in reduced ACTH levels or primary adrenal insufficiency from inflammation of the adrenal glands. Patients may have electrolyte derangement with hyponatremia and hyperkalemia as well as hypotension. Patients in an adrenal crisis require urgent medical intervention, as the condition is life-threatening.[59]

Grade 1−2 adrenal sufficiency was noticed in 2% of patients who received BMS-936559 (PD-L1 antibody).[60] Ipilimumab monotherapy caused it in 2% of patients.[23] Grade 3−4 adrenal insufficiency was noticed in 6% of patients who received the combination of pembrolizumab and ipilimumab for NSCLC.[61]

Table 11.1 shows the grades of adrenal insufficiency. Adrenal sufficiency needs to be managed with glucocorticoid replacement therapy regardless of its grade. If an adrenal crisis is suspected, IV stress-dose corticosteroids including IV hydrocortisone 100 mg or dexamethasone 4 mg should be given, as well as aggressive volume expansion and electrolyte repletion.[62] Endocrinology consultation is necessary.

Type 1 Diabetes

Type 1 diabetes induced by ICIs is extremely rare, and only a few reports have been documented. It can present as mild to moderate hyperglycemia, but diabetic ketoacidosis has also been reported.

Pembrolizumab caused grade 3−4 type 1 diabetes in less than 1% of patients with melanoma.[20] Ipilimumab plus nivolumab or nivolumab monotherapy also caused diabetic ketoacidosis in 5% of patients as a new symptom from ICI-induced inflammation.[36,63]

Table 11.1 shows grades of diabetes mellitus. Patients who develop diabetes from ICIs do not receive corticosteroids because they can worsen their hyperglycemic state. Instead, patients are managed similarly as in those with type 1 diabetes mellitus using insulin therapy.[64] The role of immunosuppressants including infliximab or mycophenolate mofetil has not been verified.

Pneumonitis

Pneumonitis is observed in less than 10% of patients treated with ICIs. Patients with pneumonitis often report mild symptoms such as shortness of breath and cough, but several severe cases have resulted in death. Any patient with suspected respiratory compromise requires further investigation and delay of ICI administration. Patients should undergo CT imaging to assess for ground glass opacities or nodular infiltrates.[56,65]

Pneumonitis has been reported in patients treated with both anti-PD1/PD-L1 and anti-CTLA4 therapy. With nivolumab treatment, grade 1−2 pneumonitis was noticed in up to 9% and grade 3−4 in 1%−3% of patients.[31,56] Similar frequencies were shown with pembrolizumab (grade 1−2 in up to 4% and grade 3−4 in 1%) with one death described in a patient with NSCLC.[13,19,23,32] Durvalumab caused it in 1% of patients.[66] Ipilimumab monotherapy resulted in pneumonitis in up to 5% of patients, although more patients reported mild dyspnea and cough.[32] Combination therapy with ipilimumab and nivolumab has the highest rate of pneumonitis with 5%−10% any grade and nearly 2% grade 3–4 events.[44] The combination of pembrolizumab plus ipilimumab and that of durvalumab plus tremelimumab caused pneumonitis in 6% and 5% of patients, respectively.[37,61] Of the patients with NSCLC who received nivolumab plus platinum-doublet chemotherapy, 13% and 7% developed grade 1–2 and grade 3–4 pneumonitis, respectively.[67] ICIs cause pneumonitis more frequently when combined with chemotherapeutics that are known causes of pneumonitis.

Table 11.1 shows grades of pneumonitis. Pneumonitis is a potentially life-threatening disease, and therefore, clinicians must have a low threshold for urgent workup and intervention. Cancer patients can develop pulmonary embolism, obstructive pneumonia, or atypical lung infections including *Pneumocystis jirovecii*, influenza, or syncytial virus, which are differential diagnoses in the setting of cancer treatment with ICIs. These life-threatening diseases need to be ruled out first. Patients in whom underlying infection is suspected should be considered for bronchoscopy with lavage.[65] Patients with grade 1 pneumonitis are usually monitored without any intervention. However, if pneumonitis does not improve and patients become symptomatic (grade 2), ICIs are temporarily discontinued and prednisone 1 mg/kg (or equivalent) should be initiated. Chest imaging study is warranted. If there is clinical improvement to grade 1, corticosteroids are tapered and ICIs are resumed. Grade 3–4 pneumonitis requires permanent discontinuation of ICIs and aggressive management with IV methylprednisolone 2–4 mg/kg (or equivalent), as well as intensive care support. If respiratory symptoms do not improve over 48 hours, infliximab should be provided. Mycophenolate mofetil is considered for refractory pneumonitis not responding to corticosteroids or infliximab.[68]

Nephritis

ICI-induced renal injury is not common. Some of histopathologic manifestations of ICI-induced renal toxicities also include lupus nephritis and granulomatous interstitial nephritis.[69,70] It has been reported in less than 1% of patients who received nivolumab monotherapy for squamous cell carcinoma of the lung[71] and 3% of patients who received nivolumab plus sunitinib or pazopanib for renal cell carcinoma.[72] The combination of nivolumab and ipilimumab causes renal failure in 8% of melanoma patients.[58] Per a report by Cortazar et al.,[73] of 13 patients who received ipilimumab, nivolumab, pembrolizumab, or the combination of nivolumab and ipilimumab, 12 patients had acute tubulointerstitial nephritis and 1 patient had thrombotic microangiopathy. One of the main characteristic was its long latency period with a relatively delayed manifestation of renal toxicity that ranges from 21 to 245 days. Transient hemodialysis was required in two patients, but two patients remained dialysis dependent. Corticosteroids are used to treat ICI-induced nephritis, and more patients return to baseline kidney function.

Table 11.1 shows grades of renal injury based on the grades of acute kidney injury. Because nephritis is not a common side effect of ICIs, no standard management protocol has been suggested. However, corticosteroids are suggested as in other ICI-induced irAEs. Supportive care including temporary or permanent hemodialysis is critical.

Pancreatitis

An elevation of amylase and lipase in patients who received ICIs has been reported in multiple studies. Among patients with Hodgkin lymphoma who received nivolumab, 4% developed severe pancreatitis, although whether these patients had abdominal pain was not specified.[74] Amylase and lipase elevation was noticed in up to 17% of patients who received nivolumab for hepatocellular carcinoma.[40] Of those who received pembrolizumab, 15% developed asymptomatic pancreatitis.[34] In this study, the definition of pancreatitis was elevated lipase or amylase. Ipilimumab, tremelimumab, and the combination of nivolumab and ipilimumab caused pancreatitis in 1%, 3%, and up to 25% of patients, respectively.[36,43,46,57]

Whether asymptomatic patients with elevated lipase or amylase are required to be treated remains unclear. In addition, the grading system for ICI-induced pancreatitis has not been established, although there are multiple grading systems for pancreatitis including BISAP score or Ranson criteria for assessing the severity of acute pancreatitis or Balthazar score for the evaluation of CT-based severity of acute pancreatitis. Clinicians generally agree that steroid treatment is recommended in patients with moderate to severe elevations of lipase or amylase. The dosage of corticosteroids or the addition of other immunosuppressants including infliximab or mycophenolate mofetil has yet to be determined in a similar way to that of other ICI-induced AEs.

Neurologic

Although neurologic side effects are not common, they can be fatal. In a retrospective study of 352 patients with melanoma treated with ICIs, neurotoxicity was observed in one study at a rate of 2.8% overall and 1%, 7%, 2%, and 14% with ipilimumab, nivolumab, pembrolizumab, and ipilimumab plus nivolumab, respectively.[75] The combination of pembrolizumab plus ipilimumab and that of durvalumab plus tremelimumab caused it in 6% and 1% of patients, respectively.[37,61] Guillain–Barre syndrome, myasthenia gravis, aseptic meningitis, autoimmune encephalitis, posterior reversible encephalopathy syndrome, enteric neuropathy, and transverse myelitis have also been reported.[76–79]

Differential diagnoses include diabetes-induced neuropathy, vitamin B12 or folate deficiency, infection including hepatitis or human immunodeficiency virus (HIV), hypothyroidism, previous heavy alcohol use, or other autoimmune diseases (e.g., vasculitis), which could also be caused by ICIs. Thorough investigation into other pathologic mechanisms must be concluded before a diagnosis of an ICI-induced neurotoxicity can be made.

For mild neurologic symptoms causing no interference with function, close monitoring for progression is advised with a low threshold to withdraw ICIs. Once patients develop any cranial nerve deficits or have interference with activities of daily living, ICIs should be withheld, and prednisolone 1 mg/kg (or equivalent) and/or pregabalin or duloxetine for pain should be initiated. If patients develop severe symptoms including respiratory compromise, patients should be admitted for intensive care support and started on methylprednisolone 2 mg/kg (or equivalent) with other workups including MRI brain/spine, lumbar puncture, and pulmonary function test. Corticosteroids are tapered slowly over 4–8 weeks.[75]

Ocular Toxicity

Both PD-1 and CTLA-4 inhibitors are reported to cause ocular AEs. These include uveitis, episcleritis, iritis, and exudative retinal detachment,[80,81] causing symptoms such as double/blurry vision, dry eye, ocular pain, photophobia, and decreased vision or acuity.[82] Incidence of ocular AEs from ipilimumab is less than 1%, and those from pembrolizumab, nivolumab, and atezolizumab are also less than 1%.[24,83,84] The combination of pembrolizumab and ipilimumab caused ocular toxicity in 6% of patients.[61] A retrospective study of patients with metastatic melanoma who received ipilimumab and developed ocular or orbital inflammation shows that four out of seven patients had orbital inflammation, two had uveitis, and one had peripheral ulcerative keratitis. These patients were managed with topical and systemic corticosteroids, and symptoms resolved with no long-term sequelae.[85] There are no standard treatment options for ocular irAEs, and clinical judgment is warranted for each case of AEs.

Cardiotoxicity

Animal models have demonstrated autoimmune myocarditis associated with PD-1/PD-L1 or CTLA-4 mechanisms: in mice, PD-1 deficiency was a predisposition to the development of myocarditis,[86,87] CTLA-4–deficient mice are known to develop severe myocarditis.[5] Based on these models, there is a theoretical concern for cardiotoxicity induced by PD-1 or CTLA-4 inhibitors.

Cardiotoxicity has been observed in patients who have received both PD-1 and CTLA-4 inhibitors, although it is not a common side effect. Two cases were reported in 2016 with cardiac electrical instability and myocarditis with a robust presence of T-cell and macrophage infiltrates.[88,89] For example, eight cases of ICI-induced cardiotoxicity were found in patients who received ipilimumab (six patients), pembrolizumab (one patient), or combination of ipilimumab and nivolumab (one patient).[89] Five out of eight patients had underlying cardiac diseases, although they were free of symptoms before the initiation of ICIs. Myocarditis, cardiomyopathy, heart failure, myocardial fibrosis, and cardiac arrest were the reported cardiotoxicities. In addition to a drop of left ventricular ejection fraction (LVEF) in six out of eight patients, left ventricular apical akinesis similar to takotsubo cardiomyopathy was also observed. Three out of six patients who had decreased LVEF returned to the baseline LVEF. Three patients died from these AEs despite corticosteroid therapy.

There is no established grading system for ICI-induced cardiotoxicity. However, for patients who have severe symptoms or a significant decrease in LVEF, corticosteroids (methylprednisolone 2 mg/kg) should be initiated as managed in other irAEs. Patients with troponinemia, elevated B-type natriuretic peptide, or decreased LVEF should be managed in an intensive care unit. If symptoms do not improve on corticosteroids, an early use of mycophenolate mofetil, infliximab, or antithymocyte globulin is indicated.

Hematologic Toxicity

Neutropenia, anemia, and thrombocytopenia are very rare side effects of ICIs. Red cell aplasia, neutropenia, pancytopenia, and hemophilia A were reported in patients who received anti–CTLA-4.[90–93] Cryoglobulinemia was reported in a patient with adenocarcinoma of the lung who received nivolumab.[94] This patient received prednisone, and the cryoglobulinemia resolved after 26 days of steroid therapy. Aplastic anemia was reported in a patient with melanoma treated with nivolumab.[95] The prevalence of hematologic disorders is summarized in Table 11.3.

All of these AEs seem to be immune mediated, and therefore, systemic corticosteroid administration is the treatment of choice. Of note, many other differential diagnoses should be ruled out first because hematologic toxicity is rare in patients receiving ICIs. Differential diagnoses include hematologic malignancies or malignant bone marrow infiltration of the tumor.

Rheumatologic and Musculoskeletal Toxicity

Patients who receive ICIs may develop arthralgias and arthritis. However, they are rarely reported and only a few cases have been documented. One of 122 patients developed severe arthralgia after receiving nivolumab,[39] and 17% of patients who received durvalumab and dabrafenib/trametinib developed mild arthralgia.[96] Another report showed that 13 patients who received nivolumab or ipilimumab as monotherapy or nivolumab plus ipilimumab developed rheumatologic irAEs such as inflammatory arthritis, synovitis, and sicca syndrome. All 13 patients received corticosteroids, and 2 patients required methotrexate and anti−TNF-α treatment.[97] It is treated in a similar way as in patients with autoimmune rheumatologic diseases of other etiologies.

SYSTEMIC ADVERSE EVENTS

Fatigue

Organ-specific toxicities from ICIs are closely monitored and aggressively treated to prevent toxicity-associated mortalities. However, the most common side effect from ICIs is fatigue. This seems to be from reactivation of the immune system causing a generalized whole body inflammation mediated by cytokine release.[12] Anti−CTLA-4 antibodies or combination of PD-1 and CTLA-4 antibodies seem to cause fatigue more often than anti−PD-1 antibodies. For example, nivolumab caused fatigue in 13%−33% of patients[31,74] and pembrolizumab in 19%−35% of patients.[19,98] Ipilimumab monotherapy caused fatigue in up to 42% of patients.[23] Nivolumab plus ipilimumab caused fatigue in 35%−38% of patients;[36,48] the combination of pembrolizumab plus ipilimumab caused fatigue in 33% of patients.[61] When ICIs are combined with chemotherapy or molecular targeted therapy, fatigue is also the most common side effect. When nivolumab is combined with platinum-doublet chemotherapy for patients with NSCLC, fatigue was reported in 71% of patients.[67] When atezolizumab was combined with bevacizumab, 40% of patients had fatigue;[99] the combination of atezolizumab, bevacizumab, and FOLFOX for colorectal cancer caused fatigue in 47% of patients.[100]

Severe fatigue for which a discontinuation of ICIs is considered is not common, but mild to moderate fatigue is commonly reported in patients receiving anti−PD-1 inhibitors or CTLA-4 inhibitors. The differential diagnoses of fatigue are vast and include endocrinopathies such as hypophysitis, adrenal insufficiency, and hypothyroidism as well as infection. These potential pathologies can cause severe morbidity/mortality as well as poor quality of life. Clinicians should rule out these first when fatigue is noticed in patients receiving ICIs.

Pyrexia

Pyrexia from ICIs is not a common side effect, but it has been well documented in several clinical studies. The pathophysiology is not well known, but it appears to be associated with cytokine release and nonspecific inflammation from reactivation of the immune system, similar to that in fatigue as described earlier. For example, 6% and 13% of patients who received nivolumab developed pyrexia as reported in two studies;[30,74] 12% of patients who received atezolizumab developed pyrexia.[42] Ipilimumab, tremelimumab, and the combination of nivolumab and ipilimumab caused pyrexia in 6%−12%, 24%−41%, and 37% of patients, respectively.[21,43,44,48,57] When an ICI is combined with other medications that have reportedly caused pyrexia, more patients developed pyrexia. For example, melanoma patients who received durvalumab, dabrafenib, and trametinib caused pyrexia in 37% of patients, and 2% of patients developed grade 3−4 toxicities leading to the discontinuation of the medications.[96] In patients who received atezolizumab and bevacizumab or atezolizumab, bevacizumab, and FOLFOX, 21% and 20% developed pyrexia, respectively.[99,100] Because neutropenia from ICIs is not common, patients with pyrexia are not likely to have neutropenic fever. Therefore, antipyretics including acetaminophen are used. However, when an ICI is combined with chemotherapy, patients with pyrexia should be managed as though they have a neutropenic fever.

Infusion Reaction

Infusion reaction is less common in patients receiving ICIs than those who receive chemotherapy. However, an infusion reaction may occur with any drug, and it has also been reported in patients receiving ICIs. For example, 9% of patients who received nivolumab developed infusion reaction.[56] Pembrolizumab, ipilimumab, and the combination of nivolumab and ipilimumab caused it in 3%, 6%, and 3% of patients, respectively.[19,58,101] Because this is a hypersensitivity reaction to the infused medication, an antihistamine or glucocorticoid should be administered.

Immunosuppressants and Infection

As discussed earlier, immune-mediated toxicities are treated with a high dose of corticosteroids. Patients having persistent side effects require a slow taper of corticosteroids. These patients can experience a series of side effects including uncontrolled serum glucose, insomnia, mood change, bone density loss, and opportunistic infections. Serum glucose may be uncontrollable in patients with underlying diabetes mellitus, and this is managed with short-acting insulin until corticosteroids are tapered off. Prophylactic proton pump inhibitors are used while patients are on corticosteroids. Patients who are on corticosteroids or other immunosuppressants for more than 4 weeks (especially, prednisone >20 mg daily or equivalent) should receive prophylactic antibiotics including trimethoprim and sulfamethoxazole, atovaquone, or pentamidine to prevent opportunistic infections including *Pneumocystis jirovecii*.[102]

Underlying Autoimmune Diseases

Autoimmune disorders originate from dysregulated immunity. Immune-related AEs due to ICIs are from uncontrolled reactivation of depressed T-cells against a patient's own tissue. This immune tolerance and autoimmunity are partly maintained by the PD-1/PD-L1 axis[103] and the CTLA-4 axis.[104] Tumor-associated antigens, neoantigens, and host tissues may share similar epitopes with cross-reactivity, which can potentiate irAEs.[105]

Therefore, there has been a fear of exacerbation or a flare of underlying autoimmune disorders when patients with autoimmune disorders receive ICIs to treat cancer, and most clinical trials have excluded patients with a history of, or active, autoimmune disorders to limit a risk of irAEs.

An analysis of patients diagnosed with metastatic melanoma in 2014 reveals that 28.3% of patients had autoimmune disorders.[106] Another report identified that 13.5% of patients with lung cancer had autoimmune disorders, and this is estimated to be 20–50 million individuals in the United States.[107] Therefore, there is an urgent need to explore the effects of ICIs on underlying autoimmune disorders to minimize the exclusion of desperate patients who could benefit from ICIs. A study of 30 melanoma patients treated with ipilimumab who had preexisting autoimmune disorders revealed that 27% of patients had exacerbations of the same disorders and 33% experienced other irAEs, requiring treatment.[108] Another study of 52 melanoma patients with underlying autoimmune diseases treated with anti–PD-1 antibodies[109] shows that 20/52 (38%) had a flare of the same autoimmune diseases requiring immunosuppression: 7/13 with rheumatoid arthritis, 3/3 with polymyalgia rheumatica, 2/2 with Sjögren syndrome, 2/2 with immune thrombocytopenic purpura, and 3/8 with psoriasis. However, no patients with gastrointestinal or neurologic autoimmune disorders showed the same disease flare. Only two patients were required to discontinue the anti–PD-1 therapy. Of 52 patients, 15 patients (29%) developed irAEs other than their underlying autoimmune disorders. The study also included 67 melanoma patients who had developed irAEs from ipilimumab, showing that 2/67 patients (3%) had a recurrence of the same ipilimumab-induced irAEs, and 23 (34%) developed new irAEs.

Whether administration of ICIs is safe in those with preexisting autoimmune diseases has not been fully explored owing to a lack of clinical data. However, analyses discussed earlier suggest that ICIs for patients with autoimmune diseases suffering from refractory malignancies would be feasible under close monitoring.[110]

Solid Organ and Stem Cell Transplantation

With the reactivation of T-cell immunity with ICI treatment, there are concerns about graft rejection or graft-versus-host-disease (GVHD) in patients who previously underwent solid organ or allogeneic stem cell transplantation. The PD-1/PD-L1 pathway is known to be critical for induction and maintenance of transplantation tolerance and prevention of chronic rejection in solid organ transplantation.[111] The interplay between donor PD-L1 and recipient PD-1 molecules counterregulates rejection activities against liver grafts.[112] In patients who received allogeneic stem cell transplantation for hematologic malignancies, excessive or persistent PD-1 expression on tumor-specific T-cells is associated with increased mortality.[113] One of the key pathways to fine-tune the degree of GVHD is the modulation of the PD-1/PD-L1 axis and associated T-cell–mediated immune responses.[114]

Whether anti–PD-1 antibodies are safe to be given to patients with solid organ or stem cell transplantation is not clear. Many case reports have demonstrated mixed results. For example, renal graft rejection,[115–117] cardiac allograft rejection,[118] and worsening of GVHD after allogeneic stem cell transplantation[119–121] have been reported. On the contrary, other case reports suggest that anti–PD-1 antibodies may be safely given to patients without graft failure[122] or AEs similar to GVHD.[122–126]

The CTLA-4 pathway activates Tregs, resulting in inhibition of T-cell–based immune surveillance. Several clinical studies have been performed, hypothesizing that modulation of the CTLA-4 pathway may adjust immune responses associated with solid organ transplantation.[127] However, the role of CTLA-4–mediated signals in solid organ transplantation has not been clearly verified. One study using a mouse model suggests that the inhibition of CTLA-4 increases the severity of GVHD mediated by CD4+ T-cells.[128] Valid concerns about the detrimental effect of CTLA-4 inhibitors have been raised when administered to those with allogeneic stem cell or solid organ transplants. Only one case report has shown graft rejection in patients treated with a combination of ipilimumab and nivolumab.[116] All other case reports favor toleration of ipilimumab in solid organ transplantation.[129–131] A phase I trial of ipilimumab (0.1 mg/kg and 3 mg/kg) for patients with a relapsed hematologic malignancy status post allogeneic stem cell transplantation demonstrated no evidence of GVHD.[132] This study was expanded to include patients treated with higher doses of ipilimumab (3 mg/kg and 10 mg/kg), in which ipilimumab caused GVHD in 4/28 patients (14%).[133]

Patients with advanced lymphoma can be treated with anti–PD-1 antibodies. Some of these patients eventually progress and ultimately receive allogeneic stem cell transplantation. There is a concern that prior PD-1 blockade may modify the safety profile and efficacy of stem cell transplantation. An international retrospective analysis of 39 patients with lymphoma previously treated with an anti–PD-1 inhibitor addressed this issue:[134] the incidence of acute GVHD at 1 year follow-up was 22%–44%, and 1-year overall

and progression-free survival rates were 89% and 76%. PD-1+ T-cells were significantly decreased with a decreased ratio of Tregs to conventional CD4 and CD8 T-cells. This demonstrates that there is an increased risk of early immune-related complications, although the posttransplant relapse rate was rather favorable.

The mixed results of ICIs in patients with solid organ and stem cell transplantation suggest that ICIs be used with extreme caution because the immune checkpoint inhibition can cause life-threatening complications.[110]

Preexisting Infectious Disease
The association of malignancy and chronic infection is well described in patients with hepatocellular carcinoma (HCC) because hepatitis B and C infections are strong risk factors for HCC. Immune system derangement in patients with hepatitis B virus (HBV), hepatitis C virus (HCV), and HIV results from immune system exhaustion as a result of chronic exposure to viral antigens. In these patients, the T-cell–mediated immune response is attenuated, and the expression of PD-1 and PD-L1 is upregulated.[135] Clinical studies have aimed to use ICIs to treat chronic HBV or HCV infection. For example, a significant decrease in hepatitis C viral load was observed when HCV was treated with nivolumab.[136] Despite promising results, there is concern about administering ICIs to patients with preexisting infections and a modified immune response.

A phase I clinical trial of tremelimumab demonstrated that patients with both inoperable HCC and HCV had a significant decrease in the hepatitis C viral load without causing intolerable side effects.[137] CheckMate-040 studied nivolumab in patients with advanced HCC and showed that nivolumab had a durable response in those with HBV or HCV, as well as in those without underlying HBV or HCV.[138,139] More studies are ongoing to assess the safety profiles of ICIs in cancer patients with chronic infections treated with ICIs.

CTLA-4 and PD-1 Combination
The combination of PD-1 and CTLA-4 inhibitors appears to cause AEs more frequently than PD-1 or CTLA-4 monotherapy as already discussed in each organ-specific toxicity. Detailed organ-specific toxicities and prevalence of the combination of PD-1 (PD-L1) and CTLA-4 are summarized in Table 11.3.

Combination of Chemotherapy and Immune Checkpoint Inhibitor
Several clinical trials are ongoing to explore the efficacy of combined ICI and chemotherapy. This combination

is based on the premise that chemotherapy is potentially immunogenic and could augment ICIs by increasing turnover of tumor-associated antigens or neoantigens.

An addition of nivolumab to platinum-doublet chemotherapy showed similar side effect profiles to those in chemotherapy alone in patients with NSCLC.[67] The most common side effect was fatigue (71%), and nausea, low appetite, and alopecia followed in 46%, 36%, and 30%, respectively. Pneumonitis was observed in 13% of patients. In a randomized, open-label, phase II study for patients with nonsquamous NSCLC,[140] patients were assigned to two groups: 60 patients received carboplatin (area under curve 5 mg/mL per min), pemetrexed (500 mg/m^2), and pembrolizumab (200 mg) and 63 patients received carboplatin and pemetrexed (the same dosages). In the chemotherapy plus pembrolizumab group, any AEs of grade 1–2, grade 3, grade 4, and grade 5 were 54%, 31%, 7%, and 2%, respectively; in the chemotherapy group, those were 65%, 19%, 3%, and 3%, respectively. Common AEs except for fatigue and nausea in both groups were anemia, rash, or diarrhea. The most common AEs of grade 3 or higher in both groups were anemia and neutropenia. These studies suggest that an addition of an ICI to chemotherapy does not cause different side effect profiles than chemotherapy without an ICI. However, this needs to be verified in other malignancies with different combinations of ICIs and chemotherapy.

Immune Checkpoint Inhibitors and Elderly Patients

Cancer is most commonly a disease of older patients. Age is a risk factor for cancer, and patients older than 65 years account for more than 60% of newly diagnosed malignancies and 70% of all cancer-related mortality.[141] However, for the sake of clinical trial design, many studies exclude elderly patients, especially those with performance status >2. Not much data are available to draw a conclusion about efficacy and side effect profiles of ICIs owing to low accrual of older patients with age-related comorbidities and poor performance status.

The immune system is gradually deteriorated with natural age advancement (immunosenescence), and this has raised a doubt about the efficacy of ICIs, as well as the expectation of mild side effect profiles in older patients. On the contrary, there is a concern about more side effects, as the incidence of autoimmune antibodies also increases with age.[142]

CheckMate 069 study compared ipilimumab plus nivolumab with ipilimumab monotherapy in melanoma patients. The rate of grade 3–4 toxicities in those older than 65 years was 52% in the ipilimumab plus nivolumab cohort and 15% in the monotherapy cohort, and in those younger than 65 years it was 54% and 26% in the combination and monotherapy cohorts, respectively, suggesting similar side effect profiles in both younger and older patients. The objective response rate was superior in younger patients (64%) to older patients (53%).[21,47] CheckMate-057, which compares nivolumab with docetaxel in patients with NSCLC, shows similar objective response rates in all the patients, patients younger than 65 years, and those who are 65–75 years old at 19.2% versus 12.4%, 17% versus 13%, and 22% versus 12%, respectively. Hazard ratios for death were 0.73 (0.59–0.89), 0.81 (0.62–1.04), and 0.63 (0.45–0.89).[143] This study does not suggest a better response in younger patients.

Many studies do not have subgroup data analyses on both safety and efficacy of ICIs in older patients; therefore, drawing a conclusion would be premature. Nevertheless, it is generally accepted that patients aged between 65 and 75 years have a similar side effect profile and efficacy from ICIs as in those younger than 65 years. It is not as clear in patients older than 75 years. Older patients do not seem to have specific age-related toxicities that are more commonly reported in this patient population.[144] Many clinicians prefer to use ICIs for patients with advanced cancer with poor performance status owing to age-related comorbidities or in those who have consumed all available systemic chemotherapy options. This is mainly due to the more tolerable side effect profiles of ICIs than chemotherapy, although the role, efficacy, and advanced age-related side effects of ICIs are not fully established.

CONCLUSION

Systemic chemotherapy has been the first treatment of choice for advanced or recurrent cancer. Chemotherapeutic regimens have been optimized over the past several decades. More recently, clinical trials of ICIs, particularly PD-1/PD-L1 and CTLA-4 inhibitors, have shown promising results for patients with disease progression on systemic chemotherapy or molecular targeted therapy. Although ICIs have relatively well-tolerated side effect profiles, they can cause severe AEs complicating treatment courses. The side effect profile ranges from generalized symptoms including fatigue to inflammation of any organ systems, mimicking autoimmune diseases: dermatitis, colitis, hepatitis, endocrinopathies including thyroid dysfunction, hypophysitis, adrenal insufficiency, and type 1 diabetes, pneumonitis, nephritis, pancreatitis, neurologic diseases, cardiotoxicity, ocular toxicity, hematologic toxicity, and rheumatologic toxicity. Oncologists may encounter difficult clinical scenarios where elderly patients with multiple comorbidities or those with other significant medical issues that can potentially complicate the treatment course are involved in cancer care. Medical oncologists are faced with the challenge of managing extensive, but not yet well-established, side effect profiles of ICIs, as well as taking care of difficult populations.

REFERENCES

1. Woo SR, Turnis ME, Goldberg MV, et al. Immune inhibitory molecules LAG-3 and PD-1 synergistically regulate T-cell function to promote tumoral immune escape. *Cancer Res.* 2012;72(4):917−927.
2. Ngiow SF, von Scheidt B, Akiba H, Yagita H, Teng MW, Smyth MJ. Anti-TIM3 antibody promotes T cell IFN-gamma-mediated antitumor immunity and suppresses established tumors. *Cancer Res.* 2011;71(10):3540−3551.
3. Le Mercier I, Chen W, Lines JL, et al. VISTA regulates the development of protective antitumor immunity. *Cancer Res.* 2014;74(7):1933−1944.
4. Spranger S, Spaapen RM, Zha Y, et al. Up-regulation of PD-L1, IDO, and T(regs) in the melanoma tumor microenvironment is driven by CD8(+) T cells. *Sci Transl Med.* 2013;5(200):200ra116.
5. Tivol EA, Borriello F, Schweitzer AN, Lynch WP, Bluestone JA, Sharpe AH. Loss of CTLA-4 leads to massive lymphoproliferation and fatal multiorgan tissue destruction, revealing a critical negative regulatory role of CTLA-4. *Immunity.* 1995;3(5):541−547.
6. Iwama S, De Remigis A, Callahan MK, Slovin SF, Wolchok JD, Caturegli P. Pituitary expression of CTLA-4 mediates hypophysitis secondary to administration of CTLA-4 blocking antibody. *Sci Transl Med.* 2014;6(230):230ra45.
7. Orlov S, Salari F, Kashat L, Walfish PG. Induction of painless thyroiditis in patients receiving programmed death 1 receptor immunotherapy for metastatic malignancies. *J Clin Endocrinol Metab.* 2015;100(5):1738−1741.
8. Weber JS, Kahler KC, Hauschild A. Management of immune-related adverse events and kinetics of response with ipilimumab. *J Clin Oncol.* 2012;30(21):2691−2697.
9. Lebbe C, O'Day S, Chiarion Sileni V, et al. *Analysis of the onset and resolution of immunerelated adverse events during treatment with ipilimumab in patients with metastatic melanoma.* October 2−4, 2008.
10. Weber JS, Hodi FS, Wolchok JD, et al. Safety profile of nivolumab monotherapy: a pooled analysis of patients with advanced melanoma. *J Clin Oncol.* 2017;35(7):785−792.
11. Horvat TZ, Adel NG, Dang TO, et al. Immune-related adverse events, need for systemic immunosuppression, and effects on survival and time to treatment failure in patients with melanoma treated with ipilimumab at memorial sloan kettering cancer center. *J Clin Oncol.* 2015;33(28):3193−3198.
12. Weber JS, Yang JC, Atkins MB, Disis ML. Toxicities of immunotherapy for the practitioner. *J Clin Oncol.* 2015;33(18):2092−2099.
13. Robert C, Long GV, Brady B, et al. Nivolumab in previously untreated melanoma without BRAF mutation. *N Engl J Med.* 2015;372(4):320−330.
14. Krenacs T, Kiszner G, Stelkovics E, et al. Collagen XVII is expressed in malignant but not in benign melanocytic tumors and it can mediate antibody induced melanoma apoptosis. *Histochem Cell Biol.* 2012;138(4):653−667.
15. Pintova S, Sidhu H, Friedlander PA, Holcombe RF. Sweet's syndrome in a patient with metastatic melanoma after ipilimumab therapy. *Melanoma Res.* 2013;23(6):498−501.
16. Joseph RW, Cappel M, Goedjen B, et al. Lichenoid dermatitis in three patients with metastatic melanoma treated with anti-PD-1 therapy. *Cancer Immunol Res.* 2015;3(1):18−22.
17. Carlos G, Anforth R, Chou S, Clements A, Fernandez-Penas P. A case of bullous pemphigoid in a patient with metastatic melanoma treated with pembrolizumab. *Melanoma Res.* 2015;25(3):265−268.
18. Weber JS, Antonia SJ, Topalian SL, et al. Safety profile of nivolumab (NIVO) in patients (pts) with advanced melanoma (MEL): a pooled analysis. *J Clin Oncol.* 2015;33(suppl 15):9018.
19. Garon EB, Rizvi NA, Hui R, et al. Pembrolizumab for the treatment of non-small-cell lung cancer. *N Engl J Med.* 2015;372(21):2018−2028.
20. Robert C, Schachter J, Long GV, et al. Pembrolizumab versus ipilimumab in advanced melanoma. *N Engl J Med.* 2015;372(26):2521−2532.
21. Hodi FS, Postow MA, Chesney JA, et al. Clinical response, progression-free survival (PFS), and safety in patients (pts) with advanced melanoma (MEL) receiving nivolumab (NIVO) combined with ipilimumab (IPI) vs IPI monotherapy in CheckMate 069 study. *J Clin Oncol.* 2015;33.
22. Eggermont AM, Chiarion-Sileni V, Grob JJ, et al. Prolonged survival in stage III melanoma with ipilimumab adjuvant therapy. *N Engl J Med.* 2016;375(19):1845−1855.
23. Hodi FS, O'Day SJ, McDermott DF, et al. Improved survival with ipilimumab in patients with metastatic melanoma. *N Engl J Med.* 2010;363(8):711−723.
24. Topalian SL, Sznol M, McDermott DF, et al. Survival, durable tumor remission, and long-term safety in patients with advanced melanoma receiving nivolumab. *J Clin Oncol.* 2014;32(10):1020−1030.

25. BLA 125377 YERVOY (ipilimumab) Injection, For Intravenous Infusionhuman Cytotoxic T-lymphocyte Antigen-4 (CTLA-4)-blocking Monoclonalantibody. https://www.accessdata.fda.gov/drugsatfda_docs/rems/Yervoy_2012-02-16_Full.pdf.

26. Ramos-Casals M, Tzioufas AG, Stone JH, Siso A, Bosch X. Treatment of primary sjogren syndrome: a systematic review. *JAMA*. 2010;304(4):452–460.

27. Spain L, Diem S, Larkin J. Management of toxicities of immune checkpoint inhibitors. *Cancer Treat Rev*. 2016; 44:51–60.

28. Kim KW, Ramaiya NH, Krajewski KM, et al. Ipilimumab-associated colitis: CT findings. *Am J Roentgenol*. 2013; 200(5):468.

29. Berman D, Parker SM, Siegel J, et al. Blockade of cytotoxic T-lymphocyte antigen-4 by ipilimumab results in dysregulation of gastrointestinal immunity in patients with advanced melanoma. *Cancer Immun*. 2010; 10:11.

30. Gettinger SN, Horn L, Gandhi L, et al. Overall survival and long-term safety of nivolumab (anti-programmed death 1 antibody, BMS-936558, ONO-4538) in patients with previously treated advanced non-small-cell lung cancer. *J Clin Oncol*. 2015;33(18):2004–2012.

31. Rizvi NA, Mazieres J, Planchard D, et al. Activity and safety of nivolumab, an anti-PD-1 immune checkpoint inhibitor, for patients with advanced, refractory squamous non-small-cell lung cancer (CheckMate 063): a phase 2, single-arm trial. *Lancet Oncol*. 2015;16(3): 257–265.

32. Weber JS, D'Angelo SP, Minor D, et al. Nivolumab versus chemotherapy in patients with advanced melanoma who progressed after anti-CTLA-4 treatment (CheckMate 037): a randomised, controlled, open-label, phase 3 trial. *Lancet Oncol*. 2015;16(4):375–384.

33. Hamid O, Robert C, Daud A, et al. Safety and tumor responses with lambrolizumab (anti-PD-1) in melanoma. *N Engl J Med*. 2013;369(2):134–144.

34. Le DT, Uram JN, Wang H, et al. PD-1 blockade in tumors with mismatch-repair deficiency. *N Engl J Med*. 2015; 372(26):2509–2520.

35. Armand P, Nagler A, Weller EA, et al. Disabling immune tolerance by programmed death-1 blockade with pidilizumab after autologous hematopoietic stem-cell transplantation for diffuse large B-cell lymphoma: results of an international phase II trial. *J Clin Oncol*. 2013; 31(33):4199–4206.

36. Sampson JH, Vlahovic G, Sahebjam S, et al. Preliminary safety and activity of nivolumab and its combination with ipilimumab in recurrent glioblastoma (GBM): CHECKMATE-143. *J Clin Oncol*. 2015;33(suppl 15): 3010.

37. Antonia SJ, Goldberg SB, Balmanoukian AS, et al. Phase ib study of MEDI4736, a programmed cell death ligand-1 (PD-L1) antibody, in combination with tremelimumab, a cytotoxic T-lymphocyte-associated protein-4 (CTLA-4) antibody, in patients (pts) with advanced NSCLC. *J Clin Oncol*. 2015;33(suppl 15):3014.

38. Johncilla M, Misdraji J, Pratt DS, et al. Ipilimumab-associated hepatitis: clinicopathologic characterization in a series of 11 cases. *Am J Surg Pathol*. 2015;39(8):1075–1084.

39. Motzer RJ, Rini BI, McDermott DF, et al. Nivolumab for metastatic renal cell carcinoma: results of a randomized phase II trial. *J Clin Oncol*. 2015;33(13):1430–1437.

40. El-Khoueiry AB, Melero I, Crocenzi TS, et al. Phase I/II safety and antitumor activity of nivolumab in patients with advanced hepatocellular carcinoma (HCC): CA209-040. *J Clin Oncol*. 2015;33:15s.

41. Segal NH, Antonia SJ, Brahmer JR, et al. Preliminary data from a multi-arm expansion study of MEDI4736, an anti-PD-L1 antibody. *J Clin Oncol*. 2014;32:5s.

42. Herbst RS, Soria JC, Kowanetz M, et al. Predictive correlates of response to the anti-PD-L1 antibody MPDL3280A in cancer patients. *Nature*. 2014;515(7528):563–567.

43. Calabro L, Morra A, Fonsatti E, et al. Efficacy and safety of an intensified schedule of tremelimumab for chemotherapy-resistant malignant mesothelioma: an open-label, single-arm, phase 2 study. *Lancet Respir Med*. 2015;3(4):301–309.

44. Calabro L, Morra A, Fonsatti E, et al. Tremelimumab for patients with chemotherapy-resistant advanced malignant mesothelioma: an open-label, single-arm, phase 2 trial. *Lancet Oncol*. 2013;14(11):1104–1111.

45. Bowyer S, Prithviraj P, Lorigan P, et al. Efficacy and toxicity of treatment with the anti-CTLA-4 antibody ipilimumab in patients with metastatic melanoma after prior anti-PD-1 therapy. *Br J Cancer*. 2016;114(10): 1084–1089.

46. Wolchok JD, Kluger H, Callahan MK, et al. Nivolumab plus ipilimumab in advanced melanoma. *N Engl J Med*. 2013;369(2):122–133.

47. Postow MA, Chesney J, Pavlick AC, et al. Nivolumab and ipilimumab versus ipilimumab in untreated melanoma. *N Engl J Med*. 2015;372(21):2006–2017.

48. Larkin J, Chiarion-Sileni V, Gonzalez R, et al. Combined nivolumab and ipilimumab or monotherapy in untreated melanoma. *N Engl J Med*. 2015;373(1):23–34.

49. Johnson PJ, McFarlane IG, Williams R. Azathioprine for long-term maintenance of remission in autoimmune hepatitis. *N Engl J Med*. 1995;333(15):958–963.

50. Chmiel KD, Suan D, Liddle C, et al. Resolution of severe ipilimumab-induced hepatitis after antithymocyte globulin therapy. *J Clin Oncol*. 2011;29(9):237.

51. Faje A. Immunotherapy and hypophysitis: clinical presentation, treatment, and biologic insights. *Pituitary*. 2016;19(1):82–92.

52. Eggermont AM, Chiarion-Sileni V, Grob JJ, et al. Adjuvant ipilimumab versus placebo after complete resection of high-risk stage III melanoma (EORTC 18071): a randomised, double-blind, phase 3 trial. *Lancet Oncol*. 2015; 16(5):522–530.

53. Ribas A, Puzanov I, Dummer R, et al. Pembrolizumab versus investigator-choice chemotherapy for ipilimumab-refractory melanoma (KEYNOTE-002): a randomised, controlled, phase 2 trial. *Lancet Oncol*. 2015;16(8): 908–918.

54. Sarnaik AA, Yu B, Yu D, et al. Extended dose ipilimumab with a peptide vaccine: immune correlates associated with clinical benefit in patients with resected high-risk stage IIIc/IV melanoma. *Clin Cancer Res.* 2011;17(4): 896–906.
55. Borodic G, Hinkle DM, Cia Y. Drug-induced graves disease from CTLA-4 receptor suppression. *Ophthal Plast Reconstr Surg.* 2011;27(4):87.
56. Topalian SL, Hodi FS, Brahmer JR, et al. Safety, activity, and immune correlates of anti-PD-1 antibody in cancer. *N Engl J Med.* 2012;366(26):2443–2454.
57. Ascierto PA, Del Vecchio M, Robert C, et al. Ipilimumab 10 mg/kg versus ipilimumab 3 mg/kg in patients with unresectable or metastatic melanoma: a randomised, double-blind, multicentre, phase 3 trial. *Lancet Oncol.* 2017;18(5):611–622.
58. Hellmann MD, Ott PA, Zugazagoitia J, et al. Nivolumab (nivo) ± ipilimumab (ipi) in advanced small-cell lung cancer (SCLC): first report of a randomized expansion cohort from CheckMate 032. *J Clin Oncol.* 2017;35.
59. Hahner S, Loeffler M, Bleicken B, et al. Epidemiology of adrenal crisis in chronic adrenal insufficiency: the need for new prevention strategies. *Eur J Endocrinol.* 2010; 162(3):597–602.
60. Brahmer JR, Tykodi SS, Chow LQ, et al. Safety and activity of anti-PD-L1 antibody in patients with advanced cancer. *N Engl J Med.* 2012;366(26):2455–2465.
61. Patnaik AM, Socinski MA, Gubens MA, et al. Phase 1 study of pembrolizumab (pembro; MK-3475) plus ipilimumab (IPI) as second-line therapy for advanced non-small cell lung cancer (NSCLC): KEYNOTE-021 cohort D. *J Clin Oncol.* 2015;35:15s.
62. Bornstein SR, Allolio B, Arlt W, et al. Diagnosis and treatment of primary adrenal insufficiency: an endocrine society clinical practice guideline. *J Clin Endocrinol Metab.* 2016;101(2):364–389.
63. Hughes J, Vudattu N, Sznol M, et al. Precipitation of autoimmune diabetes with anti-PD-1 immunotherapy. *Diabetes Care.* 2015;38(4):55.
64. Diabetes Control and Complications Trial Research Group, Nathan DM, Genuth S, et al. The effect of intensive treatment of diabetes on the development and progression of long-term complications in insulin-dependent diabetes mellitus. *N Engl J Med.* 1993; 329(14):977–986.
65. Nishino M, Sholl LM, Hodi FS, Hatabu H, Ramaiya NH. Anti-PD-1-related pneumonitis during cancer immunotherapy. *N Engl J Med.* 2015;373(3):288–290.
66. Rizvi NA, Brahmer JR, Ou S-HI, et al. Safety and clinical activity of MEDI4736, an anti-programmed cell death-ligand 1 (PD-L1) antibody, in patients with non-small cell lung cancer (NSCLC). *J Clin Oncol.* 2015;33.
67. Antonia SJ, Brahmer JR, Gettinger SN. Nivolumab (anti-PD-1; BMS-936558, ONO-4538) in combination with platinum-based doublet chemotherapy (PT-DC) in advanced non-small cell lung cancer (NSCLC). *J Clin Oncol.* 2015;32:5s.
68. Postow MA. Managing immune checkpoint-blocking antibody side effects. *Am Soc Clin Oncol Educ Book.* 2015;1:76–83.
69. Fadel F, El Karoui K, Knebelmann B. Anti-CTLA4 antibody-induced lupus nephritis. *N Engl J Med.* 2009; 361(2):211–212.
70. Thajudeen B, Madhrira M, Bracamonte E, Cranmer LD. Ipilimumab granulomatous interstitial nephritis. *Am J Ther.* 2015;22(3):84.
71. Brahmer J, Reckamp KL, Baas P, et al. Nivolumab versus docetaxel in advanced squamous-cell non-small-cell lung cancer. *N Engl J Med.* 2015;373(2):123–135.
72. Amin A, Plimack ER, Infante JR, et al. Nivolumab (anti-PD-1; BMS-936558, ONO-4538) in combination with sunitinib or pazopanib in patients (pts) with metastatic renal cell carcinoma (mRCC). *J Clin Oncol.* 2014; 32:5s.
73. Cortazar FB, Marrone KA, Troxell ML, et al. Clinicopathological features of acute kidney injury associated with immune checkpoint inhibitors. *Kidney Int.* 2016;90(3): 638–647.
74. Ansell SM, Lesokhin AM, Borrello I, et al. PD-1 blockade with nivolumab in relapsed or refractory hodgkin's lymphoma. *N Engl J Med.* 2015;372(4):311–319.
75. Spain L, Walls G, Julve M, et al. Neurotoxicity from immune-checkpoint inhibition in the treatment of melanoma: a single centre experience and review of the literature. *Ann Oncol.* 2017;28(2):377–385.
76. Maur M, Tomasello C, Frassoldati A, Dieci MV, Barbieri E, Conte P. Posterior reversible encephalopathy syndrome during ipilimumab therapy for malignant melanoma. *J Clin Oncol.* 2012;30(6):76.
77. Bhatia S, Huber BR, Upton MP, Thompson JA. Inflammatory enteric neuropathy with severe constipation after ipilimumab treatment for melanoma: a case report. *J Immunother.* 2009;32(2):203–205.
78. Wilgenhof S, Neyns B. Anti-CTLA-4 antibody-induced guillain-barre syndrome in a melanoma patient. *Ann Oncol.* 2011;22(4):991–993.
79. Wick W, Hertenstein A, Platten M. Neurological sequelae of cancer immunotherapies and targeted therapies. *Lancet Oncol.* 2016;17(12):e541.
80. Voskens C, Cavallaro A, Erdmann M, et al. Anti-cytotoxic T-cell lymphocyte antigen-4-induced regression of spinal cord metastases in association with renal failure, atypical pneumonia, vision loss, and hearing loss. *J Clin Oncol.* 2012;30(33):356.
81. Maker AV, Phan GQ, Attia P, et al. Tumor regression and autoimmunity in patients treated with cytotoxic T lymphocyte-associated antigen 4 blockade and interleukin 2: a phase I/II study. *Ann Surg Oncol.* 2005; 12(12):1005–1016.
82. Robinson MR, Chan CC, Yang JC, et al. Cytotoxic T lymphocyte-associated antigen 4 blockade in patients with metastatic melanoma: a new cause of uveitis. *J Immunother.* 2004;27(6):478–479.

83. Ribas A, Hamid O, Daud A, et al. Association of pembrolizumab with tumor response and survival among patients with advanced melanoma. *JAMA*. 2016; 315(15):1600−1609.

84. TECENTRIQ-Atezolizumab Injection, Solution. https://dailymed.nlm.nih.gov/dailymed/drugInfo.cfm?setid=6fa682c9-a312-4932-9831-f286908660ee.

85. Papavasileiou E, Prasad S, Freitag SK, Sobrin L, Lobo AM. Ipilimumab-induced ocular and orbital inflammation—A case series and review of the literature. *Ocul Immunol Inflamm*. 2016;24(2):140−146.

86. Lucas JA, Menke J, Rabacal WA, Schoen FJ, Sharpe AH, Kelley VR. Programmed death ligand 1 regulates a critical checkpoint for autoimmune myocarditis and pneumonitis in MRL mice. *J Immunol*. 2008;181(4):2513−2521.

87. Wang J, Okazaki IM, Yoshida T, et al. PD-1 deficiency results in the development of fatal myocarditis in MRL mice. *Int Immunol*. 2010;22(6):443−452.

88. Johnson DB, Balko JM, Compton ML, et al. Fulminant myocarditis with combination immune checkpoint blockade. *N Engl J Med*. 2016;375(18):1749−1755.

89. Heinzerling L, Ott PA, Hodi FS, et al. Cardiotoxicity associated with CTLA4 and PD1 blocking immunotherapy. *J Immunother Cancer*. 2016;4(1):50−60.

90. Gordon IO, Wade T, Chin K, Dickstein J, Gajewski TF. Immune-mediated red cell aplasia after anti-CTLA-4 immunotherapy for metastatic melanoma. *Cancer Immunol Immunother*. 2009;58(8):1351−1353.

91. Akhtari M, Waller EK, Jaye DL, et al. Neutropenia in a patient treated with ipilimumab (anti-CTLA-4 antibody). *J Immunother*. 2009;32(3):322−324.

92. du Rusquec P, Saint-Jean M, Brocard A, et al. Ipilimumab-induced autoimmune pancytopenia in a case of metastatic melanoma. *J Immunother*. 2014;37(6):348−350.

93. Delyon J, Mateus C, Lambert T. Hemophilia A induced by ipilimumab. *N Engl J Med*. 2011;365(18):1747−1748.

94. Pellegrino B, Musolino A, Tiseo M. Anti-PD-1-related cryoglobulinemia during treatment with nivolumab in NSCLC patient. *Ann Oncol*. 2017;28(6):1405−1406.

95. Helgadottir H, Kis L, Ljungman P, et al. Lethal aplastic anemia caused by dual immune checkpoint blockade in metastatic melanoma. *Ann Oncol*. 2017;28(7):1672.

96. Ribas A, Butler M, Lutzky J, et al. Phase I study combining anti-PD-L1 (MEDI4736) with BRAF (dabrafenib) and/or MEK (trametinib) inhibitors in advanced melanoma. *J Clin Oncol*. 2015;33:15s.

97. Cappelli LC, Gutierrez AK, Baer AN, et al. Inflammatory arthritis and sicca syndrome induced by nivolumab and ipilimumab. *Ann Rheum Dis*. 2017;76(1):43−50.

98. Robert C, Ribas A, Wolchok JD, et al. Anti-programmed-death-receptor-1 treatment with pembrolizumab in ipilimumab-refractory advanced melanoma: a randomised dose-comparison cohort of a phase 1 trial. *Lancet*. 2014;384(9948):1109−1117.

99. Sznol M, McDermott MF, Jones SF, et al. Phase ib evaluation of MPDL3280A (anti-PDL1) in combination with bevacizumab (bev) in patients (pts) with metastatic renal cell carcinoma (mRCC). *J Clin Oncol*. 2015;33:15s.

100. Bendell JC, Powderly JD, Lieu CH, et al. Safety and efficacy of MPDL3280A (anti-PDL1) in combination with bevacizumab (bev) and/or FOLFOX in patients (pts) with metastatic colorectal cancer (mCRC). *J Clin Oncol*. 2015;33:5s.

101. Momtaz P, Park V, Panageas KS, et al. Safety of infusing ipilimumab over 30 minutes. *J Clin Oncol*. 2015; 33(30):3454−3458.

102. Thomas CF, Limper AH. Pneumocystis pneumonia. *N Engl J Med*. 2004;350(24):2487−2498.

103. Prokunina L, Castillejo-Lopez C, Oberg F, et al. A regulatory polymorphism in PDCD1 is associated with susceptibility to systemic lupus erythematosus in humans. *Nat Genet*. 2002;32(4):666−669.

104. Ueda H, Howson JM, Esposito L, et al. Association of the T-cell regulatory gene CTLA4 with susceptibility to autoimmune disease. *Nature*. 2003;423(6939):506−511.

105. Snyder A, Makarov V, Merghoub T, et al. Genetic basis for clinical response to CTLA-4 blockade in melanoma. *N Engl J Med*. 2014;371(23):2189−2199.

106. Ma Q, Shilkrut M, Li M, et al. Prevalence of autoimmune comorbidities in patients with metastatic melanoma in the United States. *Value Health*. 2016;19(3):A135.

107. Khan SA, Pruitt SL, Xuan L, Gerber DE. Prevalence of autoimmune disease among patients with lung cancer: implications for immunotherapy treatment options. *JAMA Oncol*. 2016;2(11):1507−1508.

108. Johnson DB, Sullivan RJ, Ott PA, et al. Ipilimumab therapy in patients with advanced melanoma and preexisting autoimmune disorders. *JAMA Oncol*. 2016;2(2): 234−240.

109. Menzies AM, Johnson DB, Ramanujam S, et al. Anti-PD-1 therapy in patients with advanced melanoma and preexisting autoimmune disorders or major toxicity with ipilimumab. *Ann Oncol*. 2017;28(2):368−376.

110. Johnson DB, Sullivan RJ, Menzies AM. Immune checkpoint inhibitors in challenging populations. *Cancer*. 2017;123(11):1904−1911.

111. Tanaka K, Albin MJ, Yuan X, et al. PDL1 is required for peripheral transplantation tolerance and protection from chronic allograft rejection. *J Immunol*. 2007; 179(8):5204−5210.

112. Shi XL, Mancham S, Hansen BE, et al. Counter-regulation of rejection activity against human liver grafts by donor PD-L1 and recipient PD-1 interaction. *J Hepatol*. 2016; 64(6):1274−1282.

113. Schade H, Sen S, Neff CP, et al. Programmed death 1 expression on CD4+ T cells predicts mortality after allogeneic stem cell transplantation. *Biol Blood Marrow Transpl*. 2016;22(12):2172−2179.

114. Saha A, O'Connor RS, Thangavelu G, et al. Programmed death ligand-1 expression on donor T cells drives graft-versus-host disease lethality. *J Clin Invest*. 2016;126(7): 2642−2660.

115. Lipson EJ, Bagnasco SM, Moore J, et al. Tumor regression and allograft rejection after administration of anti-PD-1. *N Engl J Med*. 2016;374(9):896−898.

116. Spain L, Higgins R, Gopalakrishnan K, Turajlic S, Gore M, Larkin J. Acute renal allograft rejection after immune checkpoint inhibitor therapy for metastatic melanoma. *Ann Oncol*. 2016;27(6):1135−1137.

117. Kwatra V, Karanth NV, Priyadarshana K, Charakidis M. Pembrolizumab for metastatic melanoma in a renal allograft recipient with subsequent graft rejection and treatment response failure: a case report. *J Med Case Rep*. 2017;11(1):73.

118. Owonikoko TK, Kumar M, Yang S, et al. Cardiac allograft rejection as a complication of PD-1 checkpoint blockade for cancer immunotherapy: a case report. *Cancer Immunol Immunother*. 2017;66(1):45−50.

119. Chan TS, Khong PL, Kwong YL. Pembrolizumab for relapsed anaplastic large cell lymphoma after allogeneic haematopoietic stem cell transplantation: efficacy and safety. *Ann Hematol*. 2016;95(11):1913−1915.

120. Singh AK, Porrata LF, Aljitawi O, et al. Fatal GvHD induced by PD-1 inhibitor pembrolizumab in a patient with hodgkin's lymphoma. *Bone Marrow Transpl*. 2016; 51(9):1268−1270.

121. Kwong YL. Safety of pembrolizumab after allogeneic haematopoietic stem cell transplantation. *Ann Hematol*. 2016;95(7):1191−1192.

122. Aslan A, Aras T, Ozdemir E. Successful treatment of relapsed/refractory hodgkins lymphoma with nivolumab in a heavily pretreated patient with progressive disease after both autologous and allogeneic stem cell transplantation. *Leuk Lymphoma*. 2017;58(3):754−755.

123. Shad AT, Huo JS, Darcy C, et al. Tolerance and effectiveness of nivolumab after pediatric T-cell replete, haploidentical, bone marrow transplantation: a case report. *Pediatr Blood Cancer*. 2017;64(3). https://doi.org/10.1002/pbc.26257. Epub 2016 Sep. 21.

124. Yared JA, Hardy N, Singh Z, et al. Major clinical response to nivolumab in relapsed/refractory hodgkin lymphoma after allogeneic stem cell transplantation. *Bone Marrow Transpl*. 2016;51(6):850−852.

125. Angenendt L, Schliemann C, Lutz M, et al. Nivolumab in a patient with refractory hodgkin's lymphoma after allogeneic stem cell transplantation. *Bone Marrow Transpl*. 2016;51(3):443−445.

126. Villasboas JC, Ansell SM, Witzig TE. Targeting the PD-1 pathway in patients with relapsed classic hodgkin lymphoma following allogeneic stem cell transplant is safe and effective. *Oncotarget*. 2016;7(11): 13260−13264.

127. Ford ML, Adams AB, Pearson TC. Targeting co-stimulatory pathways: transplantation and autoimmunity. *Nat Rev Nephrol*. 2014;10(1):14−24.

128. Li J, Semple K, Suh WK, et al. Roles of CD28, CTLA4, and inducible costimulator in acute graft-versus-host disease in mice. *Biol Blood Marrow Transpl*. 2011;17(7): 962−969.

129. Herz S, Hofer T, Papapanagiotou M, et al. Checkpoint inhibitors in chronic kidney failure and an organ transplant recipient. *Eur J Cancer*. 2016;67:66−72.

130. Morales RE, Shoushtari AN, Walsh MM, Grewal P, Lipson EJ, Carvajal RD. Safety and efficacy of ipilimumab to treat advanced melanoma in the setting of liver transplantation. *J Immunother Cancer*. 2015;3. eCollection 2015.

131. Lipson EJ, Bodell MA, Kraus ES, Sharfman WH. Successful administration of ipilimumab to two kidney transplantation patients with metastatic melanoma. *J Clin Oncol*. 2014;32(19):69.

132. Bashey A, Medina B, Corringham S, et al. CTLA4 blockade with ipilimumab to treat relapse of malignancy after allogeneic hematopoietic cell transplantation. *Blood*. 2009;113(7):1581−1588.

133. Davids MS, Kim HT, Bachireddy P, et al. Ipilimumab for patients with relapse after allogeneic transplantation. *N Engl J Med*. 2016;375(2):143−153.

134. Merryman RW, Kim HT, Zinzani PL, et al. Safety and efficacy of allogeneic hematopoietic stem cell transplant after PD-1 blockade in relapsed/refractory lymphoma. *Blood*. 2017;129(10):1380−1388.

135. Kasprowicz V, Schulze Zur Wiesch J, Kuntzen T, et al. High level of PD-1 expression on hepatitis C virus (HCV)-specific CD8+ and CD4+ T cells during acute HCV infection, irrespective of clinical outcome. *J Virol*. 2008;82(6):3154−3160.

136. Gardiner D, Lalezari J, Lawitz E, et al. A randomized, double-blind, placebo-controlled assessment of BMS-936558, a fully human monoclonal antibody to programmed death-1 (PD-1), in patients with chronic hepatitis C virus infection. *PLoS One*. 2013;8(5): e63818.

137. Sangro B, Gomez-Martin C, de la Mata M, et al. A clinical trial of CTLA-4 blockade with tremelimumab in patients with hepatocellular carcinoma and chronic hepatitis C. *J Hepatol*. 2013;59(1):81−88.

138. Sangro B, Park J-W, Cruz CMD, et al. A randomized, multicenter, phase 3 study of nivolumab vs sorafenib as first-line treatment in patients (pts) with advanced hepatocellular carcinoma (HCC): CheckMate-459. *J Clin Oncol*. 2016;34.

139. Kudo M. Immune checkpoint blockade in hepatocellular carcinoma: 2017 update. *Liver Cancer*. 2016;6(1): 1−12.

140. Langer CJ, Gadgeel SM, Borghaei H, et al. Carboplatin and pemetrexed with or without pembrolizumab for advanced, non-squamous non-small-cell lung cancer: a randomised, phase 2 cohort of the open-label KEYNOTE-021 study. *Lancet Oncol.* 2016;17(11):1497−1508.

141. Berger NA, Savvides P, Koroukian SM, et al. Cancer in the elderly. *Trans Am Clin Climatol Assoc.* 2006;117:6.

142. Nagele EP, Han M, Acharya NK, DeMarshall C, Kosciuk MC, Nagele RG. Natural IgG autoantibodies are abundant and ubiquitous in human sera, and their number is influenced by age, gender, and disease. *PLoS One.* 2013;8(4):e60726.

143. Borghaei H, Paz-Ares L, Horn L, et al. Nivolumab versus docetaxel in advanced nonsquamous non-small-cell lung cancer. *N Engl J Med.* 2015;373(17):1627−1639.

144. Elias R, Morales J, Rehman Y, Khurshid H. Immune checkpoint inhibitors in older adults. *Curr Oncol Rep.* 2016;18(8):9.

CHAPTER 12

Future of Immune Checkpoint Inhibitors

ALI A. MAAWY, MD • FUMITO ITO, MD, PHD

INTRODUCTION

The field of immunotherapy has shown a dramatic transformation recently in the emergence as a new armamentarium in the battle against cancer. More specifically, immune checkpoint therapy, which targets and inhibits immune regulatory signals in the immune synapse that are often manipulated by tumors in immune evasion, has led to durable responses in significant numbers of patients.[1]

Ipilimumab, a fully human monoclonal antibody (mAb) against cytotoxic T-lymphocyte–associated protein 4 (CTLA-4) was approved by the U.S. Food and Drug Administration (FDA) in 2011 for the treatment of metastatic melanoma. Anti–CTLA-4 treatment has also been studied in nonmelanoma tumors, with an 8% partial response rate (RR) noted in patients with metastatic renal cell carcinoma (RCC) in a phase II study.[2] Anti–programmed death-1 (PD-1) (pembrolizumab and nivolumab) and programmed death ligand-1 (PD-L1) (atezolizumab, avelumab and durvalumab) have revolutionized therapy of several cancer histologies, initially in advanced melanoma but now in multiple other malignancies, such as squamous cell carcinoma of the head and neck, non–small-cell lung cancer (NSCLC), urothelial cancers, colorectal cancer, renal cell cancer, Hodgkin lymphoma, and Merkel cell carcinoma. There are currently multiple anti–PD-1, anti–PD-L1, and anti–CTLA-4 antibodies in development, which are listed in Table 12.1. As we have seen encouraging data from clinical trials showing impressive results in a subset of patients treated with anti–CTLA-4, PD-1, or PD-L1, immune checkpoint inhibitors (ICIs) became one of the most extensively investigated areas in oncology drug development. Important questions still remain; however, with regards to understanding the mechanisms of resistance, optimal combination therapies, predicting which patient population will benefit or develop immune-related adverse events (irAEs), dosing, and optimal duration of therapy.

MECHANISMS OF RESISTANCE

Although a significant number of cancer patients benefit from ICIs, only a fraction of patients achieve durable clinical responses, and many patients eventually develop therapeutic resistance after an initial response to ICIs.[3–9] The IFN-γ pathway has emerged as a key player in resistance to ICIs.[3–5] Zaretsky et al. looked at biopsy samples from four patients with metastatic melanoma who had had an initial response to anti–PD-1 therapy and later demonstrated progression with pembrolizumab and found that mutations in genes encoding for IFN receptor–associated JAK1, JAK2, or β2-microglobulin, which is a necessary component of the major histocompatibility complex (MHC) class I molecule, are associated with development of acquired resistance.[3] Peng et al. showed loss of phosphatase and tensin homolog (PTEN) gene, which enhances PI3K signaling was found to be associated with resistance to anti–PD-1 therapy in patients, and treatment with selective PI3Kβ inhibitor improved the efficacy of ICIs in preclinical models.[6] Koyama et al. demonstrated that recurrence after anti–PD-1 therapy was associated with increased expression of T-cell immunoglobulin mucin 3 (TIM-3) on T-cells, and anti–PD-1 and anti–TIM-3 improved responses in preclinical models.[7] Accumulating evidence suggests that combination therapy targeting multiple key steps of the "cancer immunity cycle" (Fig. 12.1)[10] may not only demonstrate higher efficacy but may also serve to mitigate the development of acquired resistance.

DEVELOPMENT OF EFFECTIVE COMBINATION THERAPIES

The cancer immunity cycle is a model that describes a series of multistep immune events triggered by immunogenic cell death (Fig. 12.1).[10] It commences with the release of tumor antigens that are captured, processed, and presented by antigen-presenting cells (APCs), primarily dendritic cells (DCs), to T-cells in

TABLE 12.1
Anti−CTLA-4 and Anti−PD-1/PD-L1 Antibodies (Ab)

Target	Agent	Brand Name	Antibody Class	Developer	Stage of Development
CTLA-4	Ipilimumab	Yervoy	Human IgG1	Bristol-Myers Squibb	FDA approved (melanoma)
	Tremelimumab		Human IgG2	MedImmune and Pfizer	Phase III
PD-1	Nivolumab (BMS-936558)	Opdivo	Human IgG4	Bristol-Myers Squibb	FDA approved (melanoma, NSCLC, RCC)
	Pembrolizumab (MK-3475)	Keytruda	Human IgG4	Merck	FDA approved (melanoma, NSCLC)
	MEDI0680 (AMP-514)		Human IgG4	MedImmune	Phase I
	Pidilizumab (CT-011)		Human IgG1	CureTech	Phase II
PD-L1	Durvalumab (MEDI4736)	Imfinzi	Human IgG4	MedImmune	Phase III
	Atezolizumab (MPDL-3280A)	TECENTRIQ	Human IgG1	Genentech	Phase III
	AMP-224		PD-L2 IgG2a fusion protein	Amplimmune	Phase I
	MDX-1105/ BMS-936559		Human IgG4	Bristol-Myers Squibb	Phase I
	Avelumab (MSB0010718C)	Bavencio	Human IgG1	Merck Serono	Phase II

NSCLC, non−small-cell lung cancer; *RCC*, renal cell carcinoma; *FDA*, U.S. Food and Drug Administration.

the lymph nodes. This is followed by the trafficking of T-cells, including CD8+ cytotoxic T lymphocytes (CTL), to the tumor where they can recognize and kill malignant cells, thereby releasing more cancer antigens, and further stimulate the immune response. However, during key steps of this cycle, there are negative regulators that can disrupt the cancer immunity cycle leading to evasion and progression of tumor cells. One of the primary aims of cancer immunotherapy is therefore to elicit and sustain T-cell response against the tumor by the use of combination treatments to address multiple key steps in the cancer immunity cycle.

One successful example of combination therapy is to use anti−PD-1 therapy and anti−CTLA-4 therapy as demonstrated in the CheckMate 067 trial that compared combination nivolumab and ipilimumab versus ipilimumab and nivolumab monotherapy in patients with metastatic melanoma. In this randomized, double-blinded phase III trial, 945 patients with

unresectable stage III or stage IV melanoma were randomized to one of the three treatment arms with coprimary end points being progression-free survival (PFS) and overall survival. The median PFS was 11.5 months with combination therapy, as compared with 2.9 months with ipilimumab (hazard ratio (HR) 0.42) and 6.9 months with nivolumab (HR for comparison with ipilimumab 0.57). Subgroup analysis has revealed that patients with tumors with positive PD-L1 expression have a PFS of 14 months in both nivolumab arms and 3.9 months with ipilimumab alone. However, PD-L1−negative patients seem to benefit more from the combination approach with a PFS of 11.2 versus 5.3 months with nivolumab and 2.8 months with ipilimumab. The RRs are higher for patients with tumors that have PD-L1 expression, with a RR of 72% in the combination arm versus 57.5% in the nivolumab alone arm and 21.3% in the ipilimumab group. Combination therapy, however, did cause more toxicity than either

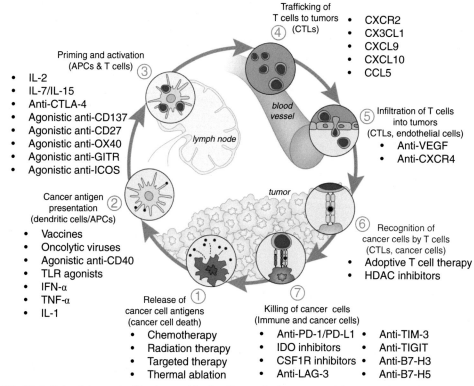

FIG. 12.1 Potential opportunities for combination therapy in the context of the cancer immunity cycle. *APC*, antigen-presenting cell; *CTL*, cytotoxic T-lymphocyte; *HDAC*, histone deacetylase; *IFN-α*, interferon alpha; *TLR*, toll-like receptor; *VEGF*, vascular endothelial growth factor. (Adapted and modified from Chen DS, Mellman I. Oncology meets immunology: the cancer-immunity cycle. *Immunity*. 2013;39(1):1—10.)

monotherapy, with grade 3—4 events in 55% of patients compared with 16.3% or 27.3% of patients treated with nivolumab or ipilimumab monotherapy, respectively. The adverse events, however, were manageable and there were no treatment-related deaths in the combination group.[11] Therapy with dual checkpoint inhibition as in the use of PD-1 and CTLA-4 inhibition in advanced melanoma is also applied to multiple types of cancer, including ovarian cancer,[12,13] RCC,[14] and NSCLC.[15]

There are clinical trials of combination treatments incorporating CTLA-4 or PD-1 inhibitors with conventional chemotherapy, radiotherapy, molecular targeted drugs such as BRAF and MEK inhibitors (vemurafenib, dabrafenib, and trametinib), PARP inhibitors (olaparib and cediranib), multikinase inhibitor (sunitinib), and immunomodulators (step 1 in Fig. 12.1). Multiple clinical trials are also underway for PD-1 inhibitors in combination with neoantigen vaccines,[16,17] oncolytic viruses[18] and agonistic anti-CD40 (step 2 in Fig. 12.1), cytokines and costimulatory immune checkpoint receptors such as 4-1BB (CD137), CD27, OX40

(CD134), glucocorticoid-induced TNFR-related protein (GITR), and inducible T-cell costimulator (ICOS) (step 3 in Fig. 12.1), angiogenesis inhibitor, anti—vascular endothelial growth factor (VEGF) (step 5 in Fig. 12.1), other coinhibitory immune checkpoint receptors such as indoleamine 2,3-dioxygenase 1 (IDO1) inhibitor, colony-stimulating factor 1 receptor (CSF1R) inhibitor, lymphocyte activation gene 3 (LAG-3) antibody,[19] TIM-3, T-cell immunoglobulin and immunoreceptor tyrosine-based inhibition motif (ITIM) domain (TIGIT), B7-H3 (CD276), and B7-H5 (V-domain Ig suppressor of T-cell activation [VISTA]) (step 7 in Fig. 12.1).

NOVEL IMMUNE CHECKPOINTS
Coinhibitory Checkpoint Molecules Such as TIM-3, LAG-3, TIGIT, B7-H3, and B7-H5
T-cell immunoglobulin mucin 3
TIM-3 is a coinhibitory receptor in the immune checkpoint pathway.[20] It is coexpressed with other inhibitory receptors and has been found on functionally exhausted cells in melanoma, NSCLC, and

follicular lymphoma.[21–23] Activation is associated with decreased production of the proinflammatory cytokines, and studies in patients with advanced melanoma showed a direct correlation between expression of TIM-3 on the surface of CD8+ T-cells and T-cell dysfunction characterized by decreased cytokine production and proliferation on antigen exposure.[22] This phenotype proved to be reversible on blockade of TIM-3 and its ligand and even more so with concurrent blockade of PD-1 and PD-L1. This has also been noted in animal models of NSCLC, which showed that an upregulation of TIM-3 is associated with resistance to PD-1 therapy.[7] Early phase trials of TIM-3 inhibitors, either as monotherapy or in combination with PD-1 blockade, for patients with advanced solid tumors are currently underway with no published results as of yet (Table 12.2).

Lymphocyte activation gene-3

LAG-3 (CD 223) is another important checkpoint belonging to the immunoglobulin superfamily and may have a synergistic effect with PD-1/PD-L1.[24] LAG-3 is a transmembrane protein that is structurally homologous to CD4, sharing about 20% of its DNA sequence and also binds MHC class II with higher affinity than CD4.[25] LAG-3 is expressed on natural killer (NK) cells, B-cells, tumor-infiltrating lymphocytes (TILs), a subset of T-cells, and DCs. LAG-3 is an inhibitory molecule and inhibits T-cell proliferation and activation. Expression is increased with T-cell activation, most prominently a few days after T-cell activation and persisting at high levels on dividing CD8+ T-cells to temper the ongoing immune response. Animal studies have demonstrated that dual blockade of PD-1 and LAG-3 significantly enhances antitumor response in comparison to either agent alone.[26]

LAG-3 has an inhibitory function on T-cells; however, on DCs, LAG-3 increases antigen presentation to cytotoxic CD8+ T-cells with an overall immunostimulatory function.[27,28] IMP321 is a soluble version of LAG-3, a 200-kDA dimeric fusion protein with immunoglobulin designed to exploit this aspect of LAG-3 function on APCs to enhance the overall immune response to tumor neoantigens. Currently, a phase I/IIa trial evaluating the combination of IMP321 and a second adjuvant with five synthetic peptides derived from tumor-associated antigens (TAAs) administered as a vaccine to patients with metastatic melanoma is underway. The combination has thus far proved safe and noted to induce CD4+ T-cell responses in all treated patients and tumor antigen-specific CD8+ T-cell responses in 81% of the patients.[29] Early phase combination studies of anti–LAG-3 antibodies (e.g., BMS-986016 [relatlimab], TSR-033, REGN3767) combined with other ICIs are ongoing.[30] MGD013 is a bispecific antibody dually targeting both LAG-3 (in tumors) and PD-1 (in T-cells), also in early phase clinical testing. Several preclinical and early clinical trials are underway assessing the use of anti–LAG-3 antibodies and IMP321 in the treatment of solid as well as hematologic malignancies (Table 12.3).

T-cell immunoglobulin and ITIM domain/CD96

TIGIT and CD96 are coinhibitory receptors that together with the costimulatory receptor CD226 (DNAM-1) form a pathway that is analogous to the CD28/CTLA-4 pathway. TIGIT is expressed on T-cells on activation and is expressed on memory T-cells, regulatory T-cells (Treg), and both follicular helper T-cells (Tfh) and Treg, and natural killer T (NKT) cells.[31,32] TIGIT is also expressed constitutively on all NK cells.[33] CD226, CD96, and TIGIT bind to CD155 and CD 112 expressed on APCs such as by DCs, T-cells, and many other cell types, including tumor cells. CD96 binds CD111 also expressed on APCs. Although CD226, TIGIT, and

TABLE 12.2
Ongoing Clinical Trials of Anti–TIM-3 Antibodies (Ab) for Hematologic and Solid Tumor Malignancies

Trial Identifier	Description	Status
NCT02817633	Phase I trial of TSR-022 (anti–TIM-3) alone or in combination with anti–PD-1 in advanced solid tumors	Recruiting
NCT02608268	Phase I/II trial of MBG453 (anti–TIM-3) alone and in combination with PDR001 (anti–PD-1) in advanced solid tumors	Recruiting
NCT03066648	Phase I/II trial of PDR001 and/or MBG453 in combination with Decitabine in patients with relapsed/refractory AML or high–risk MDS	Recruiting

AML, acute myeloid leukemia; *MDS*, myelodysplastic syndrome.

TABLE 12.3		
Ongoing Clinical Trials of Anti–LAG-3 Antibodies (Ab) for Hematologic and Solid Tumor Malignancies		
Trial Identifier	**Description**	**Status**
NCT01968109	A Phase I/IIa dose escalation and cohort expansion study of the safety, tolerability, and efficacy of anti–LAG-3 monoclonal antibody (BMS-986016) administered alone and in combination with anti–PD-1 monoclonal antibody (nivolumab, BMS-936558) in advanced solid tumors	Recruiting
NCT02460224	A phase I/II, open label, multicenter study of the safety and efficacy of LAG525 single agent and in combination with PDR001 administered to patients with advanced malignancies	Recruiting
NCT02676869	A multicenter, open label, dose escalation, phase I study in patients with unresectable or metastatic melanoma receiving IMP321 (LAG-3Ig fusion protein) as an adjunctive therapy to anti–PD-1 therapy with pembrolizumab	Recruiting
NCT00349934	A phase I study in metastatic breast carcinoma patients receiving first-line paclitaxel + IMP321	Completed, January 2010 Absence of toxicity Sustained increase/activation of APCs, NK, and CD8+ effector/memory cells 50% ORR with IMP321 and paclitaxel compared with 25% ORR with paclitaxel alone (historical data)
NCT NCT00732082	Phase I study of soluble LAG-3 (IMP321) and gemcitabine in patients with advanced pancreas cancer	Terminated, February 2010 Well-tolerated, no severe AE
NCT02061761	A phase I/IIa dose escalation and cohort expansion study of the safety, tolerability, and efficacy of anti–LAG-3 (BMS-986016) in monoclonal antibody (BMS-986016) administered alone and in combination with anti–PD-1 monoclonal antibody (nivolumab, BMS-936558) in relapsed or refractory B-cell malignancies	Recruiting
NCT03005782	A phase I, open-label, dose-escalation and cohort expansion first-in-human study of the safety, tolerability, activity, and pharmacokinetics of REGN3767 (anti–LAG-3mAb) administered alone or in combination with REGN2810 (anti–PD-1 mAb) in patients with advanced malignancies	Recruiting
NCT03219268	A phase I, first-in-human, open-label, dose-escalation study of MGD013, a bispecific DART protein that binds PD-1 and LAG-3 in patients with unresectable or metastatic neoplasms	Recruiting
NCT02966548	A phase I study of the safety, tolerability, and efficacy of anti–LAG-3 monoclonal antibody (BMS-986016) administered alone and in combination with anti–PD-1 monoclonal antibody (nivolumab, BMS-936558) in advanced solid tumors	Recruiting

Continued

TABLE 12.3

Ongoing Clinical Trials of Anti–LAG-3 Antibodies (Ab) for Hematologic and Solid Tumor Malignancies—cont'd

Trial Identifier	Description	Status
NCT03250832	A phase I dose-escalation and cohort expansion study of TSR-033, an anti–LAG-3 monoclonal antibody, alone and in combination with an anti–PD-1 in patients with advanced solid tumors	Recruiting
NCT02658981	A phase I trial of anti–LAG-3 or anti–CD137 alone and in combination with anti–PD-1 in patients with recurrent glioblastoma	Recruiting
NCT02614833	A multicentre, phase IIb, randomized, double blind, placebo-controlled study in hormone receptor–positive metastatic breast carcinoma patients receiving IMP321 versus placebo as adjunctive to a standard chemotherapy treatment regimen of paclitaxel	Recruiting
NCT02460224	Phase I/II study of LAG525 (anti–LAG-3 mAb) single agent and in combination with PDR001 in patients with advanced malignancies	Recruiting
NCT00351949	Phase I study, use of IMP321 in patients with metastatic RCC	Completed, January 2010 Safe, well-tolerated. Induction of effector memory T-cells in all patients
NCT02676869	Phase I study of IMP321 adjuvant to anti–PD-1 (pembrolizumab) therapy in unresectable or metastatic melanoma	Recruiting

AE, adverse event; *APC*, antigen-presenting cell; *DART*, dual-affinity retargeting; *ORR*, overall response rate.

CD96 each bind to CD155, they do so with strikingly different affinities.[31] The interaction of TIGIT with CD155 is of much higher affinity as compared with CD226. The higher affinity of TIGIT for CD155 compared with CD226 is analogous to the higher affinity of CTLA-4 for the B7 ligands compared with CD28, which results in competitive inhibition of CD28-driven costimulation. CD96 has intermediate affinity between TIGIT and CD226 for CD155. TIGIT regulates T-cell responses in a cell-extrinsic manner via engagement of CD155 on APCs, leading to a shift in cytokine production from IL-12 to IL-10 and dampening the overall immune response.[34] TIGIT/CD96 activation has also been shown to increase Treg suppressive capacity[35] and directly on CD4+ T-cells by decreasing IFN-γ production.[36]

Recent studies have shown a role for TIGIT and CD96 inhibition in combination with other checkpoint inhibitors. TIGIT/PD-1 coblockade in CD8+ TILs from melanoma patients has been demonstrated to enhance CD8+ T-cell expansion and cytotoxicity in response to melanoma neoantigens compared with single blockade

alone and poses an attractive target for clinical trials.[37] There is a similar rationale for targeting CD96 in combination with existing immune checkpoint blockade therapies. In multiple mouse models of cancer, anti-CD96 therapy was noted to inhibit metastasis, which was dependent on NK cells and was more effective in combination with anti–CTLA-4, anti–PD-1 blockade, or doxorubicin chemotherapy.[38] There is currently a phase I trial looking at the TIGIT inhibitor OMP313M32 in patients with locally advanced or metastatic solid tumors (NCT03119428).

B7-H3 (CD276)

B7-H3 (also known CD276) is a type I membrane protein with its sequence similar to the extracellular domain of PD-L1 (also known as B7-H1) and belongs to the B7 superfamily, a group of molecules that costimulate or downmodulate T-cell responses.[39,40] B7-H3 protein is expressed on DCs in lymphoid organs along with monocytes, T-cells, B-cells, and NK cells.[41] B7-H3 expression is significantly associated with poor outcome in patients with RCC, lung cancer, prostate cancer, colorectal carcinoma, gallbladder cancer, esophageal squamous cancer, cervical cancer, osteosarcoma, and breast cancer.[42-46]

Initially, it was reported that B7-H3 had a costimulating effect on the proliferation of both CD4+ and CD8+ T-cells. As a costimulatory molecule, B7-H3 signaling induces cellular immunity and selectively enhances IFNγ production in the presence of T-cell receptor (TCR) signaling.[47] However, accumulating evidence points to B7-H3 as a coinhibitory molecule, and it has been noted to inhibit T-cell proliferation after exposure to neoantigens by APCs.[48] In vivo preclinical model of combinatorial blockade of anti−B7-H3 together with anti−PD-1 has shown that this approach can be mutually enhancing in the treatment of established tumors.[49] Enoblituzumab (MGA271), an anti−B7-H3 antibody, is being investigated as monotherapy or in combination with other ICIs. MGD009 is a bispecific antibody that recruits T-cells (via its CD3 binding) to target B7-H3−expressing tumors (through its affinity to B7-H3) (Table 12.4).

B7-H5 or VISTA (V-domain Ig suppressor of T-cell activation)

B7-H5 or VISTA is another member of the B7 family, which is expressed on T-cells in humans but not on tumor cells.[50,51] Its signal inhibits T-cells but not B-cell proliferation and cytokine production. Therefore, VISTA inhibition promotes T-cell proliferation. JNJ-61610588 is the first fully human IgG1 anti−VISTA mAb to be tested in the clinic. Its development was terminated in August 2017 owing to business reasons. CA-170 is an oral small molecule inhibitor of PD-L1 and VISTA, which is currently being tested in a multiinstitutional phase I trial, with dose-expansion cohorts (NCT02812875).

Costimulatory Molecules: ICOS (CD278), 4-1BB (CD137), CD27, GITR, OX40 (CD134)
Inducible T-cell costimulator

ICOS (CD278) is an inducible costimulatory molecule expressed mainly on activated CD4+ T-cells following activation. It binds to an ICOS ligand expressed by B-cells, macrophages, and DCs.[52] Its function is clearly costimulatory for T-cell proliferation and cytokine secretion. However, the effects of ICOS on costimulation of T-cells appear less potent than those exerted by CD28 probably because ICOS cross-linking does not induce IL-2 production.[53] Furthermore, ICOS has been described to favor differentiation and function of Tfh, Th2, and Th17 lymphocytes, which does not lead to development of very robust immune responses.

TABLE 12.4
Ongoing Clinical Trials of Anti−B7-H3 Antibodies (Ab) for Hematologic and Solid Tumor Malignancies

Identifier	Description	Status
NCT02475213	A phase I, open-label, dose-escalation study of MGA271 in combination with pembrolizumab in patients with B7-H3−expressing melanoma, squamous cell cancer of the head and neck, non−small cell lung cancer, and other B7-H3−expressing cancers	Recruiting
NCT02628535	Phase I, first-in-human, open-label, dose-escalation study of MGD009, a humanized B7-H3 × CD3 dual-affinity retargeting (DART) protein in patients with unresectable or metastatic B7-H3−expressing neoplasms	Recruiting
NCT02381314	A phase I, open-label, dose-escalation study of MGA271 in combination with ipilimumab in patients with melanoma, non−small cell lung cancer, and other cancers	Active, not recruiting
NCT02982941	A phase I, open-label, dose-escalation study of MGA271 in pediatric patients with B7-H3−expressing relapsed or refractory solid tumors	Recruiting
NCT01391143	A phase I dose-escalation study of MGA271 in refractory cancer	Recruiting
NCT02923180	Neoadjuvant enoblituzumab (MGA271) in men with localized intermediate- and high-risk prostate cancer	Recruiting

The Tfh cells' help is critical for activation of B-cells, antibody class switching, and germinal center (GC) formation, and depletion of ICOS results in severe defects in GCs and B-cell memory.[54] In transplanted tumor models, agonistic anti—ICOS mAb do not exert a powerful immunotherapeutic effect perhaps as a result of predominant CD4 expression and because they do not aid a cytotoxic immune responses. However, under certain circumstances such as following vaccination and CTLA-4 blockade, CD4+ T-cells express ICOS, and if costimulated by the natural ligand or agonistic anti-ICOS antibodies, invigorate the CTL-mediated antitumor immune response.[55] In patients with advanced melanoma, CTLA-4 blockade with ipilimumab upregulates ICOS expression on a fraction of CD4+ T-cells. Agonistic anti—ICOS mAb are just entering clinical testing (Table 12.5).

4-1BB (CD137)

CD137 or 4-1BB is a member of the TNF receptor (TNFR) family, initially discovered as a costimulatory molecule on T cells, but can also be found on non—T-cells such as activated DCs, monocytes, neutrophils, B—cells, and NK cells.[56,57] Its ligand 4-1BBL is expressed by activated APCs, including B-cells, DCs, and macrophages. On binding to T cells, 4-1BB associates with TNFR-associated factors (TRAFs), TRAF1 and TRAF2, and activates transcription factor NF-κB and MAP-kinase pathways, resulting in proliferation, cytokine production, and survival.[58,59] In T-cells, 4-1BB engagement upregulates antiapoptotic pathways, induces proliferation and production of IFNγ and IL-2, and augment antitumor efficacy of antigen-specific T-cells.[60,61] Agonistic anti—4-1BB mAb also stimulate the cytolytic function of NK cells and enhance antitumor efficacy of DC vaccine in preclinical models.[62,63]

In mouse cancer models, especially with immunogenic tumors, agonistic 4-1BB antibody mediates regression of established tumors and generates immunologic memory with a noted increase in production of proinflammatory cytokines.[64] When a 4-1BB antibody was combined with a CTLA-4—blocking antibody in mouse cancer models, increased antitumor activity was seen, but paradoxically the toxicity of the CTLA-4 antibody appeared to be decreased, an effect which may appear to correlate with upregulation of Treg cells.[65] This may be especially useful given the severe irAEs when used in patients with advanced melanoma despite a significant clinical response. There are two 4-1BB antibodies in clinical trials, urelumab from Bristol-Myers Squibb and utomilumab (PF-05082566) from Pfizer with multiple clinical trials underway in patients with solid tumors and hematologic malignancies (NCT02845323, NCT02253992, NCT03364348, and NCT03390296). Tolcher et al. recently reported phase Ib study of utomilumab in combination with pembrolizumab in patients with advanced solid tumors and found 6/23 (26.1%) had complete or partial responses.[66]

CD27

CD27 also belongs to the TNFR family. A unique feature of CD27 among TNFR family members is its constitutive expression at significant levels on naive and memory T-cells; however, expression of CD27 is downregulated in late effector stage T-cells.[67,68] CD27 is also expressed on subsets of activated B-cells, NK cells, and hematopoietic progenitor cells. Owing to

---

TABLE 12.5

Ongoing Clinical Trials of Agonistic Anti-ICOS Antibodies (Ab) for Hematologic and Solid Tumor Malignancies

Identifier	Description	Status
NCT02520791	A phase I trial of MEDI-570 in patients with relapsed/refractory peripheral T-cell lymphoma (PTCL) follicular variant and angioimmunoblastic T-cell lymphoma (AITL)	Recruiting
NCT02723955	A phase I open-label study of GSK3359609 administered alone and in combination with anticancer agents in subjects with selected advanced solid tumors	Recruiting
NCT02904226	Phase I/II multicenter trial of ICOS agonist monoclonal antibody (mAb) JTX-2011 alone or in combination with nivolumab in adult subjects with advanced refractory solid tumor malignancies	Recruiting

ICOS, inducible T-cell costimulator.

the constitutive expression of CD27, the expression of its only known ligand, CD70, is tightly regulated. As such CD70 is only transiently expressed on activated APCs, T-cells, and NK cells under physiologic conditions.[69]

On binding to CD70, CD27 plays a key role in regulating B-cell activation and immunoglobulin synthesis. It counteracts apoptosis in activated T-cells throughout their clonal expansion and promotes their metabolism as well as the formation of memory response, thus functioning at the stages of T-cell priming, clonal expansion, and effector/memory maintenance.[70] A fully human IgG1 antibody (varlilumab) with agonistic activity against CD27 has been developed and is in active clinical trials. Varlilumab or CD-1127 promotes T-cell responses activated by TCR signaling in vitro but does not promote the function and proliferation of Tregs.[71] Multiple trials are underway investigating the use of

varlilumab in the therapy of hematologic and solid tumor malignancies (Table 12.6).

Glucocorticoid-induced TNFR-related protein

GITR belongs to the TNFR family and is expressed at low levels on resting CD4+ and CD8+ T-cells. It is upregulated 24–72 h after TCR activation and remains expressed on the lymphocyte surface for several days. In contrast, Treg cells constitutively and brightly express GITR, where it is thought to have an inhibitory function on Treg suppressive functions.[72]

GITR ligand (GITRL) is highly expressed on activated APCs and endothelial cells. On activation, GITR downstream signaling enhances T-cell proliferation and effector functions and release of proinflammatory cytokines IL-2Rα, IL-2, and IFNγ.[73] An antitumor effect of GITR stimulation has been demonstrated in multiple preclinical models with an agonistic mGITR antibody

TABLE 12.6
Ongoing Clinical Trials of Agonistic Anti-CD27 Antibodies (Ab) for Hematologic and Solid Tumor Malignancies

Identifier	Description	Status
NCT02335918	A phase I/II dose-escalation and cohort expansion study of the safety, tolerability, and efficacy of anti–CD27 antibody (varlilumab) administered in combination with anti–PD-1 (nivolumab) in advanced refractory solid tumors	Recruiting
NCT02302339	A phase II study of glembatumumab vedotin, an anti-gpNMB antibody–drug conjugate, as monotherapy or in combination with immunotherapies in patients with advanced melanoma	Recruiting
NCT02543645	A phase I/II, open-label, dose-escalation study of varlilumab (CDX-1127) in combination with atezolizumab (MPDL3280A, anti–PD-L1) in patients with advanced solid tumors	Completed on May 22, 2017. Results not reported as of yet
NCT03307746	A phase IIa study of rituximab and varlilumab in relapsed or refractory B-cell malignancies	Recruiting
NCT02924038	Pilot randomized neoadjuvant evaluation of agonist anti-CD27 monoclonal antibody varlilumab on immunologic activities of IMA950 vaccine plus poly-ICLC in patients with World Health Organization (WHO) grade 2 low-grade glioma (LGG)	Recruiting
NCT03038672	A randomized phase II study of CDX-1127 (varlilumab) in combination with nivolumab in patients with relapsed or refractory aggressive B-cell lymphomas	Recruiting
NCT02270372	A phase Ib study of ONT 10 and varlilumab in patients with advanced ovarian cancer or breast cancer	Completed on June, 2016. Results not reported as of yet

or GITRL manipulation.[74,75] Additionally, GITR agonists have demonstrated a synergistic antitumor effect when combined with vaccines, TLR (toll-like receptor) agonists, and other checkpoint inhibitors.[76,77] Recombinant forms of GITRL are also being investigated by engineering DCs to secrete a GITRL fusion protein.[77] A humanized agonistic antihuman GITR mAb (BMS-986156, TRX518, GWN323, MEDI1873, OMP-336B11, and INCAGN01876) has been developed and is being evaluated in clinical trials (Table 12.7).

OX40 (CD134)

OX40 (also known as CD134 or TNFRSF4) belongs to the TNFR family that is expressed on CD4+ and at lower levels on CD8+ T-cells 24−72 h following TCR activation.[78,79] Treg OX40 expression is upregulated on activation. Cells involved in innate immune responses such as NK, NKT cells, or neutrophils can express OX40 as well, and activation in these cells has shown a proinflammatory and prosurvival effect and enhancing function of the innate immune response. This suggests that OX40 modulation contributes not only to adaptive but also to innate immune responses.[80] In animal models, anti−OX-40 has significant antitumor activity that is augmented with the addition of other immune modulators, among them anti-CD137, anti−PD-1, and anti−CTLA-4 antibodies, as well as chemotherapy agents.[81,82]

A murine anti−OX-40 antibody, 9B-12, has been tested in a phase I trial in 30 patients, demonstrating stabilization of disease as the best response with evidence of augmented T-cell proliferation, but its use was limited by the early development of human antimurine antibodies.[83] Early phase clinical trials of humanized

TABLE 12.7

Ongoing Clinical Trials of Agonistic Anti-GITR Antibodies (Ab) for Hematologic and Solid Tumor Malignancies

Identifier	Description	Status
NCT01239134	A phase I study of TRX518 in patients with unresectable stage III or stage IV malignant melanoma or other solid tumor malignancies	Recruiting
NCT02628574	A phase I study of TRX518 in adults with advanced solid tumors	Recruiting
NCT02598960	A phase I/IIa dose-escalation and cohort expansion study for safety, tolerability, and efficacy of BMS-986156 administered alone and in combination with nivolumab (BMS-936558, anti−PD-1 monoclonal antibody) in advanced solid tumors	Recruiting
NCT02740270	A phase I/Ib open-label, multicenter, dose-escalation study of GWN323 (anti-GITR) as a single agent and in combination with PDR001 (anti−PD-1) in patients with advanced solid tumors and lymphomas	Recruiting
NCT03295942	A phase Ia open-label, dose-escalation study of the safety and pharmacokinetics of OMP-336B11 administered as a single agent to subjects with locally advanced or metastatic solid tumors	Recruiting
NCT02697591	A phase I/II, open-label, dose-escalation, safety, and tolerability study of INCAGN01876 in subjects with advanced or metastatic solid tumors	Recruiting
NCT03277352	A phase I/II safety and efficacy study of INCAGN01876 in combination with immune therapies in subjects with advanced or metastatic malignancies	Recruiting
NCT03126110	A phase I/II study exploring the safety, tolerability, and efficacy of INCAGN01876 in combination with immune therapies in subjects with advanced or metastatic malignancies	Recruiting

OX40 agonists administered as antibodies or nanoparticle encapsulated mRNA nucleotides are ongoing (e.g., PF-04518600, MEDI0562, mRNA-2416, GSK3174998, INCAGN01949). Combination studies, especially with PD-1/PD-L1 antibodies, have also started. In a recent phase I/II study, results from a study of the combination of an OX-40 antibody PF-04518600 with the PD-1 antibody, pembrolizumab, was reported.[84] Six of 23 patients had a partial or complete response, and the combination was well tolerated without significant irAEs. Interestingly, Messenheimer et al. recently reported that concomitant therapy of anti−OX-40 antibody with anti−PD-1 antibody was detrimental, whereas sequential administration of targeting OX-40, first followed by anti−PD-1 therapy, was optimal.[85] Multiple other trials are underway assessing agonistic anti−OX-40 antibodies (Table 12.8).

Targeting Killer Cell Immunoglobulin-Like Receptor and NKG2A Receptor on Natural Killer Cells

NK cell recognition of targets and its eventual cytolytic function in determining between self and nonself cells is regulated by a variety of inhibitory and activating signals, which are facilitated by NK-cell receptors.[86] The main inhibitory receptors associated with MHC class I molecules and recognition of self include killer cell immunoglobulin-like receptors (KIRs) and CD94/NKG2A specific for HLA class I histocompatibility antigen, alpha chain E (HLA-E).[87] The lack of recognition of MHC class I molecules on tumor cells by KIRs on tumor cells activates the cytotoxic activity of NK cells in fulfillment of the "missing-self" hypothesis. Self-MHC class I molecules are constitutively expressed under normal circumstances. According to the missing-self hypothesis, inhibitory KIR receptors recognize the downregulation of MHC class I molecules in virally infected or transformed self-cells, which leads to an absence of an inhibitory signal, eventually leading to cytolysis of these altered cells.[88]

Lirilumab (IPH2101) and monalizumab (IPH2201) are two IgG4 mAbs in clinical development that respectively antagonize KIR and NKG2A receptor function. In a recent study, lirilumab was administered to nine treatment-naïve patients with multiple myeloma. Unexpectedly, infusion of lirilumab resulted in rapid reduction in both NK-cell responsiveness and KIR2D expression on the NK-cell surface. In vitro assays revealed KIR2D is removed from the surface of NK cells by monocyte and neutrophil trogocytosis, with an overall reduction in NK-cell function and responsiveness. A subset of NK cells that did not have all of the KIR removed from the cell surface but retained the KIR receptor bound to lirilumab demonstrated augmented antimyeloma activity, but the overall response was significantly diminished by the contraction and reduced function of KIR2D-expressing cells.[89] Combination of KIR blockade with stimulatory cytokines, anti-TAA antibodies, or other agents reported to promote NK-cell activation such as lenalidomide could overcome the induced NK-cell hyporesponsiveness, taking advantage of KIR blockade.[90−92] Currently, multiple studies are underway assessing the use of KIR and NKG2A in the treatment of cancer (Table 12.9).

TABLE 12.8 Ongoing Clinical Trials of Agonistic Anti-OX40 Antibodies (Ab) for Solid Tumor Malignancies		
Identifier	**Description**	**Status**
NCT03092856	Phase II randomized double-blind trial of PF-04518600, an OX40 antibody, in combination with axitinib versus axitinib in immune checkpoint inhibitor−exposed patients with metastatic renal cell carcinoma.	Recruiting
NCT02559024	Phase I/Ib study of surgical resection or radiofrequency ablation (RFA) of metastatic lesions in the liver in combination with monoclonal antibody to OX40 (MEDI6469) in patients with metastatic colorectal cancer	Recruiting
NCT02410512	A phase Ib, open-label, dose-escalation study of the safety and pharmacokinetics of MOXR0916 (agonist anti−OX40 monoclonal antibody [mAb]) and atezolizumab in patients with locally advanced or metastatic solid tumors	Recruiting

TABLE 12.9

Ongoing Clinical Trials of Antibodies Targeting Killer Cell Immunoglobulin-Like Receptor (KIR) and NKG2A Receptor on Natural Killer (NK) Cell for Hematologic and Solid Tumor Malignancies

Identifier	Description	Status
NCT02399917	An open-label phase II study of lirilumab (BMS-986015) in combination with 5-azacytidine (Vidaza) for the treatment of patients with refractory/relapsed acute myeloid leukemia	Active, not recruiting
NCT02599649	Phase II combination of lirilumab and nivolumab with 5-azacitidine in patients with myelodysplastic syndromes (MDSs)	Recruiting
NCT01714739	A phase I/II study of the combination of lirilumab (anti-KIR) plus nivolumab (anti-PD-1) or lirilumab plus nivolumab and ipilimumab in advanced refractory solid tumors	Recruiting
NCT03203876	A phase I study of the safety and pharmacokinetics of anti-KIR monoclonal antibody (lirilumab, BMS-986015) in combination with anti−PD-1 monoclonal antibody (nivolumab, BMS-936558) or in combination with nivolumab and anti−CTLA-4 monoclonal antibody (ipilimumab, BMS-734016) in advanced and/or metastatic solid tumors	Recruiting
NCT01592370	Multiple phase I safety cohorts of nivolumab monotherapy or nivolumab combination regimens (including lirilumab) across relapsed/refractory hematologic malignancies	Recruiting
NCT02643550	Phase Ib/II trial of IPH2201 and cetuximab in patients with human papillomavirus (HPV) (+) and HPV (−) recurrent or metastatic squamous cell carcinoma of the head and neck	Recruiting
NCT02557516	Open-label Ib/IIa trial of a combination of monalizumab and ibrutinib in patients with relapsed, refractory, or previously untreated chronic lymphocytic leukemia	Recruiting
NCT03088059	A phase II patients with recurrent or metastatic squamous cell carcinoma of the head and neck progressing after first-line platinum-based chemotherapy. Based on potential biomarkers and molecular alterations patients will be allocated into biomarker-positive and immunotherapy cohorts	Not yet recruiting
NCT03341936	Adjuvant nivolumab and lirilumab in patients with relapsed, resectable squamous cell carcinoma of the head and neck	Recruiting
NCT02370888	A phase I clinical trial to evaluate the maximally tolerated dose (MTD), dose-limiting toxicities (DLTs), and safety profiles of increasing doses of lenalidomide after allo-HCT in AML and MDS subjects with minimal residual disease (MRD) detected by the CD34+ mixed chimerism analysis (UF-BMT-MRD-101)	Recruiting

CD40

CD40 is a tumor necrosis factor receptor superfamily member expressed on APCs including DCs, B-cells, and macrophages and is required for their activation.[93] Its ligand CD154 (CD40L) is transiently expressed on activated CD4$^+$ T-cells and promotes T-cell−dependent immunoglobulin class switching, memory B-cell development, and GC formation.[94] Ligation of CD40 on DCs induces increased surface expression of costimulatory and MHC molecules, production of proinflammatory cytokines, and enhanced T-cell triggering. CD40 ligation on resting B-cells increases antigen-presenting function and proliferation. The consequences of CD40 signaling are multifaceted and depend on the type of cell expressing CD40 and the microenvironment in which the CD40 signal is provided.

Activation of CD40 has multiple mechanisms of action, which include recruitment of immune effectors, antibody-dependent cellular cytotoxicity (ADCC), cell signaling to induce direct apoptosis or growth arrest, and most importantly, activating APCs to stimulate an anticancer immune response. This might prove useful in cancers such as pancreatic adenocarcinoma (PDAC), in which M2 macrophages promoting immune suppression predominate, and intraepithelial CD8+ T-cell infiltration is generally low.[95,96] This approach might be an important clinical advance and immunotherapeutic alternative because, thus far, checkpoint blockade has not been reported to induce reproducible objective responses in the great majority of patients with pancreatic and gastroesophageal adenocarcinoma.

Four agonistic and antagonistic anti-CD40 mAb, dacetuzumab (SGN-40) from Seattle Genetics, CP-870,893 from Pfizer, Chi Lob 7/4 from Cancer Research UK, APX005M from Apexigen, and lucatumumab from Novartis, respectively, have been investigated in early human clinical trials in a variety of lymphoid and solid tumors as monotherapies and in combination with other drugs. A 27.3% response rate was obtained with anti-CD40 (CP-870,893) plus anti−CTLA-4 (tremelimumab) in a phase I study in melanoma patients.[97] Agonistic anti-CD40 has been shown to upregulate PD-L1 in a mouse model and eventually leading to treatment resistance,[82] suggesting that higher RRs might be obtained with an agonistic anti-CD40 plus anti−PD-1 mAb. Indeed, anti-CD40 (APX005M) is currently studied in combination with anti−PD-1 (pembrolizumab) in a phase I/II trial in melanoma patients (NCT02706353).

Subsequent studies with CP-870,893 have included combinations with carboplatin and paclitaxel in solid tumor patients, with gemcitabine in PDAC and with cisplatin + pemetrexed in mesothelioma. In mesothelioma, a 40% RR was noted (6/15 patients);[98] in pancreatic cancer, an 18% RR (4/22 patients)[96]; and for the carboplatin/paclitaxel/CD40 antibody triplet, a 20% RR (6/30 patients).[99] SGN-40, or dacetuzumab, was tested in diffuse large B-cell lymphoma (DLBCL); a 9% RR was observed (4/46 patients).[100] When multiple myeloma was treated with SGN-40, the best RR was 20% with stable disease (9/44). A 12% RR was observed in non-Hodgkin lymphoma,[101] but no responses were seen in patients with chronic lymphocytic leukemia (CLL).[102] A trial of 151 patients with refractory DLBCL was conducted in which patients were randomized to receive three cycles of R-ICE (rituximab, ifosfamide, cyclophosphamide, etoposide) + dacetuzumab versus R-ICE + placebo. That trial was stopped early because of lack of a difference in RR and survival.[103] Overall, the clinical benefit from the use of dacetuzumab has been modest.

Lucatumumab is an antagonistic mAb that augments ADCC and blocks binding of CD40L with CD40, inhibiting the growth of malignant B-cells in vitro. In a phase I trial of that antibody in 26 patients with CLL, one partial response was observed.[104] In patients with multiple myeloma; one partial response was observed in 28 patients;[105] and in a subsequent trial in patients with DLBCL, the RR was 11%.[106] Overall, these data suggest that either agonistic or antagonistic antibodies directed against CD40 have very modest antitumor activity alone or in combination trials in hematologic malignancies and solid tumors.

CONCLUSION

Since the beginning of cancer immunotherapy in the 19th century, treatment options have evolved to include the use of mAbs, ICIs, genetically engineered cancer-targeting immune cells, cancer vaccines, and combination therapies that combine traditional chemotherapy with one of the aforementioned approaches to treat cancer. With the arrival of novel treatment options, a greater need for improved animal and translational models has also emerged. These include highly sophisticated mouse models of cancer, spontaneous cancer models such as the canine model, and translational models bearing transplanted human tumors such as the patient-derived xenograft (PDX) models. Together, their use will further increase our understanding of cancer biology and antitumor immunology, allow for a speedier assessment of the efficacy and safety of novel approaches, and ultimately provide a faster bench to bedside transition.

Multiple members of the immunoglobulin superfamilies or TNFRSFs are candidates for interventions to alter cell signaling in T-effector cells or Tregs and thereby mediate regression of cancer. Although it is possible that small-molecule or antibody treatments that target the pathways outlined previously will provide significant benefit for patients, recapitulating the outstanding success of PD-1/PD-L1 abrogation is a high bar to pass. Preclinical data suggest that the greatest use of many of these reagents will be in combination either with established checkpoint inhibitors such as PD-1/PD-L1 antibodies or CTLA-4 antibodies or in rational combinations that target different pathways in T-cells, Tregs, or myeloid-derived suppressor cells. Well-designed phase I and rationally conceived phase II combination trials will inform the best way to use them in a personalized immunotherapy approach to cancer. As our understanding of the processes that influence a successful antitumor immune response improves, new combinations of immunoregulatory antibodies supplemented by manipulation of novel immune signaling pathways including ion channels or complement receptors may also arise as important nodes where a positive impact may augment the efficacy of the checkpoints described herein.

REFERENCES

1. Blumenthal GM, Pazdur R. Approvals in 2016: the march of the checkpoint inhibitors. *Nat Rev Clin Oncol.* 2017; 14(3):131–132.
2. Yang JC, Hughes M, Kammula U, et al. Ipilimumab (anti-CTLA4 antibody) causes regression of metastatic renal cell cancer associated with enteritis and hypophysitis. *J Immunother (Hagerst Md 1997).* 2007;30(8):825.
3. Zaretsky JM, Garcia-Diaz A, Shin DS, et al. Mutations associated with acquired resistance to PD-1 blockade in melanoma. *N Engl J Med.* 2016;375(9):819–829.
4. Gao J, Shi LZ, Zhao H, et al. Loss of IFN-gamma pathway genes in tumor cells as a mechanism of resistance to anti-CTLA-4 therapy. *Cell.* 2016;167(2):397–404.e399.
5. Benci JL, Xu B, Qiu Y, et al. Tumor interferon signaling regulates a multigenic resistance program to immune checkpoint blockade. *Cell.* 2016;167(6):1540–1554.e1512.
6. Peng W, Chen JQ, Liu C, et al. Loss of PTEN promotes resistance to T cell-mediated immunotherapy. *Cancer Discov.* 2016;6(2):202–216.
7. Koyama S, Akbay EA, Li YY, et al. Adaptive resistance to therapeutic PD-1 blockade is associated with upregulation of alternative immune checkpoints. *Nat Commun.* 2016;7:10501.
8. George S, Miao D, Demetri GD, et al. Loss of PTEN is associated with resistance to anti-PD-1 checkpoint blockade therapy in metastatic uterine leiomyosarcoma. *Immunity.* 2017;46(2):197–204.
9. Ribas A. Adaptive immune resistance: how cancer protects from immune attack. *Cancer Discov.* 2015;5(9):915–919.
10. Chen DS, Mellman I. Oncology meets immunology: the cancer-immunity cycle. *Immunity.* 2013;39(1):1–10.
11. Larkin J, Chiarion-Sileni V, Gonzalez R, et al. Combined nivolumab and ipilimumab or monotherapy in untreated melanoma. *N Engl J Med.* 2015;373(1):23–34.
12. Bourla AB, Zamarin D. Immunotherapy: new strategies for the treatment of gynecologic malignancies. *Oncol (Willist Park).* 2016;30(1):59–66, 69.
13. Besser MJ, Shapira-Frommer R, Treves AJ, et al. Clinical responses in a phase II study using adoptive transfer of short-term cultured tumor infiltration lymphocytes in metastatic melanoma patients. *Clin Cancer Res.* 2010; 16(9):2646–2655.
14. Hammers H, Plimack E, Infante J, et al. Phase i study of nivolumab in combination with ipilimumab (ipi) in metastatic renal cell carcinoma (mrcc). *BJU Int.* 2014; 114:8.
15. Patnaik A, Socinski MA, Gubens MA, et al. Phase 1 study of pembrolizumab (pembro; MK-3475) plus ipilimumab (IPI) as second-line therapy for advanced non-small cell lung cancer (NSCLC): KEYNOTE-021 cohort D. *Journal of Clinical Oncology.* May 20, 2015;33(15):8011.
16. Ott PA, Hu Z, Keskin DB, et al. An immunogenic personal neoantigen vaccine for patients with melanoma. *Nature.* 2017;547(7662):217–221.
17. Sahin U, Derhovanessian E, Miller M, et al. Personalized RNA mutanome vaccines mobilize poly-specific therapeutic immunity against cancer. *Nature.* 2017; 547(7662):222–226.
18. Ribas A, Dummer R, Puzanov I, et al. Oncolytic virotherapy promotes intratumoral T cell infiltration and improves anti-PD-1 immunotherapy. *Cell.* 2017;170(6): 1109–1119.e1110.
19. Nguyen LT, Ohashi PS. Clinical blockade of PD1 and LAG3—potential mechanisms of action. *Nat Rev Immunol.* 2015;15(1):45.
20. Monney L, Sabatos CA, Gaglia JL, et al. Th1-specific cell surface protein Tim-3 regulates macrophage activation and severity of an autoimmune disease. *Nature.* 2002; 415(6871):536–541.
21. Yang ZZ, Grote DM, Ziesmer SC, et al. IL-12 upregulates TIM-3 expression and induces T cell exhaustion in patients with follicular B cell non-Hodgkin lymphoma. *J Clin Invest.* 2012;122(4):1271–1282.
22. Fourcade J, Sun Z, Benallaoua M, et al. Upregulation of Tim-3 and PD-1 expression is associated with tumor antigen-specific CD8+ T cell dysfunction in melanoma patients. *J Exp Med.* 2010;207(10):2175–2186.
23. Gao X, Zhu Y, Li G, et al. TIM-3 expression characterizes regulatory T cells in tumor tissues and is associated with lung cancer progression. *PLoS One.* 2012;7(2):e30676.
24. Woo S-R, Turnis ME, Goldberg MV, et al. Immune inhibitory molecules LAG-3 and PD-1 synergistically regulate T-cell function to promote tumoral immune escape. *Cancer Res.* 2012;72(4):917–927.
25. Triebel F, Jitsukawa S, Baixeras E, et al. LAG-3, a novel lymphocyte activation gene closely related to CD4. *J Exp Med.* 1990;171(5):1393–1405.
26. Matsuzaki J, Gnjatic S, Mhawech-Fauceglia P, et al. Tumor-infiltrating NY-ESO-1–specific CD8+ T cells are negatively regulated by LAG-3 and PD-1 in human ovarian cancer. *Proc Natl Acad Sci.* 2010; 107(17):7875–7880.
27. El Mir S, Triebel F. A soluble lymphocyte activation gene-3 molecule used as a vaccine adjuvant elicits greater humoral and cellular immune responses to both particulate and soluble antigens. *J Immunol.* 2000;164(11): 5583–5589.
28. Andreae S, Piras F, Burdin N, Triebel F. Maturation and activation of dendritic cells induced by lymphocyte activation gene-3 (CD223). *J Immunol.* 2002;168(8): 3874–3880.

29. Legat A, Maby-El Hajjami H, Baumgaertner P, et al. Vaccination with LAG-3Ig (IMP321) and peptides induces specific CD4 and CD8 T-cell responses in metastatic melanoma patients—report of a phase I/IIa clinical trial. *Clin Cancer Res.* 2016;22(6):1330–1340.

30. Ascierto PA, Melero I, Bhatia S, et al. Initial efficacy of anti-lymphocyte activation gene-3 (anti—LAG-3; BMS-986016) in combination with nivolumab (nivo) in pts with melanoma (MEL) previously treated with anti—PD-1/PD-L1 therapy. *J Clin Oncol.* 2017;35(suppl 15):9520.

31. Yu X, Harden K, Gonzalez LC, et al. The surface protein TIGIT suppresses T cell activation by promoting the generation of mature immunoregulatory dendritic cells. *Nat Immunol.* 2009;10(1):48–57.

32. Joller N, Hafler JP, Brynedal B, et al. Cutting edge: TIGIT has T cell-intrinsic inhibitory functions. *J Immunol.* 2011;186(3):1338–1342.

33. Stanietsky N, Simic H, Arapovic J, et al. The interaction of TIGIT with PVR and PVRL2 inhibits human NK cell cytotoxicity. *Proc Natl Acad Sci.* 2009;106(42):17858–17863.

34. Dougall WC, Kurtulus S, Smyth MJ, Anderson AC. TIGIT and CD96: new checkpoint receptor targets for cancer immunotherapy. *Immunol Rev.* 2017;276(1):112–120.

35. Joller N, Lozano E, Burkett PR, et al. Treg cells expressing the coinhibitory molecule TIGIT selectively inhibit proinflammatory Th1 and Th17 cell responses. *Immunity.* 2014;40(4):569–581.

36. Lozano E, Dominguez-Villar M, Kuchroo V, Hafler DA. The TIGIT/CD226 axis regulates human T cell function. *J Immunol.* 2012;188(8):3869–3875.

37. Chauvin J-M, Pagliano O, Fourcade J, et al. TIGIT and PD-1 impair tumor antigen—specific CD8+ T cells in melanoma patients. *J Clin Investig.* 2015;125(5):2046.

38. Blake SJ, Stannard K, Liu J, et al. Suppression of metastases using a new lymphocyte checkpoint target for cancer immunotherapy. *Cancer Discov.* 2016;6(4):446–459.

39. Sun M, Richards S, Prasad DV, Mai XM, Rudensky A, Dong C. Characterization of mouse and human B7-H3 genes. *J Immunol.* 2002;168(12):6294–6297.

40. Leitner J, Klauser C, Pickl WF, et al. B7-H3 is a potent inhibitor of human T-cell activation: no evidence for B7-H3 and TREML2 interaction. *Eur J Immunol.* 2009;39(7):1754–1764.

41. Steinberger P, Majdic O, Derdak SV, et al. Molecular characterization of human 4Ig-B7-H3, a member of the B7 family with four Ig-like domains. *J Immunol.* 2004;172(4):2352–2359.

42. Zhao J, Lei T, Xu C, et al. MicroRNA-187, down-regulated in clear cell renal cell carcinoma and associated with lower survival, inhibits cell growth and migration though targeting B7-H3. *Biochem Biophys Res Commun.* 2013;438(2):439–444.

43. Wu S, Zhao X, Wu S, et al. Overexpression of B7-H3 correlates with aggressive clinicopathological characteristics in non-small cell lung cancer. *Oncotarget.* 2016;7(49):81750.

44. Fan H, Zhu J-H, Yao X-Q. Prognostic significance of B7-H3 expression in patients with colorectal cancer: a meta-analysis. *Pak J Med Sci.* 2016;32(6):1568.

45. Bachawal SV, Jensen KC, Wilson KE, Tian L, Lutz AM, Willmann JK. Breast cancer detection by B7-H3—Targeted ultrasound molecular imaging. *Cancer Res.* 2015;75(12):2501–2509.

46. Liu C, Zang X, Huang H, et al. The expression of B7-H3 and B7-H4 in human gallbladder carcinoma and their clinical implications. *Eur Rev Med Pharmacol Sci.* 2016;20(21):4466–4473.

47. Chapoval AI, Ni J, Lau JS, et al. B7-H3: a costimulatory molecule for T cell activation and IFN-[gamma] production. *Nat Immunol.* 2001;2(3):269.

48. Suh W-K, Gajewska BU, Okada H, et al. The B7 family member B7-H3 preferentially down-regulates T helper type 1-mediated immune responses. *Nat Immunol.* 2003;4(9):899.

49. Lee YH, Martin-Orozco N, Zheng P, et al. Inhibition of the B7-H3 immune checkpoint limits tumor growth by enhancing cytotoxic lymphocyte function. *Cell Res.* 2017;27(8):1034–1045.

50. Zhu Y, Yao S, Iliopoulou BP, et al. B7-H5 costimulates human T cells via CD28H. *Nat Commun.* 2013;4:2043.

51. Wang L, Rubinstein R, Lines JL, et al. VISTA, a novel mouse Ig superfamily ligand that negatively regulates T cell responses. *J Exp Med.* 2011;208(3):577–592.

52. Simpson TR, Quezada SA, Allison JP. Regulation of CD4 T cell activation and effector function by inducible costimulator (ICOS). *Curr Opin Immunol.* 2010;22(3):326–332.

53. Choi YS, Kageyama R, Eto D, et al. ICOS receptor instructs T follicular helper cell versus effector cell differentiation via induction of the transcriptional repressor Bcl6. *Immunity.* 2011;34(6):932–946.

54. McAdam AJ, Greenwald RJ, Levin MA, et al. ICOS is critical for CD40-mediated antibody class switching. *Nature.* 2001;409(6816):102–105.

55. Fan X, Quezada SA, Sepulveda MA, Sharma P, Allison JP. Engagement of the ICOS pathway markedly enhances efficacy of CTLA-4 blockade in cancer immunotherapy. *J Exp Med.* 2014;211(4):715–725.

56. Schoenbrunn A, Frentsch M, Kohler S, et al. A converse 4-1BB and CD40 ligand expression pattern delineates activated regulatory T cells (Treg) and conventional T cells enabling direct isolation of alloantigen-reactive natural Foxp3+ Treg. *J Immunol.* 2012;189(12):5985–5994.

57. Vinay DS, Kwon BS. 4-1BB signaling beyond T cells. *Cell Mol Immunol.* 2011;8(4):281–284.

58. Martinez-Forero I, Azpilikueta A, Bolanos-Mateo E, et al. T cell costimulation with anti-CD137 monoclonal antibodies is mediated by K63-polyubiquitin-dependent signals from endosomes. *J Immunol.* 2013;190(12):6694–6706.

59. McPherson AJ, Snell LM, Mak TW, Watts TH. Opposing roles for TRAF1 in the alternative versus classical NF-kappaB pathway in T cells. *J Biol Chem.* 2012;287(27):23010–23019.

60. Watts TH. TNF/TNFR family members in costimulation of T cell responses. *Annu Rev Immunol.* 2005;23:23–68.

61. Li Q, Carr A, Ito F, Teitz-Tennenbaum S, Chang AE. Polarization effects of 4-1BB during CD28 costimulation in generating tumor-reactive T cells for cancer immunotherapy. *Cancer Res.* 2003;63(10):2546–2552.

62. Ito F, Li Q, Shreiner AB, et al. Anti-CD137 monoclonal antibody administration augments the antitumor efficacy of dendritic cell-based vaccines. *Cancer Res.* 2004;64(22):8411–8419.

63. Zhu BQ, Ju SW, Shu YQ. CD137 enhances cytotoxicity of CD3(+)CD56(+) cells and their capacities to induce CD4(+) Th1 responses. *Biomed Pharmacother.* 2009;63(7):509–516.

64. Melero I, Shuford WW, Newby SA, et al. Monoclonal antibodies against the 4-1BB T-cell activation molecule eradicate established tumors. *Nat Med.* 1997;3(6):682–685.

65. Kocak E, Lute K, Chang X, et al. Combination therapy with anti–CTL antigen-4 and anti-4-1BB antibodies enhances cancer immunity and reduces autoimmunity. *Cancer Res.* 2006;66(14):7276–7284.

66. Tolcher AW, Sznol M, Hu-Lieskovan S, et al. Phase Ib study of utomilumab (PF-05082566), a 4-1BB/CD137 agonist, in combination with pembrolizumab (MK-3475) in patients with advanced solid tumors. *Clin Cancer Res.* 2017;23(18):5349–5357.

67. Van Lier R, Borst J, Vroom TM, et al. Tissue distribution and biochemical and functional properties of Tp55 (CD27), a novel T cell differentiation antigen. *J Immunol.* 1987;139(5):1589–1596.

68. Gattinoni L, Klebanoff CA, Palmer DC, et al. Acquisition of full effector function in vitro paradoxically impairs the in vivo antitumor efficacy of adoptively transferred CD8+ T cells. *J Clin Invest.* 2005;115(6):1616–1626.

69. Borst J, Hendriks J, Xiao Y. CD27 and CD70 in T cell and B cell activation. *Curr Opin Immunol.* 2005;17(3):275–281.

70. Denoeud J, Moser M. Role of CD27/CD70 pathway of activation in immunity and tolerance. *J Leukoc Biol.* 2011;89(2):195–203.

71. Song D-G, Ye Q, Poussin M, Harms GM, Figini M, Powell DJ. CD27 costimulation augments the survival and antitumor activity of redirected human T cells in vivo. *Blood.* 2012;119(3):696–706.

72. MacHugh R, Piccirilo C, Young D, Shevach E, Collins M, Byrne C. CD4CD25 immunoregulatory T cells: gene expression analysis reveals a functional role for the glucocorticoid-induced TNF receptor. *Immunity.* 2002;16:311–323.

73. Nocentini G, Riccardi C. GITR: a multifaceted regulator of immunity belonging to the tumor necrosis factor receptor superfamily. *Eur J Immunol.* 2005;35(4):1016–1022.

74. Ko K, Yamazaki S, Nakamura K, et al. Treatment of advanced tumors with agonistic anti-GITR mAb and its effects on tumor-infiltrating Foxp3+ CD25+ CD4+ regulatory T cells. *J Exp Med.* 2005;202(7):885–891.

75. Cohen AD, Schaer DA, Liu C, et al. Agonist anti-GITR monoclonal antibody induces melanoma tumor immunity in mice by altering regulatory T cell stability and intra-tumor accumulation. *PLoS One.* 2010;5(5):e10436.

76. Cohen AD, Diab A, Perales M-A, et al. Agonist anti-GITR antibody enhances vaccine-induced CD8+ T-cell responses and tumor immunity. *Cancer Res.* 2006;66(9):4904–4912.

77. Pruitt SK, Boczkowski D, de Rosa N, et al. Enhancement of anti-tumor immunity through local modulation of CTLA-4 and GITR by dendritic cells. *Eur J Immunol.* 2011;41(12):3553–3563.

78. Mallett S, Fossum S, Barclay AN. Characterization of the MRC OX40 antigen of activated CD4 positive T lymphocytes—a molecule related to nerve growth factor receptor. *Embo J.* 1990;9(4):1063.

79. Croft M. Control of immunity by the TNFR-related molecule OX40 (CD134). *Annu Rev Immunol.* 2009;28:57–78.

80. Karulf M, Kelly A, Weinberg AD, Gold JA. OX40 ligand regulates inflammation and mortality in the innate immune response to sepsis. *J Immunol.* 2010;185(8):4856–4862.

81. Hirschhorn-Cymerman D, Rizzuto GA, Merghoub T, et al. OX40 engagement and chemotherapy combination provides potent antitumor immunity with concomitant regulatory T cell apoptosis. *J Exp Med.* 2009;206(5):1103–1116.

82. Zippelius A, Schreiner J, Herzig P, Müller P. Induced PD-L1 expression mediates acquired resistance to agonistic anti-CD40 treatment. *Cancer Immunol Res.* 2015;3(3):236–244.

83. Curti BD, Kovacsovics-Bankowski M, Morris N, et al. OX40 is a potent immune-stimulating target in late-stage cancer patients. *Cancer Res.* 2013;73(24):7189–7198.

84. Hamid O, Thompson JA, Diab A, et al. First in human (FIH) study of an OX40 agonist monoclonal antibody (mAb) PF-04518600 (PF-8600) in adult patients (pts) with select advanced solid tumors: preliminary safety and pharmacokinetic (PK)/pharmacodynamic results. *Am Soc Clin Oncol.* 2016;34.

85. Messenheimer DJ, Jensen SM, Afentoulis ME, et al. Timing of PD-1 blockade is critical to effective combination immunotherapy with anti-OX40. *Clin Cancer Res.* 2017;23(20):6165–6177.

86. Radaev S, Sun PD. Structure and function of natural killer cell surface receptors. *Annu Rev Biophysics Biomol Struct.* 2003;32(1):93–114.

87. Parham P, Moffett A. How did variable NK-cell receptors and MHC class I ligands influence immunity, reproduction and human evolution? *Nat Rev Immunol.* 2013;13(2):133.

88. Kärre K. Natural killer cell recognition of missing self. *Nat Immunol.* 2008;9(5):477.

89. Carlsten M, Korde N, Kotecha R, et al. Checkpoint inhibition of KIR2D with the monoclonal antibody IPH2101 induces contraction and hyporesponsiveness of NK-cells in patients with myeloma. *Clin Cancer Res.* 2016;22:clincanres.1108.2016.

90. Benson DM, Cohen AD, Jagannath S, et al. A phase I trial of the anti-KIR antibody IPH2101 and lenalidomide in patients with relapsed/refractory multiple myeloma. *Clin Cancer Res.* 2015;21(18):4055−4061.

91. Nijhof IS, van Bueren JJL, van Kessel B, et al. Daratumumab-mediated lysis of primary multiple myeloma cells is enhanced in combination with the human anti-KIR antibody IPH2102 and lenalidomide. *Haematologica.* 2015;100(2):263−268.

92. Ardolino M, Azimi CS, Iannello A, et al. Cytokine therapy reverses NK cell anergy in MHC-deficient tumors. *J Clin Investig.* 2014;124(11):4781.

93. Clark EA, Ledbetter JA. Activation of human B cells mediated through two distinct cell surface differentiation antigens, Bp35 and Bp50. *Proc Natl Acad Sci.* 1986;83(12):4494−4498.

94. Noelle RJ, Roy M, Shepherd DM, Stamenkovic I, Ledbetter JA, Aruffo AA. 39-kDa protein on activated helper T cells binds CD40 and transduces the signal for cognate activation of B cells. *Proc Natl Acad Sci.* 1992;89(14):6550−6554.

95. Beatty GL, Chiorean EG, Fishman MP, et al. CD40 agonists alter tumor stroma and show efficacy against pancreatic carcinoma in mice and humans. *Science.* 2011;331(6024):1612−1616.

96. Beatty GL, Torigian DA, Chiorean EG, et al. A phase I study of an agonist CD40 monoclonal antibody (CP-870,893) in combination with gemcitabine in patients with advanced pancreatic ductal adenocarcinoma. *Clin Cancer Res.* 2013;19:clincanres.1320.2013.

97. Bajor DL, Mick R, Riese MJ, et al. Abstract CT137: combination of agonistic CD40 monoclonal antibody CP-870,893 and anti-CTLA-4 antibody tremelimumab in patients with metastatic melanoma. *AACR.* 2015;75.

98. Ridge JP, Di Rosa F, Matzinger P. A conditioned dendritic cell can be a temporal bridge between a CD4+ T-helper and a T-killer cell. *Nature.* 1998;393(6684):474.

99. Nowak A, Cook A, McDonnell A, et al. A phase 1b clinical trial of the CD40-activating antibody CP-870,893 in combination with cisplatin and pemetrexed in malignant pleural mesothelioma. *Ann Oncol.* 2015;26(12):2483−2490.

100. Hussein M, Berenson JR, Niesvizky R, et al. A phase I multidose study of dacetuzumab (SGN-40; humanized anti-CD40 monoclonal antibody) in patients with multiple myeloma. *Haematologica.* 2010;95(5):845−848.

101. Advani R, Forero-Torres A, Furman RR, et al. Phase I study of the humanized anti-CD40 monoclonal antibody dacetuzumab in refractory or recurrent non-Hodgkin's lymphoma. *J Clin Oncol.* 2009;27(26):4371−4377.

102. Furman RR, Forero-Torres A, Shustov A, Drachman JG. A phase I study of dacetuzumab (SGN-40, a humanized anti-CD40 monoclonal antibody) in patients with chronic lymphocytic leukemia. *Leuk Lymphoma.* 2010;51(2):228−235.

103. Forero-Torres A, Bartlett N, Beaven A, et al. Pilot study of dacetuzumab in combination with rituximab and gemcitabine for relapsed or refractory diffuse large B-cell lymphoma. *Leuk Lymphoma.* 2013;54(2):277−283.

104. Byrd JC, Kipps TJ, Flinn IW, et al. Phase I study of the anti-CD40 humanized monoclonal antibody lucatumumab (HCD122) in relapsed chronic lymphocytic leukemia. *Leuk Lymphoma.* 2012;53(11):2136−2142.

105. Bensinger W, Maziarz RT, Jagannath S, et al. A phase 1 study of lucatumumab, a fully human anti-CD40 antagonist monoclonal antibody administered intravenously to patients with relapsed or refractory multiple myeloma. *Br J Haematol.* 2012;159(1):58−66.

106. Fanale M, Assouline S, Kuruvilla J, et al. Phase IA/II, multicentre, open-label study of the CD40 antagonistic monoclonal antibody lucatumumab in adult patients with advanced non-Hodgkin or Hodgkin lymphoma. *Br J Haematol.* 2014;164(2):258−265.

Index

Note: Page numbers followed by "f" indicate figures, "t" indicate tables.

Printed in the United States
By Bookmasters